Surgical Management of Advanced Pelvic Cancer

Surgical Management of Advanced Pelvic Cancer

Edited by Michael E. Kelly and Desmond C. Winter

St. Vincent's University Hospital
Dublin, Ireland

WILEY Blackwell

This edition first published 2022
© 2022 John Wiley & Sons Ltd

All rights reserved. No part of this publication may be reproduced, stored in a retrieval system, or transmitted, in any form or by any means, electronic, mechanical, photocopying, recording or otherwise, except as permitted by law. Advice on how to obtain permission to reuse material from this title is available at http://www.wiley.com/go/permissions.

The right of Michael E. Kelly and Desmond C. Winter to be identified as the authors of the editorial material in this work has been asserted in accordance with law.

Registered Office(s)
John Wiley & Sons, Inc., 111 River Street, Hoboken, NJ 07030, USA
John Wiley & Sons Ltd, The Atrium, Southern Gate, Chichester, West Sussex, PO19 8SQ, UK

Editorial Office
9600 Garsington Road, Oxford, OX4 2DQ, UK

For details of our global editorial offices, customer services, and more information about Wiley products visit us at www.wiley.com.

Wiley also publishes its books in a variety of electronic formats and by print-on-demand. Some content that appears in standard print versions of this book may not be available in other formats.

Limit of Liability/Disclaimer of Warranty
The contents of this work are intended to further general scientific research, understanding, and discussion only and are not intended and should not be relied upon as recommending or promoting scientific method, diagnosis, or treatment by physicians for any particular patient. In view of ongoing research, equipment modifications, changes in governmental regulations, and the constant flow of information relating to the use of medicines, equipment, and devices, the reader is urged to review and evaluate the information provided in the package insert or instructions for each medicine, equipment, or device for, among other things, any changes in the instructions or indication of usage and for added warnings and precautions. While the publisher and authors have used their best efforts in preparing this work, they make no representations or warranties with respect to the accuracy or completeness of the contents of this work and specifically disclaim all warranties, including without limitation any implied warranties of merchantability or fitness for a particular purpose. No warranty may be created or extended by sales representatives, written sales materials, or promotional statements for this work. The fact that an organization, website, or product is referred to in this work as a citation and/or potential source of further information does not mean that the publisher and authors endorse the information or services the organization, website, or product may provide or recommendations it may make. This work is sold with the understanding that the publisher is not engaged in rendering professional services. The advice and strategies contained herein may not be suitable for your situation. You should consult with a specialist where appropriate. Further, readers should be aware that websites listed in this work may have changed or disappeared between when this work was written and when it is read. Neither the publisher nor authors shall be liable for any loss of profit or any other commercial damages, including but not limited to special, incidental, consequential, or other damages.

Library of Congress Cataloging-in-Publication data applied for

ISBN: 9781119518402

Cover design by Wiley
Cover image: © Getty Images/Stephen Welstead

Set in 9.5/12.5pt STIXTwoText by Straive, Pondicherry, India
Printed and bound by CPI Group (UK) Ltd, Croydon, CR0 4YY

C091024_290921

Contents

List of Contributors *viii*
Preface *xiii*

1 **From Early Pioneers to the PelvEx Collaborative** *1*
Éanna J. Ryan and P. Ronan O'Connell

2 **The Role of the Multidisciplinary Team in the Management of Locally Advanced and Recurrent Rectal Cancer** *12*
Dennis P. Schaap, Joost Nederend, Harm J.T. Rutten, and Jacobus W.A. Burger

3 **Preoperative Assessment of Tumor Anatomy and Surgical Resectability** *17*
Akash M. Mehta, David Burling, and John T. Jenkins

4 **Neoadjuvant Therapy Options for Advanced Rectal Cancer** *32*
Alexandra Zaborowski, Paul Kelly, and Brian Bird

5 **Preoperative Optimization Prior to Exenteration** *45*
Marta Climent and Miguel Pera

6 **Patient Positioning and Surgical Technology** *52*
Ben Creavin, Michael E. Kelly, and Desmond C. Winter

7 **Intraoperative Assessment of Resectability and Operative Strategy** *62*
Rory Kokelaar, Dean Harris, and Martyn Evans

8 **Anterior Pelvic Exenteration** *73*
Jan W.A. Hagemans, Jan M. van Rees, Joost Rothbarth, Cornelis Verhoef, and Jacobus W.A. Burger

9 **Posterior Pelvic Exenteration** *85*
Werner Hohenberger, Maximilian Brunner, and Susanne Merkel

10 **Total Pelvic Exenteration** *90*
Satish K. Warrier, Andrew C. Lynch, and Alexander G. Heriot

11 **Extended Exenterative Resections Involving Bone** *97*
    Timothy Chittleborough, Gordon Beadel, and Frank Frizelle

12 **Exenterative Resections Involving Vascular and Pelvic Sidewall Structures** *110*
    Brian K. Bednarski and George J. Chang

13 **Extended Exenterative Resections for Recurrent Neoplasm** *120*
    Peter Sagar

14 **Pelvic Exenteration in the Setting of Peritoneal Disease** *127*
    Niels Kok, Arend Aalbers, and Geerard Beets

15 **Minimally Invasive Pelvic Exenteration** *132*
    Danielle Collins, Christos Kontovounisios, Shahnawaz Rasheed, and Paris Tekkis

16 **Stoma Considerations Following Exenteration** *138*
    Gabrielle H. van Ramshorst and Jurriaan B. Tuynman

17 **Reconstructive Techniques Following Pelvic Exenteration** *149*
    Dimitrios Patsouras, Alexis Schizas, and Mark George

18 **Minimizing Morbidity from Pelvic Exenteration** *158*
    Meara Dean, Alex Colquhoun, Peter Featherstone, Nicola S. Fearnhead, and R. Justin Davies

19 **Crisis Management** *170*
    Henrik Kidmose Christensen, Mette Møller Sørensen, and Victor Jilbert Verwaal

20 **Quality of Life and Patient-Reported Outcome Measures Following Pelvic Exenteration** *177*
    Daniel Steffens, Cherry Koh, and Michael Solomon

21 **Adjuvant Therapy Options after Pelvic Exenteration for Advanced Rectal Cancer** *194*
    Ka On Lam, Jeremy Yip, and Wai Lun Law

22 **Adjuvant Therapy Options after Pelvic Exenteration for Gynecological Malignancy** *205*
    Nisha Jagasia

23 **Adjuvant Therapy Options for Urological Neoplasms** *214*
    Gregory J. Nason, Clare O'Connell, and Paul K. Hegarty

24 **The Role of Re-irradiation for Locally Recurrent Rectal Cancer** *223*
    Johannes H.W. de Wilt and Jacobus W.A. Burger

25 **Palliative Pelvic Exenteration** *230*
    Hidde M. Kroon and Tarik Sammour

26 **Outcomes of Pelvic Exenteration for Locally Advanced and Recurrent Rectal Cancer** *243*
Awad M. Jarrar and Scott R. Steele

27 **Outcomes Following Exenteration for Urological Neoplasms** *255*
Frank McDermott, Ian Daniels, Neil Smart, and John McGrath

28 **Outcomes Following Exenteration for Gynecological Neoplasms** *265*
Päivi Kannisto, Fredrik Liedberg, and Marie-Louise Lydrup

29 **Mesenchymal and Non-Epithelial Tumors of the Pelvis** *283*
Eugenia Schwarzkopf and Patrick Boland

Index *298*

List of Contributors

Arend Aalbers, MD
Netherlands Cancer Institute, Amsterdam,
The Netherlands

Gordon Beadel, MB, FRACS
Department of Orthopedic Surgery, Christchurch
Hospital, Christchurch, New Zealand

Brian K. Bednarski, MD, MEd, FACS
Department of Surgical Oncology, University
of Texas MD Anderson Cancer Center,
Houston, Texas, USA

Geerard Beets, MD, PhD
Netherlands Cancer Institute, Amsterdam,
The Netherlands

Brian Bird, BA, MB, FRCPI
Department of Medical Oncology
Bons Secours, Cork, Ireland

Patrick Boland, MD, FRCS(I), FRCS
Orthopaedic Service, Department of Surgery
at Memorial Sloan Kettering Cancer Center,
New York; City, USA

Maximilian Brunner, MD
Department of Surgery, University Hospital
Erlangen, Friedrich-Alexander-Universität
Erlangen-Nürnberg, Erlangen, Germany

Jacobus W.A. Burger, MD, PhD
Department of Surgery, Catharina Hospital
Eindhoven, The Netherlands

David Burling, MBBS MRCP FRCR
Department of Gastro-Intestinal Radiology,
Complex Cancer Clinic, St. Mark's Hospital,
London, UK

George J. Chang, MD, MS
Department of Surgical Oncology, University
of Texas MD Anderson Cancer Center,
Houston, Texas, USA

Timothy Chittleborough, MBBS, DMedSc, FRACS
Colorectal Surgery Unit, The Royal
Melbourne Hospital, Melbourne, Victoria,
Australia

Henrik Kidmose Christensen, MD
Aarhus University Hospital, Denmark

Marta Climent, MD, PhD
Department of Surgery, Bellvitge University
Hospital, Barcelona, Spain

Danielle Collins, MB, MD, FRCSI
Edinburgh Colorectal Unit, Western General
Hospital, Edinburgh, UK

Alex Colquhoun, MD, FRCS(Urol)
Department of Surgery, Cambridge University
Hospitals NHS Foundation Trust, Cambridge,
UK

Ben Creavin, MB, MD, MRCSI
St. Vincent's University Hospital,
Dublin, Ireland

List of Contributors

Ian Daniels, FRCS
Exeter Surgical Health Service Research Unit (HeSRU)/University of Exeter Medical School, Exeter, UK

R. Justin Davies, MA, MB MChir, LRCP, FRCS, FEBS, FASCRS
Department of Surgery, Cambridge University Hospitals NHS Foundation Trust, Cambridge, UK

Meara Dean, MBBS (Hons), MPH, MSurg, FRACS, FRCS
Department of Surgery, Cambridge University Hospitals NHS Foundation Trust, Cambridge, UK

Martyn Evans, BM, MPhil, FRCS
Department of Surgery, Morriston Hospital, Swansea, Wales, UK

Nicola S. Fearnhead, BM, DM, FRCS
Department of Surgery, Cambridge University Hospitals NHS Foundation Trust, Cambridge, UK

Peter Featherstone, MB, BSc(Hons), MRCP, FRCA, FFICM
Department of Intensive Care Medicine and Anaesthesia, Cambridge University Hospitals NHS Foundation Trust, Cambridge, UK

Frank Frizelle, MBChB, MMedSci, FRACS, FACS, FASCRS, FNZMA, FRCSI (Hon)
Department of Surgery, University of Otago and Christchurch Hospital, Christchurch, New Zealand

Mark George, BSc, MS, FRCS
Department of Colorectal Surgery, St. Thomas' Hospital, London, UK

Jan W.A. Hagemans, MD
Department of Surgery, Erasmus MC, Rotterdam, The Netherlands

Dean Harris, MD, FRCS
Department of Surgery, Morriston Hospital, Swansea, Wales, UK

Paul K. Hegarty, MD, FRCS Urol
Department of Urology, Mater Hospital, Cork, Ireland

Alexander G. Heriot, MB, MA, MD, MBA, FRCSEd, FRACS
Department of Surgical Oncology, Peter MacCallum Cancer Centre, Melbourne, Australia

Werner Hohenberger, MD
Department of Surgery, University Hospital Erlangen, Friedrich-Alexander-Universität Erlangen-Nürnberg, Erlangen, Germany

Nisha Jagasia, MB, FRANZCOG, CGO, GradDipPallC
Department of Gynecological Oncology, Mater Adults Hospital, Brisbane, Australia

Awad M. Jarrar, MD
Department of Colorectal Surgery, Cleveland Clinic, Cleveland, OH, USA

John T. Jenkins, BSc MD FRCS FEBC
Department of Surgery, Complex Cancer Clinic, St. Mark's Hospital, London, UK

Päivi Kannisto, MD, PhD
Department of Obstetrics and Gynecology, Skåne University Hospital, Lund, Sweden

Michael E. Kelly, BA, MB, MCh, EBSQ (Coloproctology), FRCSI
Department of Colorectal Surgery, St. Vincent's University Hospital, Dublin, Ireland

Paul Kelly, BA, MB, FFRCSI
Department of Radiation Oncology Bons Secours, Cork, Ireland

Cherry Koh, MB (Hons), MS, FRACS
Surgical Outcomes Research Centre (SOuRCe); RPA Institute of Academic Surgery; Department of Colorectal Surgery, Royal Prince Alfred Hospital, Sydney, New South Wales, Australia; Discipline of Surgery, Central Clinical School, Sydney Medical School, University of Sydney, Sydney, New South Wales, Australia

List of Contributors

Niels Kok, MD, PhD
Netherlands Cancer Institute, Amsterdam,
The Netherlands

Rory Kokelaar, MA, MEd, MRCS
Department of Surgery, Morriston Hospital,
Swansea, Wales, UK

**Christos Kontovounisios, MD, PhD,
FACS, FRCS**
Department of Colorectal Surgery,
Chelsea and Westminster NHS Foundation
Trust, London, UK; Department of Surgery
and Cancer, Imperial College, London,
UK; Department of Colorectal Surgery,
Royal Marsden Hospital,
London, UK

Hidde M. Kroon, MD, PhD
Colorectal Unit, Department of Surgery,
Royal Adelaide Hospital, Adelaide,
Australia; Faculty of Health and Medical
Science, School of Medicine, University of
Adelaide, Adelaide, Australia

**Ka On Lam, MBBS(HK), FRCR, FHKCR,
FHKAM (Radiology)**
Department of Clinical Oncology, Faculty of
Medicine, University of Hong Kong,
Hong Kong

**Wai Lun Law, MB, MS, FRCSEd, FCSHK, FHKAM
(Surgery)**
Department of Surgery, Faculty of Medicine,
University of Hong Kong, Hong Kong

Fredrik Liedberg, MD, PhD
Institution of Translational Medicine, Lund
University, Malmö, Sweden; Department of
Urology, Skåne University Hospital, Malmö,
Sweden

Marie-Louise Lydrup, MD, PhD
Division of Surgery, Department of Clinical
Sciences, Lund University, Skåne University
Hospital, Malmö, Sweden

**Andrew C. Lynch, MBChB, MMedSci, FRACS,
FCSSANZ**
Department of Surgical Oncology, Peter
MacCallum Cancer Centre, Melbourne, Australia

Frank McDermott, MD, FRCS
Exeter Surgical Health Service Research
Unit (HeSRU)/University of Exeter Medical
School, Exeter, UK

John McGrath, FRCS
Exeter Surgical Health Service Research
Unit (HeSRU)/University of Exeter Medical
School, Exeter, UK

Akash M. Mehta, MD
Department of Surgery, Complex
Cancer Clinic, St. Mark's Hospital,
London, UK

Susanne Merkel, MD
Department of Surgery, University Hospital
Erlangen, Friedrich-Alexander-Universität
Erlangen-Nürnberg, Erlangen, Germany

Gregory J. Nason, MSc, FRCS Urol, FEBU
Division of Uro-Oncology, University of
Toronto, Ontario, Canada

Joost Nederend, MD, PhD
Department of Radiology, Catharina Hospital
Eindhoven, The Netherlands

Clare O'Connell, MSc, MRCSI
Department of Urology, Tallaght University
Hospital, Dublin 24, Ireland

Dimitrios Patsouras, MSc, PhD, FRCS
Department of Colorectal Surgery,
St. Thomas' Hospital, London, UK

**Shahnawaz Rasheed, BClinSci, MBBS,
DIC, PhD, FRCS**
Department of Colorectal Surgery, Royal
Marsden Hospital, London, UK

P. Ronan O'Connell, MD, FRCSI, FRCS Eng, FRCPS Glas, FRCS Edin
Department of Surgery, St. Vincent's University Hospital, Dublin, Ireland; Royal College of Surgeons in Ireland, Dublin, Ireland

Miguel Pera, MD, PhD
Hospital del Mar Universidad Autónoma de Barcelona, Spain

Joost Rothbarth, MD, PhD
Department of Surgery, Erasmus MC, Rotterdam, The Netherlands

Harm J.T. Rutten, MD, PhD
Department of Surgery, Catharina Hospital Eindhoven, The Netherlands

Éanna J. Ryan, MB, MD, MRCSI
Department of Surgery, St. Vincent's University Hospital, Dublin, Ireland

Peter Sagar, MD, FRCS, FRCPS (Hon), FASCRS (Hon)
The John Goligher Department of Colorectal Surgery, St. James's University Hospital, Leeds, UK; University of Leeds, Leeds, UK

Tarik Sammour, BHB, MB, FRACS, CSSANZ, PhD
Colorectal Unit, Department of Surgery, Royal Adelaide Hospital, Adelaide, Australia; Faculty of Health and Medical Science, School of Medicine, University of Adelaide, Adelaide, Australia

Dennis. P. Schaap, MD
Department of Surgery, Catharina Hospital Eindhoven, The Netherlands

Alexis Schizas, MSc, MD, FRCS
Department of Colorectal Surgery, St. Thomas' Hospital, London, UK

Eugenia Schwarzkopf, MD
Orthopaedic Service, Department of Surgery at Memorial Sloan Kettering Cancer Center, New York; City, USA

Neil Smart, MB, FRCSEd
Exeter Surgical Health Service Research Unit (HeSRU)/University of Exeter Medical School, Exeter, UK

Michael Solomon, DMed, DMedSc, MSc, FRACS, FRCSI
Surgical Outcomes Research Centre (SOuRCe); RPA Institute of Academic Surgery; Department of Colorectal Surgery, Royal Prince Alfred Hospital, Sydney, New South Wales, Australia; Discipline of Surgery, Central Clinical School, Sydney Medical School, University of Sydney, Sydney, New South Wales, Australia

Mette Møller Sørensen, MD, PhD
Aarhus University Hospital, Denmark

Scott R. Steele, MD, MBA
Department of Colorectal Surgery, Cleveland Clinic, Cleveland, OH, USA

Daniel Steffens, BPhty (Hons), PhD
Surgical Outcomes Research Centre (SOuRCe), Royal Prince Alfred Hospital, Sydney, New South Wales, Australia

Paris Tekkis, BMedSci, BM, MD, HonD, FRCS
Department of Colorectal Surgery, Chelsea and Westminster NHS Foundation Trust, London, UK; Department of Surgery and Cancer, Imperial College, London, UK; Department of Colorectal Surgery, Royal Marsden Hospital, London, UK

Jurriaan B. Tuynman, MD, PhD
Department of Surgery, Amsterdam UMC, Amsterdam, The Netherlands

Gabrielle H. van Ramshorst, MD, PhD
Department of Gastrointestinal Surgery, Ghent University Hospital, Ghent, Belgium

Jan M. van Rees, MD
Department of Surgery, Erasmus MC, Rotterdam, The Netherlands

Cornelis Verhoef, MD, PhD
Department of Surgery, Erasmus MC, Rotterdam, The Netherlands

Victor Jilbert Verwaal MD
Aarhus University Hospital, Denmark

Satish K. Warrier, MBBS, MS, FRACS
Department of Surgical Oncology, Peter MacCallum Cancer Centre, Melbourne, Australia

Johannes H.W. de Wilt, MD, PhD
Department of Surgery, Radboud University Hospital, Nijmegen, The Netherlands

Desmond C. Winter, MB, FRCSI, MD, FRCS (Gen)
Department of Colorectal Surgery, St. Vincent's University Hospital, Dublin, Ireland

Jeremy Yip, MBBS(HK), FRCSEd, FCSHK, FHKAM (Surgery)
Department of Surgery, Faculty of Medicine, University of Hong Kong, Hong Kong

Alexandra Zaborowski, BA, MB, MRCSI
St. Vincent's University Hospital, Dublin, Ireland

Preface

The management of advanced pelvic malignancies has evolved substantially over the last few decades. This book aims to outline all aspects of patient care, from perioperative decision-making and prehabilitation, to treatment strategies, operative approaches, and more. The topics discussed are succinctly covered by experts from around the world. Key recommendations and references highlight international consensus on optimal treatment planning.

This book is only possible by the immense effort and involvement of the entire PelvEx Collaborative network. First established in 2015, PelvEx has grown to include over one-hundred institutions across the globe. Our mission is to provide a platform for clinical studies and trials to improve perioperative and survival outcomes, while ensuring better quality of life for patients with advanced pelvic malignancy. We would like to thank everyone involved in PelvEx, the contributors who have made this book possible, and you for reading it. We hope you find it useful and informative.

Michael E. Kelly & Desmond C. Winter
On Behalf of the *PelvEx Collaborative*

1

From Early Pioneers to the PelvEx Collaborative

Éanna J. Ryan[1] and P. Ronan O'Connell[1,2]

[1] Department of Surgery, St. Vincent's University Hospital, Dublin, Ireland
[2] Royal College of Surgeons in Ireland, Dublin, Ireland

Background

Pelvic exenteration, involving radical multivisceral resection of the pelvic organs, represents the best treatment option. The first report of pelvic exenteration was in 1948 by Alexander Brunschwig of the Memorial Hospital (New York USA), as a palliative procedure for cervical cancer [1]. Due to high morbidity and mortality rates many considered palliative exenteration too radical, and it was performed only in a small number of centers in North America [2].

Technologic advancements, surgical innovations, and improved perioperative care facilitated the evolution of safer and more radical exenterative techniques for the treatment of advanced gastrointestinal and urogynecological malignancies [3]. Worldwide collaborative data [4, 5] have demonstrated that a negative resection margin is crucial in predicting survival and quality of life after surgery. Carefully selected patients who undergo en-bloc resection of contiguously involved anatomic structures with R0 resection margins can expect good long-term survival with acceptable levels of morbidity [4, 5].

The Pioneers

Eugene M. Bricker (Columbia, USA), a contemporary of Brunschwig, had been independently performing exenterative procedures beginning in 1940 [6]. Due to adverse outcomes and the interruption of World War II, his experience remained unpublished [6]. Jesse E. Thompson (Dallas, USA), one of the founders of vascular surgery as a subspecialty, and Chester W. Howe (Boston, USA) reported the first case of "complete pelvic evisceration" for locally advanced rectal cancer (LARC) in 1950. Other early advocates of the concept included Lyon H. Appleby (Vancouver, Canada), who performed a procedure he termed a "proctocystectomy" [7], and Edgar S. Brintnall (a general and vascular surgeon) and Rubin H. Flocks (an early urologist from Iowa, USA), who termed their procedure "pelvic viscerectomy" [8].

Brunschwig's Operation

While elsewhere PE was being developed principally for patients with LARC, in New York, Alexander Brunschwig was performing PE as

---

Surgical Management of Advanced Pelvic Cancer, First Edition.
Edited by Michael E. Kelly and Desmond C. Winter.
© 2022 John Wiley & Sons Ltd. Published 2022 by John Wiley & Sons Ltd.

a palliative procedure for locally advanced gynecologic malignancies. Before the introduction of PE, the prognosis for locally advanced cervical cancer was particularly poor. External beam radiation therapy was the mainstay of management. Local extension commonly occurred and cure rates were as low as 20% for primary disease [9]. Forty percent of deaths were the result of advanced disease confined to the pelvis [10]. Patients with end-stage malignancy suffered refractory pain, as well as intestinal and ureteric obstruction as major complications [11, 12].

Brunschwig, who had been among the first to report a one-stage radical pancreaticoduodenectomy in 1937 [1, 13], observed that PE was a "procedure of desperation since all other attempts to control the disease had failed." Initially his only selection criterion was that disease must be "confined to the pelvis." Interestingly, "not a single patient refused the operation even after detailed explanation of the procedure and the complications associated with surgery" [1]. The operative approach was similair (Figure 1.1).

Although Many surgeons were critical, considering it "a thoughtless form of mutilation, with limited chance of success for palliation, much less cure" [14]. In the earliest series, the survival outcomes were poor, with one in every three operations resulting in perioperative mortality [1, 15]. In Brunschwig's 1948 article, he reported operating on 22 patients with 5 deaths. [4].

By 1950, Bricker was also investigating the role of PE in the management of cervical cancer. His first patient, despite widespread local invasion, had a disease-free survival of 42 years [6]. The suitability of PE for the management of cervical and other gynecological cancers was later confirmed by Brunschwig in several series [16, 17]. In the ensuing decades, several units (mostly in North America) increasingly performed PE for advanced cancer of the vulva [18], ovary [19], and prostate [20], and for pelvic sarcoma [21]. The first documented non-malignant application for PE was for management of severe radiation necrosis of several pelvic organs in 1951. This remained a relatively common indication for PE until more contemporary radiation therapies became available [22].

Evolution in Pelvic Exenterative Surgery

Urinary Reconstruction

The key challenge in extended pelvic resection was urinary tract reconstruction. Though urinary diversion techniques had been described since 1852, leakage and infection issues resulted in many modifications in technique over the last century [23]. In 1909, Verhoogan and De Graeuwe (Brussels, Belgium) implanted ureters into an isolated segment of terminal ileum draining via an appendicostomy [24]. However, isolated ileal segments temporarily fell out of use [25]. Over the next three decades, Robert C. Coffey (Oregan, USA) experimented with various methods of bladder substitution by implanting ureters into the residual colon [26, 27]. Although he presented his outcomes outcomes in 1925 they were never published because "exposure of the ureters and kidneys to the fecal stream often led to sepsis, hyperchloremic acidosis, and kidney failure" [24]. Brunschwig's favored technique of "wet colostomy" was essentially reproduction of Coffey's method and suffered from the same shortcomings [22].

Other pioneers interested in this type of surgery had also attempted the creation of artificial bladders from bowel or alternatively developing cutaneous ureterostomies [22]. Appleby (Vancouver, Canada) examined the possibility of transferring both ureters to an intact cecum draining through a sigmoid colostomy, but with limited effect [7]. Similarly, Bricker created a diversion that involved isolation of a cecal segment "to be drained intermittently of urine through a catheter" [6]. Gilchrist and colleagues reported attaining successful

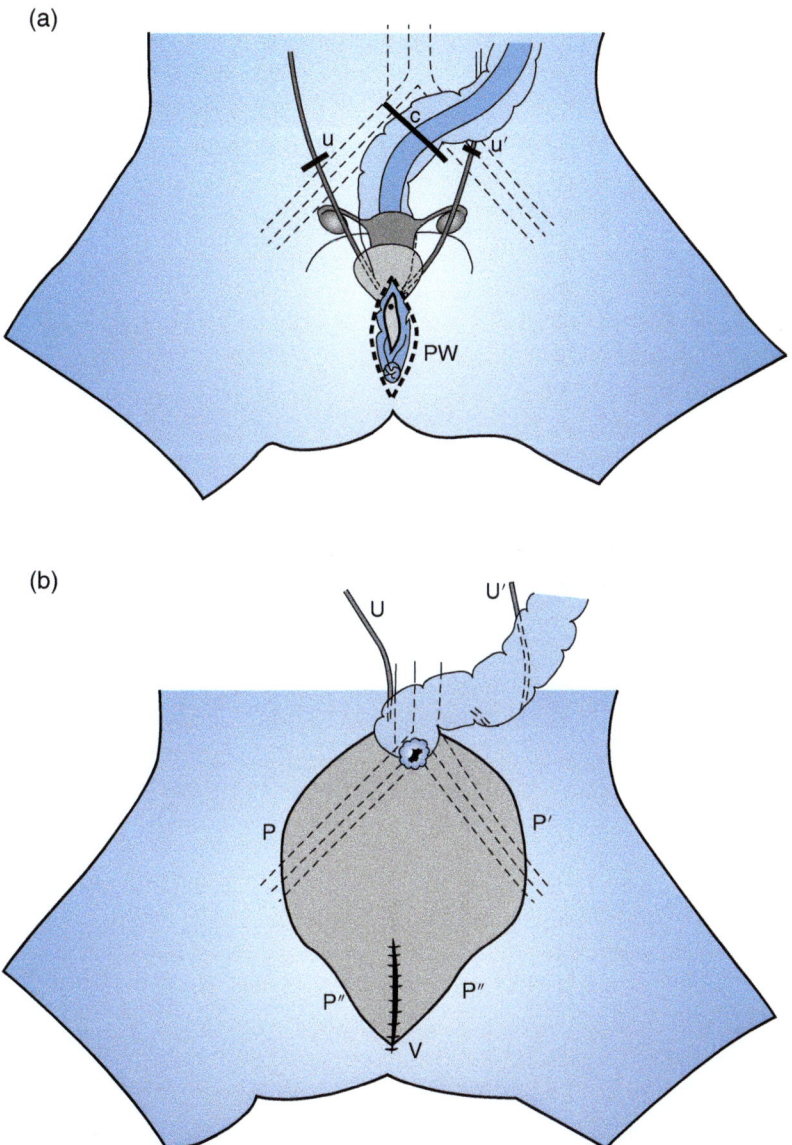

Figure 1.1 (a) Levels of transection of the ureters (U) and colon (C) and incision encompassing the vulva (V) and anus (PW) from Brunschwig's original article. (b) Conditions at end of operation, indicating areas of peritonectomy (shaded area, P, P', Pl", and Pl'''). Midline colostomy is shown with both ureters (U and U') implanted into the colon a short distance above colostomy. Copyright © 1948 American Cancer Society. *Source:* Reproduced with permission from John Wiley & Sons Ltd. [1].

continence with the construction of an intra-abdominal reservoir from isolated cecum draining via the terminal ileum [28]. However, Bricker was unable to duplicate these results and chronic leakage of urine frustrated clinicians and patients alike (Figure 1.2) [29].

The Koenig–Rutzen Bag

In 1944, Alfred Strauss (Chicago, USA) encouraged a young engineering student named Koenig who had an ileostomy following colectomy for ulcerative colitis to develop an

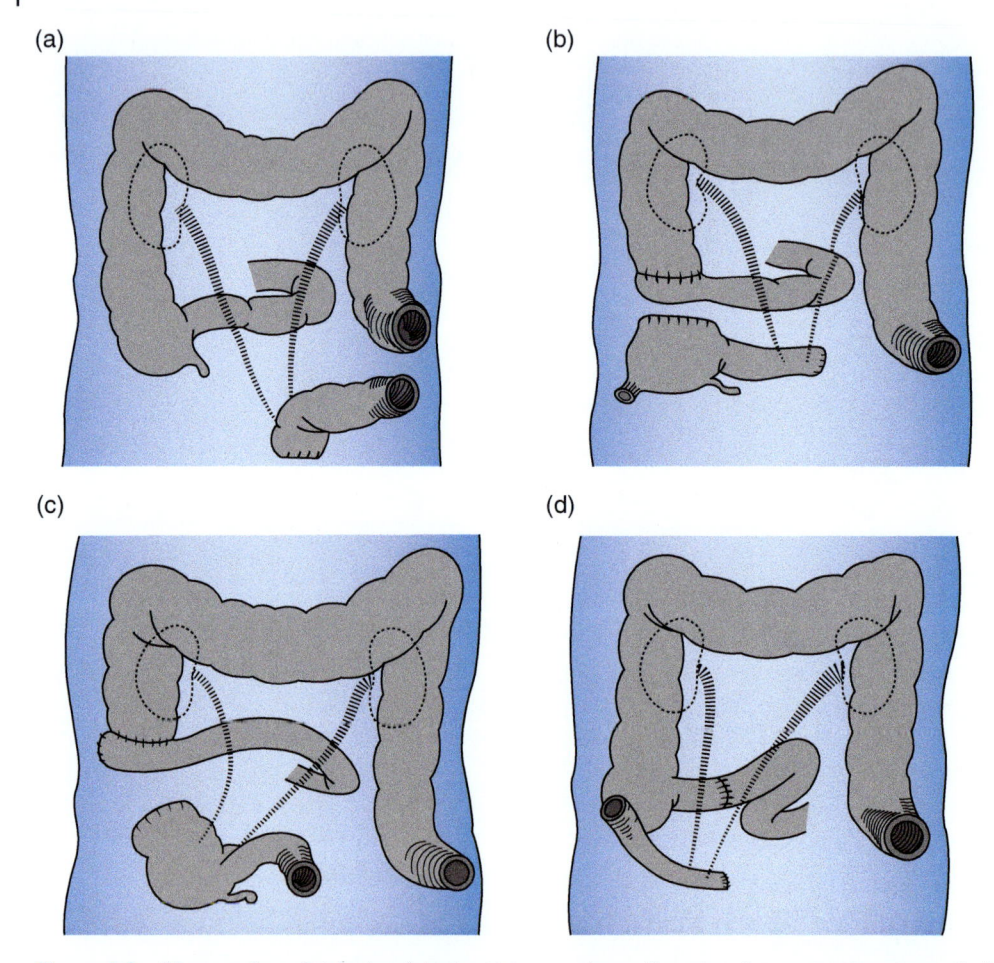

Figure 1.2 Diagram from Bricker's original article on urinary diversion demonstrating the evolution of various intestinal reconstruction techniques, including bilateral ureteric anastomosis to an isolated segment of sigmoid colon (A), terminal ileum with cecal reservoir (B), cecum with terminal ileum for urinary drainage tract (C), and contemporary ileal conduit (D). Copyright © 1950 Surgical Clinics of North America. *Source:* Reproduced with permission from Elsevier [29].

ileostomy appliance. Koenig designed a slender bag with a circular faceplate to accommodate the stoma. This was held in place with a latex sealant, Koenig formed a commercial partnership with Rutzen and the device was known as the Koenig–Rutzen bag. When Bricker heard of the device, he and his colleagues began to direct their efforts toward refining the construction of the uretero-ileal conduit [24].

Evolution of the Uretero-Ileal Conduit

By the late 1950s, the ileal conduit became the established urinary diversion technique, and the high mortality and morbidity rates associated with pelvic exenteration began to decline [30]. In particular the procedure avoided the complications of implanting ureters into an intact colon and could be fashioned from ileum that was undisturbed by any pre-existing radiotherapeutic field [31]. Despite these benefits, the complex nature of exenterative surgery made significant postoperative complications associated with urinary diversion were considered unavoidable, particularly the development of urinary fistulas [15, 32]. Brunschwig observed that, in patients who survived > 5 years "the most frequent subsequent cause of death is the deterioration of the diverted urinary tract" [33]. He advocated continuous surveillance of the urinary diversion and for the early use of temporary or permanent nephrostomy tubes for any evidence of obstruction [33].

Today, en-bloc cystectomy is required in approximately half of all patients undergoing pelvic exenteration [34–37]. Despite much progress, postoperative urological complications remain a major cause of morbidity, prolonging hospital admission and impacting on quality of life [35]. Major complication rates between 9 and 24% are reported, with urinary leak rates occurring in 7–16% of patient [35–37]. Newer techniques for continent urinary diversion, such as the internal ileal pouch reservoir [38, 39], remain controversial. Alternatives like the Indiana pouch and the Miami pouch are suitable in highly selected patients [40, 41].

Subspecialization and Partial Exenteration

The synchronous abdomino-perineal pelvic exenteration performed by the majority of exenterative units today was adapted from the technique for LARC described by Schmitz (Chicago, USA) in 1959 [42]. Over time it was recognized that the malignancy did not always extend to all of the adjacent pelvic organs. Consequently, partial exenteration was described, preserving urinary and/or rectal function. The later part of the twentieth century also saw the intensification of surgical subspecialization, driven in part by returning surgical veterans from World War II who had gained experience in specialties such as orthopedics and plastic and reconstructive surgery. The rapid subspecialization that ensued, combined with major advances in perioperative care, including intensive care and cardiac monitoring contributed to the progress seen in exenterative surgery (Figure 1.3) [2].

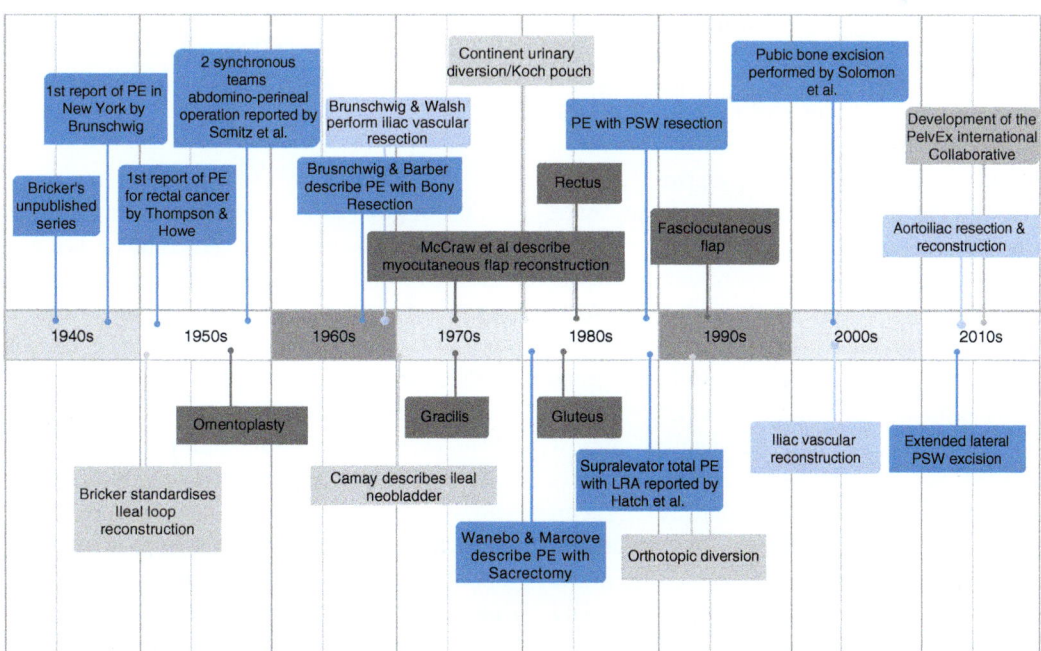

Figure 1.3 Evolution of pelvic exenterative surgery.

Composite Pelvic Exenterations

The development of compartmentalization of the pelvis and of partial exenteration resulted in more targeted approaches Bone resection was necessary for tumors involving the sacrum, coccyx, ischium, pubic symphysis, and/or ischiopubic rami [2]. Recent collaborative data show that bone resection (where needed) along with R0 margins are the most important factors influencing overall survival following PE for LRRC [5]. Disease proximal to the S1/S2 level was considered unresectable in many centers, and this represents another challenge [43–46].

Brunschwig and Barber reported a series of 28 patients, perioperative mortality was 29%, with five-year survival of 15% [47]. These initial outcomes discouraged many from pursing en-bloc bone resection. Research and better operative techniques developed for the management of sacral chordomas rekindled interest in composite PE in the 1980s [48]. Wanebo and Marcove (Charlottesville, USA) described the abdominal-trans-sacral approach for resecting LARC with sacral extension in 1981 (Figure 1.4) [49]. The initial dissection of the intrapelvic organs was accomplished through the traditional anterior approach followed by resection of the sacrum with the patient repositioned lying prone [46, 49]. Takagi and colleagues (Nagoya, Japan) encountered no postoperative mortality with this technique [50].

These outcomes stimulated research into the role of composite sacral resection for LARC and led to various units undertaking more radical resections, reporting morbidity rates between 40 and 91%, with < 5% perioperative mortality and five-year survival of almost 50% [51–55]. In recent years, specialist units developed techniques for en-bloc partial sacral resection. Hemisacrectomy, a procedure involving resection of the anterior cortex of the sacrum to preserve the sacral nerve roots, and segmental sacrectomy are alternatives [55–59].

Lateral Pelvic Sidewall Resection

Brunschwig and Walsh described "resection of the great veins of the lateral pelvic wall" to gain clearance for advanced gynecological tumors in the late 1940s [60]. However, extension of pelvic cancer into the pelvic sidewall was traditionally been considered contraindication to resection. Due to the technical difficulty of safely attaining an R0 resection margin. Efforts at vascular reconstruction were hampered by the procedure being frequently preformed in a grossly contaminated and often previously heavily irradiated field [61]. Due to these poor early outcomes, few undertook such radical resections until very recently [62].

Contemporary studies have reported en-bloc resection of the pelvic sidewall for both locally advance and recurrent rectal cancer involving the lateral pelvic neurovasculature with good outcomes [63]. Similarly, extended lateral wall resection is possible in advanced gynecological tumors [64]. Some units are providing "higher and wider" resections for tumors involving the common and external iliac vessels [65, 66] and extending to the sciatic nerve and ischial bone [2, 57, 67]. Reported R0 resection rates range from 38 to 58%, with no perioperative mortality, and 96–100% long-term graft patency [65, 66].

Perineal Reconstruction

In the original series, after the exenteration was performed, the pelvis was generally packed and allowed to heal by secondary intention. Later, surgeons closed the perineum in two layers, to prevent the small intestine prolapsing into the pelvic cavity [1]. In recent decades, various techniques for filling the "dead-space" have been examined. The omental pedicle flap was reported as an adjunct in keeping the small bowel and urinary conduit from prolapsing into the pelvic cavity, with the hope of reducing fistula rates [68, 69]. In addition, the use of mesh reconstruction of the pelvic inlet, colonic advancement, and locoregional myocutaneous flaps have been advocated with varying degrees

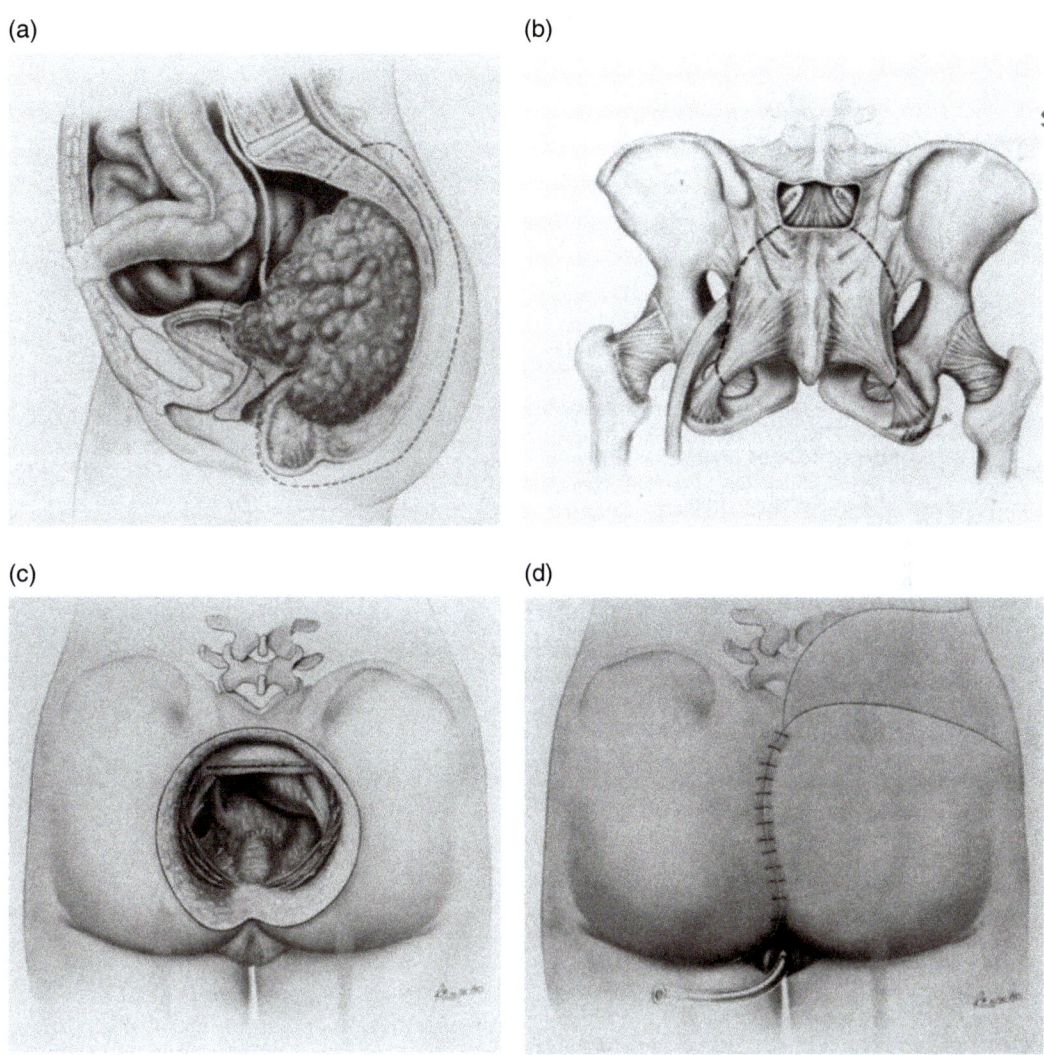

Figure 1.4 Diagrams from the first description by Wanebo and Marcove of abdomino-prone sacral resection showing the extent of resection required for recurrence of rectal cancer in the posterior compartment (A), lines of transection of the sacrum from the posterior approach (B), the operative defect after sacral resection (C), and rotational skin flaps for wound closure (D). Copyright © 1981 J.B. Lippincott Company. *Source:* Reproduced with permission from Wolters Kluwer [49].

of success (Figure 1.5) [70–72]. The use of flaps in particular was an important development that simultaneously allowed closure of perineal wounds not amenable to primary closure and transfer of viable tissue into the pelvis to decrease septic and perineal complications [73, 74]. Moreover, myocutaneous flaps may be used to construct a neovagina [75, 76].

Future Directions

The ability to perform radical and extended pelvic cancer surgery is the only potentially curative treatment for patients with locally advanced or recurrent pelvic tumors.

Better diagnostics and chemotherapeutics are likely to be "key" in personalizing

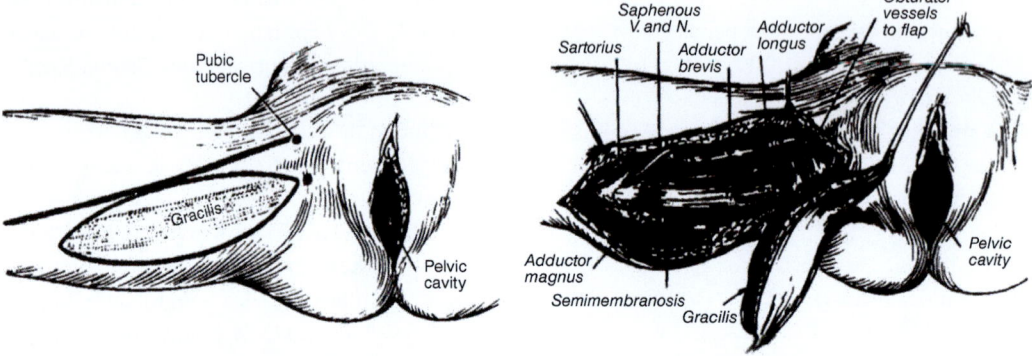

Figure 1.5 Gracilis myocutaneous flap for reconstruction of the perineum after PE as described by McCraw et al. in 1976. Copyright © 1976 Plastic & Reconstructive Surgery. *Source:* Reproduced with permission from Wolters Kluwer [70].

patient care, improving survival, or converting unresectable disease to resectable. In addition, there is growing research on quality-of-life outcome data following extended radical surgery. This is increasingly becoming as important an outcome measure as survival. The PelvEx Collaborative, offers an unique opportunity to prospectively assess exenterative outcomes, refine treatment options and further improve the management of advanced pelvic malignacies.

References

1. Brunschwig, A. (1948). Complete excision of pelvic viscera for advanced carcinoma; a one-stage abdominoperineal operation with end colostomy and bilateral ureteral implantation into the colon above the colostomy. *Cancer* 1 (2): 177–183.
2. Brown, K.G.M., Solomon, M.J., and Koh, C.E. (2017). Pelvic exenteration surgery: the evolution of radical surgical techniques for advanced and recurrent pelvic malignancy. *Dis. Colon Rectum* 60 (7): 745–754.
3. Harji, D.P., Griffiths, B., McArthur, D.R., and Sagar, P.M. (2013). Surgery for recurrent rectal cancer: higher and wider? *Colorectal Dis.* 15 (2): 139–145.
4. PelvEx Collaborative (2019). Surgical and survival outcomes following pelvic exenteration for locally advanced primary rectal cancer: results from an international collaboration. *Ann. Surg.* 269 (2): 315–321.
5. PelvEx Collaborative (2018). Factors affecting outcomes following pelvic exenteration for locally recurrent rectal cancer. *Br. J. Surg.* 105 (6): 650–657.
6. Bricker, E. (1994). Evolution of radical pelvic surgery. *Surg. Clin. North Am.* 3: 197–203.
7. Appleby, L.H. (1950). Proctocystectomy. *Am. J. Surg.* 79 (1): 57–60.
8. Brintnall, E. and Flocks, R. (1950). En masse pelvic viscerectomy with uretero-intestinal anastomosis. *AMA Arch. Surg.* 61 (5): 851–868.
9. Morris, J.M. and Meigs, J.V. (1950). Carcinoma of the cervix; statistical evaluation of 1,938 cases and results of treatment. *Surg. Gynecol. Obstetr.* 90 (2): 135–150.
10. Parsons, L. and Bell, J.W. (1950). An evaluation of the pelvic exenteration operation. *Cancer* 3 (2): 205–213.
11. Kenny, M. (1947). Relief of pain in intractable cancer of the pelvis. *Br. Med. J.* 2 (4534): 862.

12 Weinberg, A. and Kaiser, J.B. (1950). Pelvic evisceration for advanced persistent or recurrent carcinoma of the cervix. *J. Obstetr. Gynaecol. Br. Empire* 57 (4): 605–607.

13 Whipple, A.O., Parsons, W.B., and Mullins, C.R. (1935). Treatment of carcinoma of the ampulla of vater. *Ann. Surg.* 102 (4): 763–779.

14 Boronow, R.C. (2008). Remembering Alexander Brunschwig, MD (1901–1969). *Gynecol. Oncol.* 111 (2): S2–S8.

15 Parsons, L. and Leadbetter, W.F. (1950). Urologic aspects of radical pelvic surgery. *New Engl. J. Med.* 242 (20): 774–779.

16 Brunschwig, A. and Daniel, W. (1954). Total and anterior pelvic exenteration. I. Report of results based upon 315 operations. *Surg. Gynecol. Obstetr.* 99 (3): 324–330.

17 Brunschwig, A. (1954). What can surgery accomplish in recurrent carcinoma of the cervix? *American Journal of Obstetrics and Gynecology* 68 (3): 776–780.

18 Brunschwig, A. and Daniel, W. (1956). Pelvic exenterations for advanced carcinoma of the vulva. *Am. J. Obstetr. Gynecol.* 72 (3): 489–496.

19 Barber, H. and Brunschwig, A. (1965). Pelvic exenteration for locally advanced and recurrent ovarian cancer. Review of 22 cases. *Surgery* 58 (6): 935.

20 McCullough, D.L. and Leadbetter, W.F. (1972). Radical pelvic surgery for locally extensive carcinoma of the prostate. *J. Urol.* 108 (6): 939–943.

21 Marshall, V.F. (1956). Pelvic exenteration for polypoid myosarcoma (sarcoma botryoides) of the urinary bladder of an infant. *Cancer* 9 (3): 620–621.

22 Brunschwig, A. (1951). Partial or complete pelvic exenteration for extensive irradiation necrosis of pelvic viscera in the female. *Surg. Gynecol. Obstet.* 93 (4): 431–438.

23 Beer, E. (1929). Total cystectomy and partial prostatectomy for infiltrating carcinoma of the neck of the bladder: report of eight operated cases. *Ann. Surg.* 90 (5): 864–885.

24 Lopez, M.J., Petros, J.G., and Augustinos, P. (1999). Development and evolution of pelvic exenteration: historical notes. *Semin. Surg. Oncol.* 17 (3): 47–151.

25 Hinman, F. and Belt, A.E. (1922). An experimental study of ureteroduodenostomy. *JAMA* 79 (23): 1917–1924.

26 Coffey, R. (1911). Physiologic implantation of the severed ureter or common bile-duct into the intestine. *JAMA* 56 (6): 397–403.

27 Coffey, R. (1925). A technique for simultaneous implantation of the right and left ureters into the pelvic colon which does not obstruct the ureters or disturb kidney function. *Northwest Med.* 24: 211–214.

28 Gilchrist, R., Merricks, J.W., Hamlin, H.H., and Rieger, I. (1950). Construction of a substitute bladder and urethra. *Surg. Gynecol. Obstet.* 90 (6): 752–760.

29 Bricker, E.M. (1950). Bladder substitution after pelvic evisceration. *Surg. Clin. North Am.* 30 (5): 1511–1521.

30 Eiseman, B. and Bricker, E.M. (1952). Electrolyte absorption following bilateral uretero-enterostomy into an isolated intestinal segment. *Ann. Surg.* 136 (5): 761.

31 Klinge, F.W. and Bricker, E.M. (1953). The evacuation of urine by ileal segments in man. *Ann. Surg.* 137 (1): 36–40.

32 Wrigley, J.V., Prem, K.A., and Fraley, E.E. (1976). Pelvic exenteration: complications of urinary diversion. *J. Urol.* 116 (4): 428–430.

33 Brunschwig, A. and Barber, H.R. (1968). Secondary and tertiary rediversion of the urinary tract: a study based upon 72 cases among 840 pelvic exenterations for advanced cancer. *JAMA* 203 (9): 617–620.

34 Harris, C.A., Solomon, M.J., Heriot, A.G. et al. (2016). The outcomes and patterns of treatment failure after surgery for locally recurrent rectal cancer. *Ann. Surg.* 264 (2): 323–329.

35 Teixeira, S., Ferenschild, F., Solomon, M. et al. (2012). Urological leaks after pelvic exenterations comparing formation of

colonic and ileal conduits. *Eur. J. Surg. Oncol.* 38 (4): 361–366.

36 Houvenaeghel, G., Moutardier, V., Karsenty, G. et al. (2004). Major complications of urinary diversion after pelvic exenteration for gynecologic malignancies: a 23-year mono-institutional experience in 124 patients. *Gynecol. Oncol.* 92 (2): 680–683.

37 Stotland, P.K., Moozar, K., Cardella, J.A. et al. (2009). Urologic complications of composite resection following combined modality treatment of colorectal cancer. *Ann. Surg. Oncol.* 16 (10): 2759–2764.

38 Kock, N., Nilson, A., Nilsson, L. et al. (1982). Urinary diversion via a continent ileal reservoir: clinical results in 12 patients. *J. Urol.* 128 (3): 469–475.

39 Skinner, D.G., Boyd, S.D., and Lieskovsky, G. (1984). Clinical experience with the Kock continent ileal reservoir for urinary diversion. *J. Urol.* 132 (6): 1101–1107.

40 Urh, A., Soliman, P.T., Schmeler, K.M. et al. (2013). Postoperative outcomes after continent versus incontinent urinary diversion at the time of pelvic exenteration for gynecologic malignancies. *Gynecol. Oncol.* 129 (3): 580–585.

41 Solomon, M.J., Austin, K.K., Masya, L., and Lee, P. (2015). Pubic bone excision and perineal urethrectomy for radical anterior compartment excision during pelvic exenteration. *Dis. Colon Rectum* 58 (11): 1114–1119.

42 Schmitz, H.E., Schmitz, R.L., Smith, C.J., and Molitor, J.J. (1959). The technique of synchronous (two team) abdominoperineal pelvic exenteration. *Surg. Gynecol. Obstet.* 14 (4): 613–617.

43 Wanebo, H.J., Koness, R.J., Vezeridis, M.P. et al. (1994). Pelvic resection of recurrent rectal cancer. *Ann. Surg.* 220 (4): 586–595; discussion 595-7.

44 Sugarbaker, P.H. (1982). Partial sacrectomy for en bloc excision of rectal cancer with posterior fixation. *Dis. Colon Rectum* 25 (7): 708–711.

45 Wanebo, H.J., Antoniuk, P., Koness, R.J. et al. (1999). Pelvic resection of recurrent rectal cancer. *Dis. Colon Rectum* 42 (11): 1438–1448.

46 Pawlik, T.M., Skibber, J.M., and Rodriguez-Bigas, M.A. (2006). Pelvic exenteration for advanced pelvic malignancies. *Ann. Surg. Oncol.* 13 (5): 612–623.

47 Brunschwig, A. and Barber, H.R. (1969). Pelvic exenteration combined with resection of segments of bony pelvis. *Surgery* 65 (3): 417–420.

48 Stener, B. and Gunterberg, B. (1978). High amputation of the sacrum for extirpation of tumors. Principles and technique. *Spine* 3 (4): 351–366.

49 Wanebo, H.J. and Marcove, R.C. (1981). Abdominal sacral resection of locally recurrent rectal cancer. *Ann. Surg.* 194 (4): 458.

50 Takagi, H., Morimoto, T., Kato, T. et al. (1983). Pelvic exenteration combined with sacral resection for recurrent rectal cancer. *J. Surg. Oncol.* 24 (3): 161–166.

51 Sagar, P., Gonsalves, S., Heath, R. et al. (2009). Composite abdominosacral resection for recurrent rectal cancer. *Br. J. Surg.* 96 (2): 191–196.

52 Bosman, S., Vermeer, T., Dudink, R. et al. (2014). Abdominosacral resection: long-term outcome in 86 patients with locally advanced or locally recurrent rectal cancer. *Eur. J. Surg. Oncol.* 40 (6): 699–705.

53 Colibaseanu, D.T., Dozois, E.J., Mathis, K.L. et al. (2014). Extended sacropelvic resection for locally recurrent rectal cancer: can it be done safely and with good oncologic outcomes? *Dis. Colon Rectum* 57 (1): 47–55.

54 Yamada, K., Ishizawa, T., Niwa, K. et al. (2002). Pelvic exenteration and sacral resection for locally advanced primary and recurrent rectal cancer. *Dis. Colon Rectum* 45 (8): 1078–1084.

55 Milne, T., Solomon, M.J., Lee, P. et al. (2013). Assessing the impact of a sacral resection on morbidity and survival after extended radical surgery for locally recurrent rectal cancer. *Ann. Surg.* 258 (6): 1007–1013.

56 Evans, M., Harji, D., Sagar, P. et al. (2013). Partial anterior sacrectomy with nerve preservation to treat LARC. *Colorectal Dis.* 15 (6): e336–e339.

57 Shaikh, I., Aston, W., Hellawell, G. et al. (2014). Extended lateral pelvic sidewall excision (ELSiE): an approach to optimize complete resection rates in locally advanced or recurrent anorectal cancer involving the pelvic sidewall. *Tech. Coloproctol.* 18 (12): 1161–1168.

58 Brown, K., Solomon, M., Austin, K. et al. (2016). Posterior high sacral segmental disconnection prior to anterior en bloc exenteration for recurrent rectal cancer. *Tech. Coloproctol.* 20 (6): 401–404.

59 Solomon, M.J., Tan, K.-K., Bromilow, R.G. et al. (2014). Sacrectomy via the abdominal approach during pelvic exenteration. *Dis. Colon Rectum* 57 (2): 272–277.

60 Brunschwig, A. and Walsh, T.S. (1949). Resection of the great veins on the lateral pelvic wall. *Surg. Gynecol. Obstet.* 88 (4): 498.

61 Barber, H. and Brunschwig, A. (1967). Excision of major blood vessels at the periphery of the pelvis in patients receiving pelvic exenteration: common and/or iliac arteries and veins 1947 to 1964. *Surgery* 62 (3): 426.

62 Mirnezami, A.H., Sagar, P.M., Kavanagh, D. et al. (2010). Clinical algorithms for the surgical management of locally recurrent rectal cancer. *Dis. Colon Rectum* 53 (9): 1248–1257.

63 Austin, K.K. and Solomon, M.J. (2009). Pelvic exenteration with en bloc iliac vessel resection for lateral pelvic wall involvement. *Dis. Colon Rectum* 52 (7): 1223–1233.

64 Höckel, M. (2008). Laterally extended endopelvic resection (LEER) – principles and practice. *Gynecol. Oncol.* 111 (2): S13–S17.

65 Abdelsattar, Z.M., Mathis, K.L., Colibaseanu, D.T. et al. (2013). Surgery for locally advanced recurrent colorectal cancer involving the aortoiliac axis: can we achieve R0 resection and long-term survival? *Dis. Colon Rectum* 56 (6): 711–716.

66 Brown, K.G., Koh, C.E., Solomon, M.J. et al. (2015). Outcomes after en bloc iliac vessel excision and reconstruction during pelvic exenteration. *Dis. Colon Rectum* 58 (9): 850–856.

67 Solomon, M., Brown, K., Koh, C. et al. (2015). Lateral pelvic compartment excision during pelvic exenteration. *Br. J. Surg.* 102 (13): 1710–1717.

68 Clark, D.G., Daniel, W.W., and Brunschwig, A. (1962). Intestinal fistulas following pelvic exenteration. *Am. J. Obstet. Gynecol.* 84 (2): 187–191.

69 Schoenberg, H.W. and Mikuta, J.J. (1973). Technique for preventing urinary fistulas following pelvic exenteration and ureteroileostomy. *J. Urol.* 110 (3): 294–295.

70 McCraw, J.B., Massey, F.M., Shanklin, K.D., and Horton, C.E. (1976). Vaginal reconstruction with gracilis myocutaneous flaps. *Plast. Reconstr. Surg.* 58 (2): 176–183.

71 Palmer, J., Vernon, C., Cummings, B., and Moffat, F. (1983). Gracilis myocutaneous flap for reconstructing perineal defects resulting from radiation and radical surgery. *Can. J. Surg.* 26 (6): 510–512.

72 Shaw, A. and Futrell, J. (1978). Cure of chronic perineal sinus with gluteus maximus flap. *Surg. Gynecol. Obstet.* 147 (3): 417–420.

73 Temple, W.J. and Ketcham, A.S. (1982). The closure of large pelvic defects by extended compound tensor fascia lata and inferior gluteal myocutaneous flaps. *Am. J. Clin. Oncol.* 5 (6): 573–577.

74 Chessin, D.B., Hartley, J., Cohen, A.M. et al. (2005). Rectus flap reconstruction decreases perineal wound complications after pelvic chemoradiation and surgery: a cohort study. *Ann. Surg. Oncol.* 12 (2): 104–110.

75 Pursell, S.H., Day, T.G. Jr., and Tobin, G.R. (1990). Distally based rectus abdominis flap for reconstruction in radical gynecologic procedures. *Gynecol. Oncol.* 37 (2): 234–238.

76 Benson, C., Soisson, A.P., Carlson, J. et al. (1993). Neovaginal reconstruction with a rectus abdominis myocutaneous flap. *Obstet. Gynecol.* 81 (5 (Pt 2)): 871–875.

2

The Role of the Multidisciplinary Team in the Management of Locally Advanced and Recurrent Rectal Cancer

Dennis P. Schaap[1], Joost Nederend[2], Harm J.T. Rutten[1], and Jacobus W.A. Burger[1]

[1] *Department of Surgery, Catharina Hospital Eindhoven, The Netherlands*
[2] *Department of Radiology, Catharina Hospital Eindhoven, The Netherlands*

Background

Multidisciplinary team meetings (MDTMs) have been implemented to deal with the complexity of cancer care [1]. The aim of these meetings is to provide a structured discussion platform to plan patient care [2–7]. The goal is to benefit from the collective knowledge of all specialties in order to optimize staging, treatment, and follow-up. Furthermore, it can facilitate assessment for patients' inclusion in clinical trials.

The organization of the MDTM is time consuming and comes with costs. Delaying decisions until the MDTM has taken place can sometimes delay treatment. MDTM results in a significant change in diagnosis or treatment planning, ranging from 18.5 to 36% and 11.0 to 14.5% respectively [8–14]. The role of adequate preoperative tumor staging and discussion in an MDTM resulted in more patients receiving neoadjuvant treatment, increased local control, and R0 resections [15].

The governing body for the quality of care for patients with cancer in the Netherlands is the Stichting voor Oncologische Samenwerking (Foundation for Oncological Collaboration, SONCOS) [16]. SONCOS represents 29 national societies involved in cancer care, including the Society for Medical Oncology, the Society of Surgical Oncology, and the Society of Radiation Oncology. SONCOS delivers a yearly report stating the conditions that must be fulfilled by any multidisciplinary team caring for cancer patients. Dutch physicians are obliged to adhere to these conditions. Furthermore, all Dutch medical centers have agreed to standardize data registry with a national database to monitor the effect of changes in treatment strategy on quality measurements as shown in Figure 2.1. Hence, factors improving the quality of care can be identified and applied easily in order to improve patient outcome. MDTMs across the Netherlands can deal with the majority of patients with pelvic cancer from gastroenterological, urological, or gynecological origin. However, patients with locally advanced and recurrent pelvic cancer should be discussed in a specialized MDTM [16].

Complex Pelvic Cancer MDTM

Patients with locally advanced primary and recurrent pelvic cancers are associated with a higher risk of local recurrence, distant

Surgical Management of Advanced Pelvic Cancer, First Edition.
Edited by Michael E. Kelly and Desmond C. Winter.
© 2022 John Wiley & Sons Ltd. Published 2022 by John Wiley & Sons Ltd.

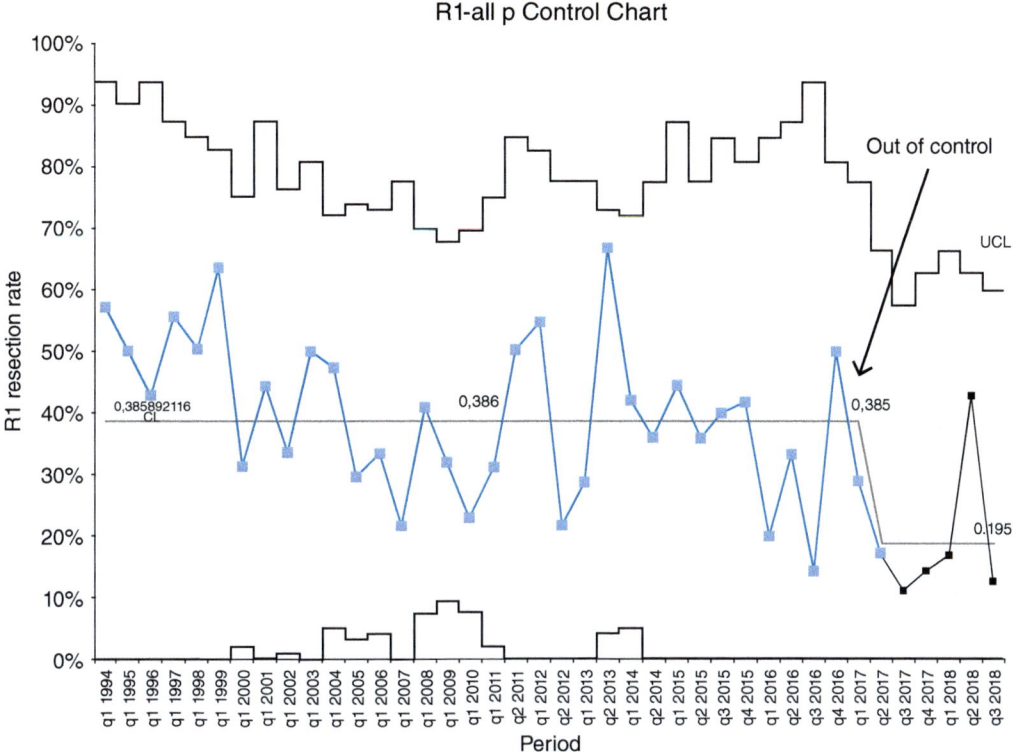

Figure 2.1 National registries help to monitor outcome. In this control chart for proportions, a decrease in R+ resection rate seems to be statistically significant and leads to differences in the mean R+ resection rate. This moment (referred to as 'out of control') coincides with the change of preoperative treatment in locally recurrent pelvic cancer patients (unpublished data). CL, Control limit; UCL, upper control limit.

metastases, and poor survival. Furthermore, these complex pelvic tumors require several specialties for an accurate preoperative evaluation, neoadjuvant and/or adjuvant therapy with a multidisciplinary surgical approach, (Table 2.1). Preoperative treatments providing downstaging are essential to both increase the chance of radical resections and prevent unnecessarily extensive resections that lead to impairment. Centralization is warranted, to identify those patients who require this specialized care.

In order to work toward a situation in which all patients with locally advanced cancers are discussed in a complex cancer MDTM, it is essential that it is easily accessible for physicians outside the specialized center.

Staging, Restaging, and Pathological Assessment

Staging

Radiologic assessment of local and distant disease in the setting of advanced pelvic cancer can be challenging. Therefore all diagnostic imaging is assessed by radiologists and nuclear medicine physicians with specific expertise in cancer imaging prior to the MDTM. An expert radiologist familiar with surgical principles may anticipate the expected organ involvement. Regular contact in the oncological network ensures that referring hospitals know which scan sequences and modalities that are required.

Table 2.1 Differences between hospitals caring for "regular" colorectal cancer patients and hospitals caring for locally advanced and recurrent pelvic cancer patients (Example from The Netherlands).

Regular care for colorectal cancer	Specialized pelvic cancer care
Consultants with special interest in colorectal cancer	Consultants with special interest in locally advanced and pelvic cancer
Two radiologists	Two radiologists with verifiable expertise in evaluation of locally advanced and recurrent pelvic cancer, before and after neoadjuvant treatment
Two surgeons	Two surgeons with verifiable technical expertise in treatment of locally advanced and recurrent pelvic cancer. At least one surgeon with expertise in treatment of stage 4 colorectal cancer
One pathologist	Pathologist with specific expertise in evaluation of specimens of the pelvis and effects of neoadjuvant therapy
One radiation oncologist	Radiation oncologist with expertise in treatment of locally advanced and recurrent pelvic cancer. Expertise in IORT = Intra-operative radiotherapy
One medical oncologist	Medical oncologist with specific expertise in curative treatment of patients with locally advanced and recurrent pelvic cancer
	Extra: Oncological urologist with expertise in urinary deviation
	Extra: Oncological gynecologist with expertise in postoperative care and recovery
	Extra: plastic and reconstructive surgeon with expertise in reconstruction of large oncological defects
24/7 intervention radiology	Experience with acquiring tissue from the pelvis and placing drains in the pelvis, including transgluteal approaches
Stomatherapy nurse clinic	Stomatherapy nurse experienced in care of urinary stoma
protocol for referral for IORT	Provides IORT
MDTM operates according to national guideline	MDTM discusses many patients that cannot be treated according to national guideline
Includes all patients in Dutch Surgical Colorectal Audit (DSCA)	Includes only T4 in audit. Registers all patients in prospective databases, compares with other T4/locally recurrent rectal cancer (LRRC) centers, and publishes results

Restaging

In patients who receive neoadjuvant treatment, response evaluation can be challenging due to the difficulties in distinguishing between malignant and fibrotic changes. Visualizing and assessing complete remission or downsizing of the tumor after neoadjuvant treatment, may alter the surgical planning in highly selected cases the surgical planning. Complete remission after (chemo)radiation cannot be predicted reliably with non-invasive imaging techniques, because of the spatial limitations to detecting microscopic tumor residue [17]. Even magnetic resonance imaging (MRI) can result in false positive predictions. Addition of diffusion-weighted imaging (DWI) to standard MRI makes detection more accurate. Overall, an experienced radiologist with considerable expertise is an essential part of the complex cancer MDTM [18–20].

Pathological Assessment

All resected specimens should be examined by an experienced histopathologist and results must be discussed in the complex cancer MDTM. The role of the pathologist includes advanced pelvic cancer specimen quality, lymph node and margin status. Reporting these findings should be done by the use of structured reports [21–22].

Complex Cancer MDTM Outcomes

All participants should have ample experience with this complex and heterogeneous group of patients. In the case of a treatment plan with curative intent, the surgeon proposes a strategy with as little harm as possible. This proposal often includes induction therapy with chemotherapy, radiotherapy, or both. The medical oncologist and radiation oncologist usually want specific aspects clarified, often involving prior medical history or imaging. The radiologist is frequently asked to specify some aspects of scans that were presented earlier. In cases of non-curative treatment, the initiative lies with the medical oncologist. The possibilities for enrolment in a clinical trial should be discussed, and when enrolment is possible, the relevant trial will be included in the MDTM outcome advice. The discussion on an individual patient ends with the chair declaring what he or she thinks the consensus of the MDTM is, after which the secretary notes the final conclusion.

Summary Box
• Increased complexity of modern cancer care requires a multidisciplinary approach. • Combining the knowledge of different specificities makes the MDTM an excellent learning environment enhance cancer care. • A lack of defined protocols in locally advanced and recurrent pelvic cancer endorses the necessity for a centralized multidisciplinary approach.

References

1. Fennell, M.L., Prabhu Das, I., Clauser, S. et al. (2010). The organization of multidisciplinary care teams: modeling internal and external influences on cancer care quality. *J. Natl Cancer Inst. Monogr* 2010 (40): 72–80.
2. Kelly, S.L., Jackson, J.E., Hickey, B.E. et al. (2013). Multidisciplinary clinic care improves adherence to best practice in head and neck cancer. *Am. J. Otolaryngol* 34 (1): 57–60.
3. Korman, H., Lanni, T.J., Shah, C. et al. (2013). Impact of a prostate multidisciplinary clinic program on patient treatment decisions and on adherence to NCCN guidelines: the William Beaumont Hospital experience. *Am. J. Clin. Oncol* 36 (2): 121–125.
4. Prades, J., Remue, E., van Hoof, E., and Borras, J.M. (2015). Is it worth reorganising cancer services on the basis of multidisciplinary teams (MDTs)? A systematic review of the objectives and organisation of MDTs and their impact on patient outcomes. *Health Policy* 119 (4): 464–474.
5. Raine, R., Wallace, I., Nic a' Bháird, C. et al. (2014). Improving the effectiveness of multidisciplinary team meetings for patients with chronic diseases: a prospective observational study. *Health Serv. Deliv. Res.* 2.37.

6 Taplin, S.H., Weaver, S., Salas, E. et al. (2015). Reviewing cancer care team effectiveness. *J. Oncol. Pract* 11 (3): 239–246.
7 Fleissig, A., Jenkins, V., Catt, S., and Fallowfield, L. (2006). Multidisciplinary teams in cancer care: are they effective in the UK? *Lancet Oncol* 7 (11): 935–943.
8 Kurpad, R., Kim, W., Rathmell, W.K. et al. (2011). A multidisciplinary approach to the management of urologic malignancies: does it influence diagnostic and treatment decisions? *Urol. Oncol.Semin. Orig. Invest* 29 (4): 378–382.
9 Oxenberg, J., Papenfuss, W., Esemuede, I. et al. (2015). Multidisciplinary cancer conferences for gastrointestinal malignancies result in measureable treatment changes: a prospective study of 149 consecutive patients. *Ann. Surg. Oncol* 22 (5): 1533–1539.
10 Snelgrove, R.C., Subendran, J., Jhaveri, K. et al. (2015). Effect of multidisciplinary cancer conference on treatment plan for patients with primary rectal cancer. *Dis. Colon Rectum* 58 (7): 653–658.
11 van Hagen, P., Spaander, M.C.W., van der Gaast, A. et al. (2013). Impact of a multidisciplinary tumour board meeting for upper-GI malignancies on clinical decision making: a prospective cohort study. *Int. J. Clin. Oncol* 18 (2): 214–219.
12 Wheless, S.A., McKinney, K.A., and Zanation, A.M. (2010). A prospective study of the clinical impact of a multidisciplinary head and neck tumor board. *Otolaryngol. Head Neck Surg.* 143 (5): 650–654.
13 Jung, S.M., Hong, Y.S., Kim, T.W. et al. (2018). Impact of a multidisciplinary team approach for managing advanced and recurrent colorectal cancer. *World J. Surg* 42 (7): 2227–2233.
14 Pillay, B., Wootten, A.C., Crowe, H. et al. (2016). The impact of multidisciplinary team meetings on patient assessment, management and outcomes in oncology settings: a systematic review of the literature. *Cancer Treatm. Rev* 42: 56–72.
15 Palmer, G., Martling, A., Cedermark, B., and Holm, T. (2011). Preoperative tumour staging with multidisciplinary team assessment improves the outcome in locally advanced primary rectal cancer. *Colorectal Dis* 13 (12): 1361–1369.
16 Samenwerking SO. Normeringsrapport SONCOS 2018, versie 6. Utrecht: SONCOS.
17 Barbaro, B., Fiorucci, C., Tebala, C. et al. (2009). Locally advanced rectal cancer: MR imaging in prediction of response after preoperative chemotherapy and radiation therapy. *Radiology* 250 (3): 730–739.
18 Curvo-Semedo, L., Lambregts, D.M.J., Maas, M. et al. (2012). Diffusion-weighted MRI in rectal cancer: apparent diffusion coefficient as a potential noninvasive marker of tumor aggressiveness. *J. Magn. Reson. Imaging* 35 (6): 1365–1371.
19 Kim, S.H., Lee, J.M., Hong, S.H. et al. (2009). Locally advanced rectal cancer: added value of diffusion-weighted MR imaging in the evaluation of tumor response to neoadjuvant chemo- and radiation therapy. *Radiology* 253 (1): 116–125.
20 Lambregts, D.M., Vandecaveye, V., Barbaro, B. et al. (2011). Diffusion-weighted MRI for selection of complete responders after chemoradiation for locally advanced rectal cancer: a multicenter study. *Ann. Surg. Oncol* 18 (8): 2224–2231.
21 Loughrey MB, Quirke P, Shepherd NA (2014). Standards and datasets for reporting cancers. Dataset for colorectal cancer histopathology reports. London: Royal College of Pathologists.
22 von Karsa, L., Patnick, J., Segnan, N. et al. (2013). European guidelines for quality assurance in colorectal cancer screening and diagnosis: overview and introduction to the full supplement publication. *Endoscopy* 45 (1): 51–59.

3

Preoperative Assessment of Tumor Anatomy and Surgical Resectability

Akash M. Mehta[1], David Burling[2], and John T. Jenkins[1]

[1] Department of Surgery, Complex Cancer Clinic, St. Mark's Hospital, London, UK
[2] Department of Gastro-Intestinal Radiology, Complex Cancer Clinic, St. Mark's Hospital, London, UK

Background

Advanced pelvic cancers including locally advanced primary rectal cancers extending beyond the normal anatomical planes (beyond the total mesorectal excision (TME) plane or primary rectal beyond TME (PR-bTME)), pelvic recurrences of previously treated cancer including recurrent rectal cancer (RRC), and recurrent squamous cell cancer (SCC) of the anus with or without colorectal peritoneal metastasis (CPM) need specialist management [1, 2].

Various exenterative techniques have evolved to address the specific anatomical and surgical challenges posed by advanced pelvic cancers [3–5]. These techniques combine visceral soft-tissue resection with bony excision to achieve a complete pathological (R0) resection of the cancer surrounded by a rim of uninvolved tissue [2]. Disease threatening or involving the sacrum can be excised utilizing either a subperiosteal approach, partial sacrectomy, or, in selected cases with superficial involvement of the anterior cortex of the proximal sacrum, high subcortical sacral resection (HiSS) [6–8]. Cancer involvement of the lateral compartment structures including the greater sciatic notch and piriformis muscle was traditionally considered unresectable. However, in recent years surgical techniques have been refined to optimize R0 resection, including lateral pelvic compartment excision using approaches from both inside and outside the true pelvis; laterally extended endopelvic resection (LEER); and extended lateral pelvic sidewall excision (ELSiE) [9–14]. Disease extending anteriorly into the retropubic space can also be excised by penile base excision with partial pubic bone resection when involved [15, 16].

The goal of exenterative surgery is achieving microscopically complete tumor clearance (≥ 1 mm microscopically clear resection margins), termed R0 resection. Five-year survival rates of up to 65% are achievable in patients undergoing R0 resection [17–20], while survival rates after R1 or R2 resections are significantly lower [21–23]. Consequently, R0 resection is currently considered the primary determinant of surgical outcome for advanced pelvic cancer. Furthermore, for curative intent surgery, only R0 resection will confer sufficient overall patient benefit to meaningfully outweigh the risk and morbidity of attempted resection.

To help achieve R0 resection, radiological assessment of advanced pelvic cancer should first accurately delineate the cancer margins, distinguishing viable tumor from scar tissue resulting from previous surgery or (chemo)

Surgical Management of Advanced Pelvic Cancer, First Edition.
Edited by Michael E. Kelly and Desmond C. Winter.
© 2022 John Wiley & Sons Ltd. Published 2022 by John Wiley & Sons Ltd.

radiotherapy, and "healthy" (uninvolved) adjacent structures. The radiologist must then create and communicate a clear roadmap for resection using surgically relevant planes to ensure R0 resection while preserving uninvolved organs. Finally, radiologists must ensure accurate and timely identification of extrapelvic metastases which could influence decision-making on whether (and when) to offer surgery. This chapter provides a more detailed review of current practice for preoperative assessment of tumor anatomy and resectability.

Cancer Anatomy and Resectability

There are several methods for assessing cancer anatomy and resectability. Examination under anesthetic (EUA) is a common method for determining whether the cancer is adherent to adjacent structures. While palpation may help the surgeon estimate R0 resectability, radiological assessment is the main determinant of whether a cancer can be completely excised with a microscopically clear margin.

Overall, radiological assessment of cancer anatomy provides more accurate assessment of margins and the relationship to adjacent structures than EUA [24]. The radiological modalities commonly utilized include magnetic resonance imaging (MRI), computed tomography (CT), and positron-emission tomography (PET). Advanced pelvic cancer surgery is complex and its radiological assessment is individualized according to the type of cancer, patient factors (e.g. tolerance, comorbidity, frailty, and metastatic disease), and location in the pelvis.

For low pelvic cancers with a distal margin threatening the preservation of the anal canal or anterior compartment structures (prostate/ seminal vesicles in men; vagina and uterus in women) endorectal ultrasound (ERUS), when performed by experienced practitioners, can provide complementary information to assist decision-making. The small volume of mesorectal fat between the distal rectum and anterior mesorectal margin can limit accuracy of MRI for detecting transmural extension of the tumor and anterior margin involvement by low rectal cancers.

Several retrospective studies correlating preoperative MRI staging of the circumferential resection margin (CRM) with histological CRM involvement have demonstrated decreased reliability of MRI for patients with low, anterior rectal cancer, with MRI mostly overestimating CRM involvement [25, 26]. In the authors' experience, if MRI shows convincing involvement of anterior structures by cancer, total pelvic exenteration or posterior exenteration is recommended, to achieve R0 resection. However, where involvement of the anterior margin is equivocal, we recommend ERUS when feasible [27, 28]. In one study including 32 patients with anterior rectal cancers, MRI and ERUS had equivalent positive and negative predictive values of 66.6 and 95.6% respectively [27]. A recent retrospective study of 24 patients observed that use of ERUS as an adjunct to MRI improved diagnostic accuracy for anterior margin involvement [29]. ERUS can also provide an accurate assessment of distal cancer margin in relation to the puborectalis muscle when considering intersphincteric dissection and preservation of the anal canal. However, clinically reliable ERUS requires experience of both endoluminal ultrasound and rigid sigmoidoscopy to optimize probe position and scan interpretation [30].

PET-CT provides complementary information on tumor function and activity [31]. PET-CT is frequently used in complex cancer patients as a complementary test to CT and liver MRI, particularly for exclusion of metastatic disease in uncommon sites or to help troubleshoot uncertain imaging findings, for example helping distinguish tumor from scar tissue or presence of nodal involvement. PET-CT utility is limited by poor spatial resolution, anatomical mismatch between sites of disease and displayed metabolic activity (due to patient movement or bowel peristalsis), and false positives generated by sites of inflammation or tissue healing [32].

Radiological Assessment of Cancer Anatomy by MRI

T2-weighted MRI is the reference standard for assessment of tumor anatomy and resectability. There are two main radiological approaches for interpretation and reporting.

The first is tumor categorization according to the pelvic compartments affected, which can help determine patient prognosis. Various tumor categorization systems have been proposed and are summarized in Table 3.1. The Mayo Clinic classification is based on the presence of symptoms and the number of sites of fixation of the tumor to surrounding pelvic structures [33]; the Yamada classification describes broad categories of localized, sacral, and lateral fixation [34]; and the Wanebo classification is based on the UICC TNM system distinguishing bony or ligamentous pelvic involvement from non-bony fixation [35]. The Memorial Sloan Kettering classification distinguishes four pelvic compartments [36], while the Royal Marsden Hospital classification distinguishes seven compartments [37]. Some of these systems have attempted to prognosticate

Table 3.1 Existing classification systems for pelvic compartments.

Group	Criteria for classification	Definitions	
Mayo Clinic	Symptoms	S0	Asymptomatic
		S1	Symptomatic without pain
		S2	Symptomatic with pain
	Tumor fixation	F0	No fixation
		F1	Fixation to one point
		F2	Fixation to two points
		F3	Fixation to more than two points
Yamada	Pattern of pelvic fixation	Localized	Invasion to adjacent pelvic organs/tissues
		Sacral invasive	Invasion to lower sacrum (≥ S3), coccyx, periosteum
		Lateral invasive	Invasion to sciatic nerve, greater sciatic notch, pelvic sidewall, upper sacrum (S1/2)
Wanebo	Stages	TR1	Limited invasion of muscularis
		TR2	Full thickness invasion of muscularis propria
		TR3	Anastomotic recurrence penetrating beyond bowel wall into perirectal soft tissue
		TR4	Invasion into adjacent organs without fixation
		TR5	Invasion of bony/ligamentous pelvis
Memorial Sloan Kettering	Anatomic region	Axial	Anastomotic, mesorectal, perirectal soft tissue, perineum
		Anterior	Genitourinary tract
		Posterior	Sacrum and presacral fascia
		Lateral	Soft tissues of the pelvic sidewall and lateral bony pelvis

(Continued)

Table 3.1 (Continued)

Group	Criteria for classification	Definitions	
Royal Marsden Hospital	Planes of dissection on MRI	Central	(Neo)rectum
			Intraluminal recurrence
			Perirectal fat or mesorectal, extraluminal recurrence
		PR	Rectovesical pouch or recto-uterine pouch of Douglas
		AA PR	Ureters and iliac vessels above peritoneal reflection
			Sigmoid colon
			Small bowel
			Lateral sidewall fascia
		AB PR	Genito-urinary tract
		Lateral	Ureters
			Iliac vessels distal to iliac bifurcation
			Lateral pelvic lymph nodes
			Sciatic nerve
			Sciatic notch
			S1/2 nerve roots
			Piriformis or obturator internus muscles
		Posterior	Coccyx
			Presacral fascia
			Sacrum
			Retrosacral space
		Inferior	Levator ani muscles
			External sphincter complex
			Perineal scar
			Ischio-anal fossa

as well, although any associations with survival outcomes must be interpreted with caution, as the different institutions had different patient populations and markedly variable R0 resection rates. Moreover, prognostication based on a compartment-based classification is inherently subject to institutional views of which cancers are resectable according to availability of expertise at that time and not necessarily considering newer surgical techniques [6, 9, 11]. The emergence and implementation of these new techniques has changed opinion on which cancers are resectable and shifted the emphasis away from relying on compartment-based radiological assessment alone. Indeed, most compartment-based approaches were designed and validated retrospectively, i.e. after exenterative surgery had already been performed [37].

The second radiological reporting approach utilized by the authors of this chapter provides a roadmap for surgical excision, whereby a highly experienced radiologist reports a detailed and unambiguous roadmap for en-bloc excision of the locally advanced cancer. Such a roadmap will be complemented by accurate exclusion of extrapelvic metastases and incorporate surgically relevant information such as significant coexisting pathology or findings which may challenge the surgical approach. In the authors' experience, radiologists who personally review and examine patients and then communicate scan findings in the outpatient clinic, alongside their surgical and nursing colleagues, develop much greater insight into patient management and surgical approaches.

The following principles may help guide radiologists to provide roadmaps for advanced pelvic cancer:

- The radiologically derived roadmap for R0 excision is generally tailored to the maximum disease extent identified on sequential MRI, even in the context of downstaging from neoadjuvant treatment. This principle is based on the knowledge that radiologically occult microscopic foci of viable tumor cells may persist beyond the downstaged tumor margins, (e.g. peritumoral scar tissue) which could lead to R1 resection if resection were based on post-treatment imaging alone [38–43]. Consequently, fibrosis in direct contact with the tumor on post-treatment imaging should be regarded as potential tumor extension and therefore incorporated in the planned surgical resection [38, 42, 44–55].
- Each radiological roadmap is created by the radiology team in close co-operation with the surgical team. The roadmap is tailored to the individual patient based on their anatomy, tumor extent, and comorbidity. The detailed description of excision planes and margins should be based on (distance to) intraoperatively assessable and fixed anatomical landmarks, including sacral promontory, ischial tuberosity, ischial spine, piriformis muscle, sacral foramina and nerve roots, sacral ligaments (sacrotuberous, sacrospinous, and ischiococcygeal), gluteal muscles, bifurcation of aorta/common iliac vessels, and origin of the superior gluteal artery (SGA). In practice, the authors of this chapter use the term SLAM ("sacral ligaments and muscle") to describe the intimately related sacrotuberous, sacrospinous, and ischiococcygeus complex.
- "BONVUE" or "a good view" is a helpful acronym which can be used to remind the team to include a description of bones, organs, nerves, vessels, ureters, and extra (tumor sites).

The key feature of the roadmap approach is that, in contrast to traditional compartment-based reporting, this system addresses the extent of involvement and resection of individual structures potentially at risk and/or which need to be resected in order to obtain an adequate margin. The structures that are systematically assessed to build the roadmap, with the corresponding surgical considerations, are listed in Table 3.2. For any given patient, a roadmap is constructed based on assessment of the relevant elements in Table 3.2 and their surgical counterparts, which, when combined together, form the definitive surgical strategy.

Case Study

A 32-year-old female patient presented to her local hospital with a perforated PR-bTME and underwent an emergency laparotomy and fashioning of a defunctioning colostomy prior to downsizing with a combination of radiotherapy and systemic chemotherapy. A diagnostic laparoscopy performed after completion of neoadjuvant treatment showed no evidence of peritoneal metastatic disease. T2-weighted MRI was obtained prior to initiation of neoadjuvant therapy and to evaluate response approximately 12 weeks after completion of neoadjuvant treatment. A compartment-based report from the referring unit using a published structure [37] is summarized as follows:

- Above peritoneal reflection: disease present at the level of the peritoneal reflection with likely compromise of the right ureter
- Below peritoneal reflection, anterior: suspected ovarian involvement with involvement of uterus and right adnexal tissues

Table 3.2 The St. Mark's roadmap approach for assessment of pelvic tumor anatomy and resection margins.

Category	Structures and assessment	Surgical considerations
Visceral structures	Rectum Uterus/vagina Prostate/seminal vesicles Bladder Base of penis	APER +/− excision of seminal vesicles +/− penile base excision Posterior/total pelvic exenteration
Ureters	Involvement relative to ureteric orifice	Partial ureterectomy +/− reimplantation/reconstruction
Vessels	Common/external iliac arteries	Vascular resection +/− reconstruction
	Internal iliac arteries: involvement relative to origin of SGA	Ligation proximal/distal to origin of SGA
Bony/ligamentous pelvis	Pubic bones + symphysis	Pubic bone resection
Sacrum and presacral fascia	Height of most proximal involvement relative to sacral promontory	Extent of subperiosteal dissection + level of sacral transection
	Depth of cortical involvement	Subperiosteal dissection HiSS Full thickness sacrectomy
	Width of involvement relative to sacral foramina	Width of HiSS or asymmetrical sacrectomy
Sacropelvic ligaments and ischial spines	Involvement of sacrospinous/sacrotuberous/ischiococcygeal ligaments (SLAM) + lateral extent relative to ischial spine	Resection of SLAM ELSiE
	Depth of involvement of ischial spine	ELSiE +/− extension into/toward acetabulum
Nerves	L5/S1 nerve roots	Resection of lumbosacral trunk with motor deficit
	S2/3/4 nerve roots	Resection with sensory deficit
	Main trunk of sciatic nerve in sciatic notch	Preservation or partial/total excision (as part of ELSiE)
Muscles	Obturator internus	Resection as part of sidewall excision
	Piriformis	Medial aspect resected transabdominally (Sub)total resection requires ELSiE

APER, Abdomino-perineal excision of the rectum;
SLAM, term denoting the complex of sacropelvic ligaments: sacrospinous, sacrotuberous, and ischiococcygeal;
SGA, superior gluteal artery;
ELSiE, extended lateral sidewall excision;
HiSS, high subcortical sacral resection.

- Posterior: tumor infiltration of presacral fascia (S1–S5) without cortical invasion; S1/2 nerve roots clear
- Lateral: tumor infiltration of pelvic sidewall fascia with sparing of internal and external iliac vessels; sacrotuberous and sacrospinous ligaments spared but right piriformis muscle infiltrated by tumor
- Infralevator: tumor involvement of right levator
- Anterior urogenital area/perineum/retropubic space: unaffected

In its conclusion, the compartment-based report states that resection would require removal of the tumor from the anterior compartment above and below the peritoneal reflection, posterior compartment from S1 down, right lateral compartment, and right infralevator compartment.

This compartment-based approach provides information on tumor extent, provides prognostic information, and helps determine if the local surgical team has the requisite skills to proceed with excision [36, 37].

In the roadmap approach, the relevant components from Table 3.2 were assessed and "translated" into a proposed surgical plan shown in Table 3.3 and Figures 3.1–3.7.

Table 3.3 Construction of the roadmap for R0 resection in patient 1.

Category	Structures and assessment	Surgical considerations	Figures
Sacrum and presacral fascia	Presacral fluid collection surrounded by rim of fibrosis, starting 38 mm from sacral promontory	Subperiosteal dissection from promontory down to point of sacral transection 38 mm distally (S1/2 junction)	3.1
	No discernible plain between presacral fibrosis and anterior sacral cortex	Full thickness sacrectomy	3.1
Nerves	Right L5 nerve root free and separate from tumor	Preservation of right L5 nerve root with resection of S1 nerve root leading to partial motor deficit	3.2
	No discernible plain between right S1 nerve root and tumor/fibrosis		
Sacropelvic ligaments and ischial spines	Right SLAM complex grossly involved by tumor including insertion into ischial spine	Right ELSiE taking the tip of the ischial spine	3.3
Muscles	Distal aspect of right obturator internus muscle undistinguishable from tumor/fibrosis	Resection of distal aspect of right obturator internus as part of ELSiE	
	Right piriformis muscle grossly tethered by tumor/fibrosis	Resection of right piriformis as part of ELSiE	3.4
Vessels	Tumor extending to origin of right SGA	Right internal iliac ligation proximal to SGA origin	3.5
Visceral structures	Primary rectal tumor tethering uterus and both ovaries	Total pelvic exenteration preferable but bladder preservation possible (to be discussed with patient)	3.6
	Bladder not directly involved but completely denervated due to required S1/2 sacrectomy		
Ureters	Distal right ureter indistinguishable from tumor/fibrosis	If bladder to be preserved: Proximal division of right ureter at level of pelvic brim, distal division just proximal to the ureterovesical junction Right ureteric reimplantation	3.7

Ultimately, the road map constructed by this multidisciplinary approach was for high sacrectomy with right ELSiE and either posterior exenteration (with the patient accepting a non-functional bladder) and right ureteric reimplantation or total pelvic exenteration. The detailed report proposed was as follows: en-bloc high sacrectomy at the S1/2 junction by dissecting down in the subperiosteal plane from the sacral promontory for 38 mm before transecting the sacrum, taking care to preserve the right L5 nerve root but including the S1 nerve root in the resection. Along the right pelvic sidewall, the internal iliac artery should be ligated proximal to the origin of the SGA and excised with the specimen. The abdominal dissection should stop at the upper level of the sciatic notch to avoid breaching the structures which need to be resected as part of the ELSiE. From the prone position, on the right side all gluteal tissues should be mobilized off the posterior aspect of the SLAM and piriformis muscle to the tip of the ischial spine; after transection of the ischial spine, the distal aspect of the obturator internus muscle should be excised.

This roadmap was strictly followed intraoperatively and a total pelvic exenteration with en-bloc S1/2 sacrectomy and right ELSiE was performed, resulting in R0 resection and very limited impact on patient mobility.

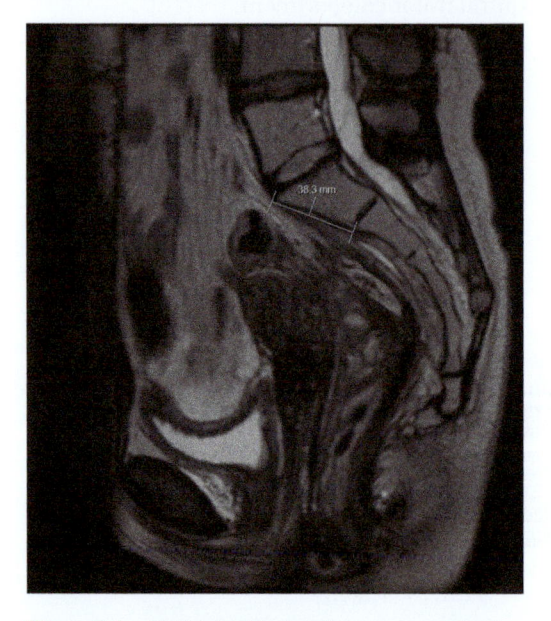

Figure 3.1 Sagittal MRI showing presacral fluid collection surrounded by a thick rim of fibrosis abutting the anterior sacral cortex; the extent of subperiosteal dissection to the level of planned sacral transection is indicated.

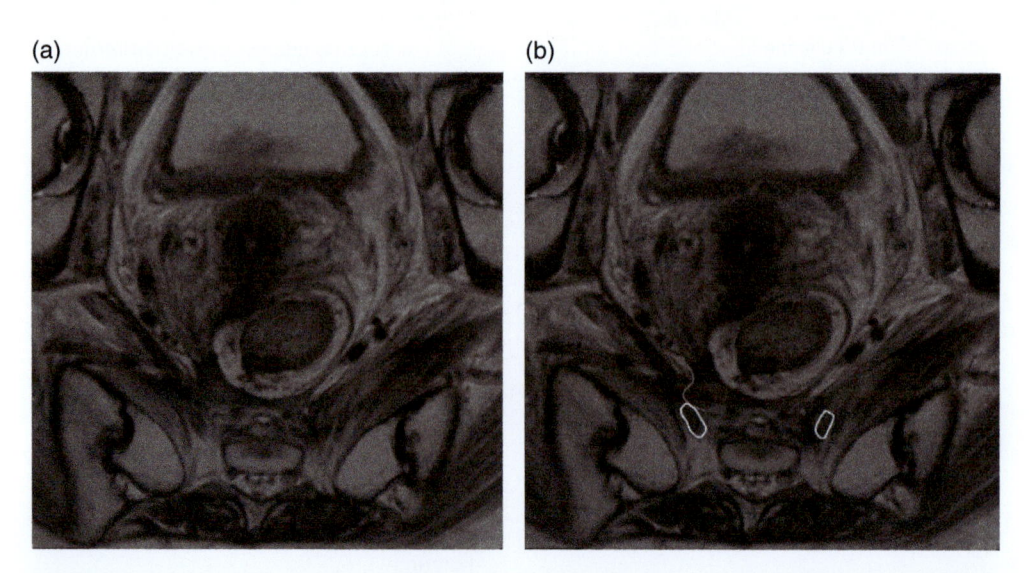

Figure 3.2 (a) Axial MRI at the level of S1 nerve roots. (b) Right S1 nerve root clearly inseparable from edge of tumor.

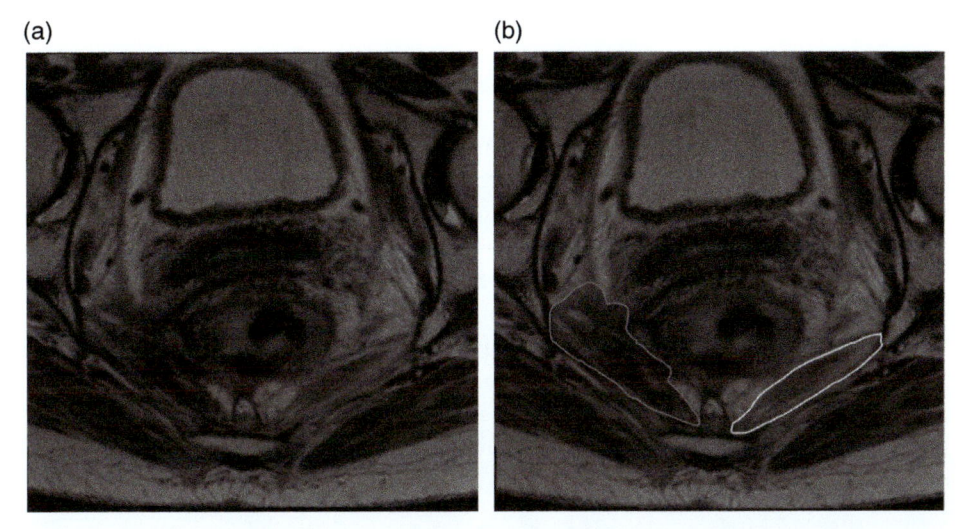

Figure 3.3 (a) Axial MRI at the level of ischial spine. (b) Gross involvement of the right SLAM complex to its insertion at the tip of the right ischial spine by tumor compared to a normal left SLAM.

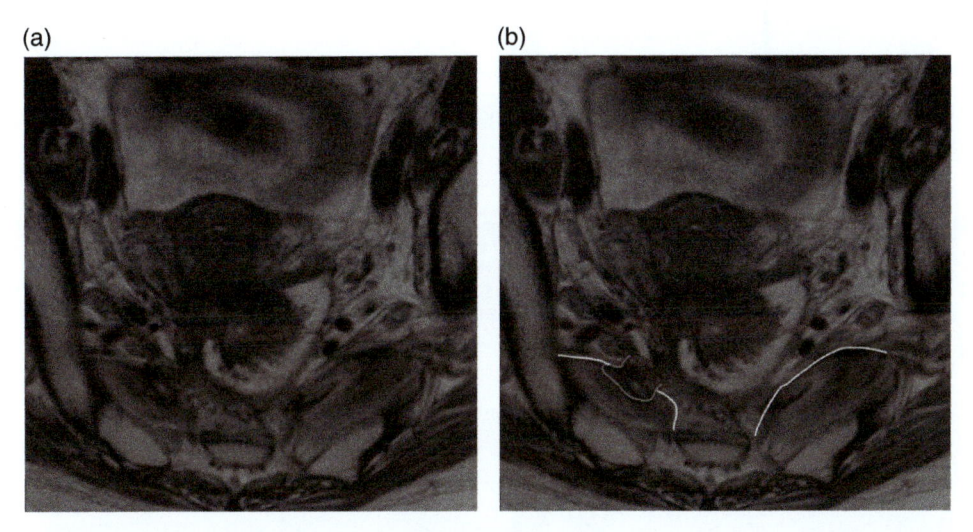

Figure 3.4 (a) Axial MRI at the level of the piriformis muscle. (b) The anterior edge of the left piriformis is smooth, but the right piriformis is clearly infiltrated by tumor.

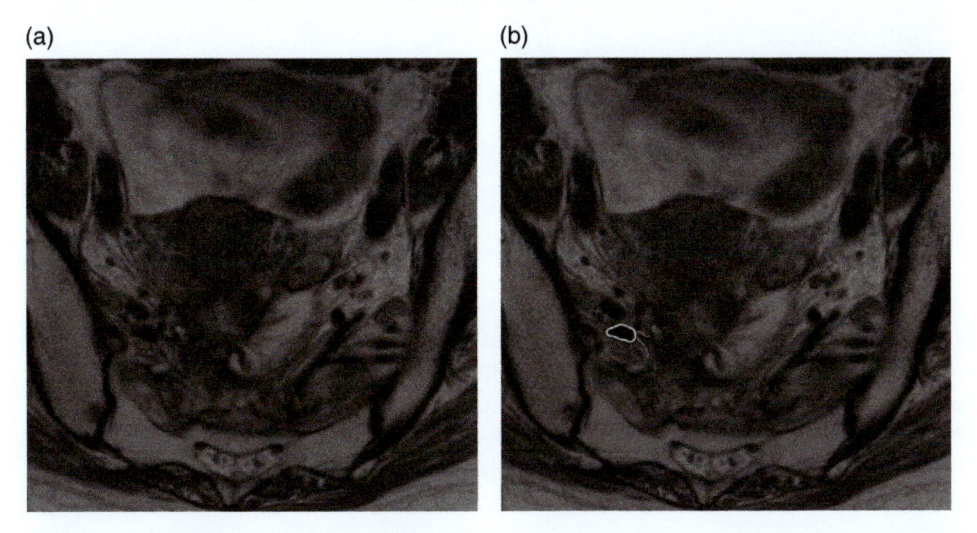

Figure 3.5 (a) Axial MRI at the level of the SGA. (b) A "tongue" of tumor clearly extending toward the medial aspect of the right SGA.

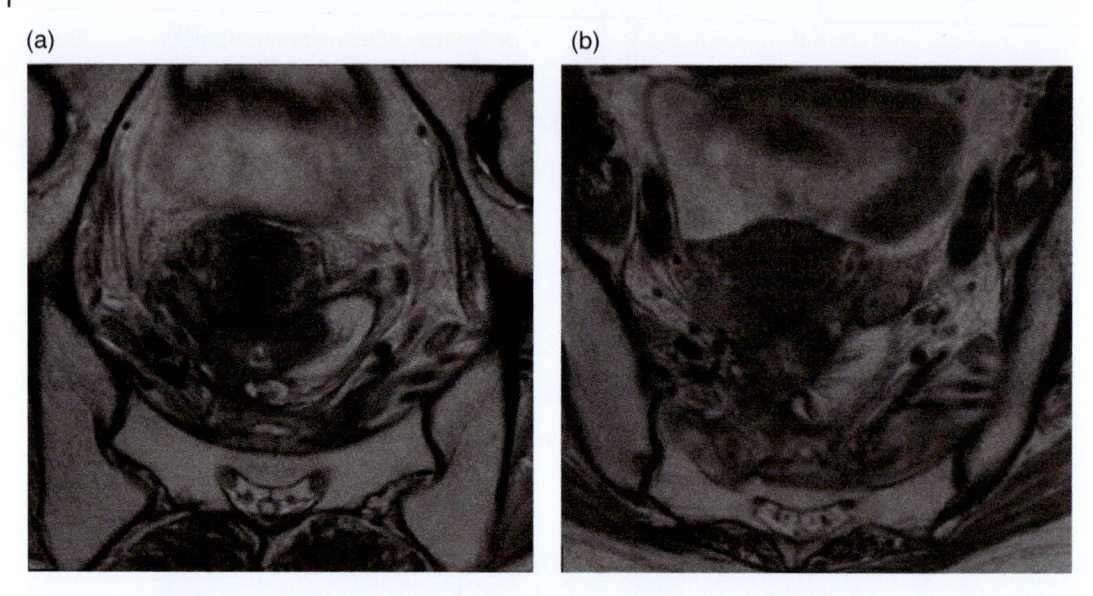

Figure 3.6 Coronal MRI showing tethering of the uterus and rectum by tumor/fibrosis.

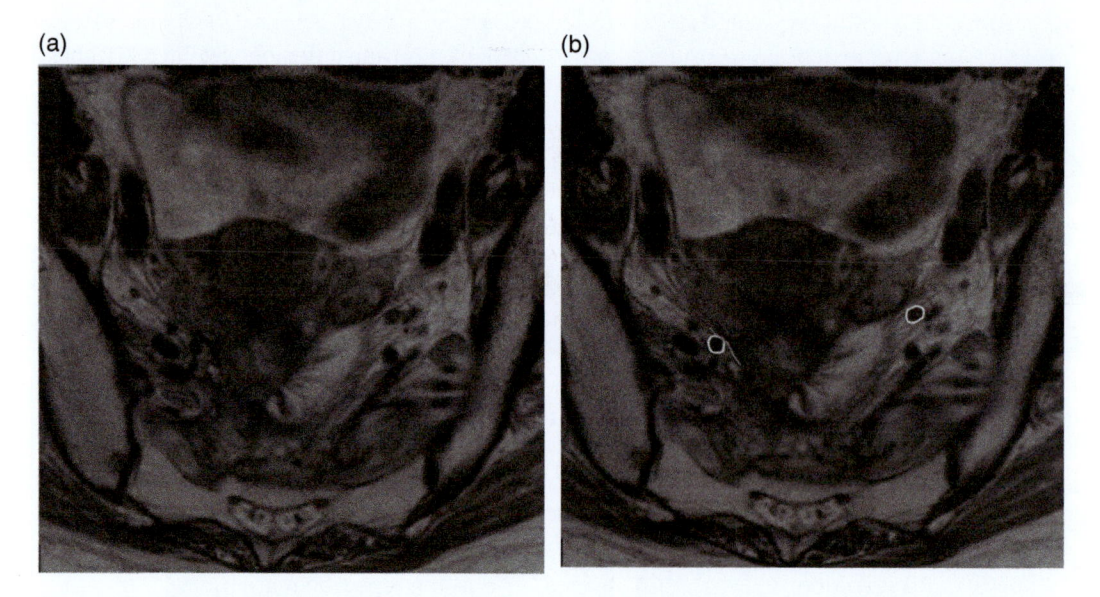

Figure 3.7 (a) Axial MRI at the level of the distal ureters. (b) The right ureter is clearly in direct contact with the edge of tumor/fibrosis; note the clear asymmetry in position of the ureters due to tethering by the tumor to the right of the midline.

Radiological Assessment of Metastatic Disease

Approximately 50% of patients with RRC will have metachronous metastatic disease at the time of diagnosis of pelvic recurrence [56]. CT examination of the chest, abdomen, and pelvis is the primary technique for identification of metastatic disease [43]. PET-CT utilizing fluorodeoxyglucose (FDG) can occasionally be helpful in troubleshooting indeterminate lesions such as borderline enlarged para-aortic or inguinal nodes or for detection of CT occult disease. Some centers routinely use PET-CT for initial assessment of all patients with advanced pelvic tumors, as it can alter management by detection of multifocal metastases [57–59]. In one study, the use of PET in preoperative staging of patients with RRC was identified as an independent predictor of overall survival after R0 resection [60]. However, the evidence supporting routine use of PET-CT for evaluation of recurrent colorectal cancer is limited [61–63]. A meta-analysis of the role of PET in staging patients with recurrent colorectal cancer found a pooled sensitivity and specificity for detection of distant metastases of 91 and 83% respectively, and 97 and 98% for detection of liver metastases alone [64]. However, there was significant heterogeneity among included studies. Overall, the consensus in many centers, including the authors of this chapter, is that PET-CT should be used selectively in the following circumstances: to troubleshoot indeterminate findings from conventional imaging such as scar versus tumor in the postoperative pelvis or for assessment of borderline enlarged lymph nodes; to help exclude CT occult metastatic disease (for example bony and brain metastases) in patients with extensive malignancy or where a tumor is associated with poor prognostic features; and when assessing response of metastatic disease to chemotherapy and/or radiotherapy.

For liver metastases, MRI is the most accurate and preferred modality and also provides useful anatomical information regarding suitability for radiofrequency ablation or excision [61].

For peritoneal metastases, the main role of imaging is assessment of the number, volume, and distribution of peritoneal disease and extraperitoneal metastases. The Peritoneal Cancer Index (PCI) is the most widely used method of estimating the tumor burden [65–71]. However, CT consistently underestimates PCI [72], with only 11% sensitivity for nodules smaller than 0.5 mm [73]. Overall accuracy of CT for detection of peritoneal lesions in the nine abdomino-pelvic regions has been estimated at 51–88% [74]. MRI has been shown to correctly predict surgical PCI in 91% of patients [72] and diffusion-weighted MRI has a sensitivity and specificity of 90 and 95.5% respectively for depicting peritoneal metastases in gynecological malignancy [75]. In the authors' experience, most "CT and MRI occult" metastases measuring 5 mm diameter or more are retrospectively visible on scan review and there is considerable interobserver variability when reporting peritoneal metastases.

Summary Box

- Preoperative staging should address local tumor anatomy as well as systemic spread.
- Preoperative staging of tumor anatomy should be aimed at maximizing the probability of R0 resection.
- MRI-based radiology, with selective additional use of ERUS, is the mainstay of assessment of tumor anatomy.
- The roadmap approach to serial MRI provides detailed assessment of structures involved or threatened by tumor and of adjacent unaffected structures which will form the resection margin.

References

1 de Wilt, J.H., Vermaas, M., Ferenschild, F.T., and Verhoef, C. (2007). Management of locally advanced primary and recurrent rectal cancer. *Clin. Colon Rectal Surg.* 20: 255–263.

2 Warrier, S.K., Heriot, A.G., and Lynch, A.C. (2016). Surgery for locally recurrent rectal cancer: tips, tricks, and pitfalls. *Clin. Colon Rectal Surg.* 29: 114–122.

3 Harji, D.P., Griffiths, B., McArthur, D.R., and Sagar, P.M. (2012). Current UK management of locally recurrent rectal cancer. *Color. Dis.* 14: 1479–1482.

4 Helewa, R.M. and Park, J. (2016). Surgery for locally advanced T4 rectal cancer: strategies and techniques. *Clin. Colon Rectal Surg.* 29: 106–113.

5 Brunschwig, A. (1948). Complete excision of pelvic viscera for advanced carcinoma; a one-stage abdominoperineal operation with end colostomy and bilateral ureteral implantation into the colon above the colostomy. *Cancer* 1: 177–183.

6 Shaikh, I., Holloway, I., Aston, W. et al. (2016). High subcortical sacrectomy: a novel approach to facilitate complete resection of locally advanced and recurrent rectal cancer with high (S1–S2) sacral extension. *Color. Dis.* 18: 386–392.

7 Milne, T., Solomon, M.J., Lee, P. et al. (2013). Assessing the impact of a sacral resection on morbidity and survival after extended radical surgery for locally recurrent rectal cancer. *Ann. Surg.* 258: 1007–1013.

8 Melton, G.B., Paty, P.B., Boland, P.J. et al. (2006). Sacral resection for recurrent rectal cancer: analysis of morbidity and treatment results. *Dis. Colon Rectum* 49: 1099–1107.

9 Shaikh, I., Aston, W., Hellawell, G. et al. (2014). Extended lateral pelvic sidewall excision (ELSiE): an approach to optimize complete resection rates in locally advanced or recurrent anorectal cancer involving the pelvic sidewall. *Tech. Coloproctol.* 18: 1161–1168.

10 Shaikh, I.A. and Jenkins, J.T. (2017). Extended pelvic side wall excision for locally advanced rectal cancers. *World J. Gastroenterol.* 23: 8261–8262.

11 Solomon, M.J., Brown, K.G., Koh, C.E. et al. (2015). Lateral pelvic compartment excision during pelvic exenteration. *Br. J. Surg.* 102: 1710–1717.

12 Austin, K.K. and Solomon, M.J. (2009). Pelvic exenteration with en bloc iliac vessel resection for lateral pelvic wall involvement. *Dis. Colon Rectum* 52: 1223–1233.

13 Hockel, M. (2015). Long-term experience with (laterally) extended endopelvic resection (LEER) in relapsed pelvic malignancies. *Curr. Oncol. Rep.* 17: 435.

14 Hockel, M. (2008). Laterally extended endopelvic resection (LEER) – principles and practice. *Gynecol. Oncol.* 111: S13–S17.

15 Solomon, M.J., Austin, K.K., Masya, L., and Lee, P. (2015). Pubic bone excision and perineal urethrectomy for radical anterior compartment excision during pelvic exenteration. *Dis. Colon Rectum* 58: 1114–1119.

16 Mehta, A.M., Hellawell, G., Burling, D. et al. (2018). Transperineal retropubic approach in total pelvic exenteration for advanced and recurrent colorectal and anal cancer involving the penile base: technique and outcomes. *Tech. Coloproctol.* 22: 663–671.

17 Bhangu, A., Ali, S.M., Brown, G. et al. (2014). Indications and outcome of pelvic exenteration for locally advanced primary and recurrent rectal cancer. *Ann. Surg.* 259: 315–322.

18 Heriot, A.G., Byrne, C.M., Lee, P. et al. (2008). Extended radical resection: the choice for locally recurrent rectal cancer. *Dis. Colon Rectum* 51: 284–291.

19 Hansen, M.H., Balteskard, L., Dorum, L.M. et al. (2009). Locally recurrent rectal cancer in Norway. *Br. J. Surg.* 96: 1176–1182.

20 Nielsen, M.B., Rasmussen, P.C., Lindegaard, J.C., and Laurberg, S. (2012). A 10-year experience of total pelvic exenteration for primary advanced and locally recurrent rectal cancer based on a prospective database. *Color. Dis.* 14: 1076–1083.

21 Bhangu, A., Ali, S.M., Darzi, A. et al. (2012). Meta-analysis of survival based on resection margin status following surgery for recurrent rectal cancer. *Color. Dis.* 14: 1457–1466.

22 PelvEx Collaborative (2019). Surgical and survival outcomes following pelvic exenteration for locally advanced primary rectal cancer: results from an international collaboration. *Ann. Surg.* 269 (2): 315–321.

23 PelvEx Collaborative (2018). Factors affecting outcomes following pelvic exenteration for locally recurrent rectal cancer. *Br. J. Surg.* 105: 650–657.

24 Georgiou, P.A., Tekkis, P.P., and Brown, G. (2011). Pelvic colorectal recurrence: crucial role of radiologists in oncologic and surgical treatment options. *Cancer Imaging* 11: S103–S111.

25 Peschaud, F., Cuenod, C.A., Benoist, S. et al. (2005). Accuracy of magnetic resonance imaging in rectal cancer depends on location of the tumor. *Dis. Colon Rectum* 48: 1603–1609.

26 Kim, Y.W., Cha, S.W., Pyo, J. et al. (2009). Factors related to preoperative assessment of the circumferential resection margin and the extent of mesorectal invasion by magnetic resonance imaging in rectal cancer: a prospective comparison study. *World J. Surg.* 33: 1952–1960.

27 Granero-Castro, P., Munoz, E., Frasson, M. et al. (2014). Evaluation of mesorectal fascia in mid and low anterior rectal cancer using endorectal ultrasound is feasible and reliable: a comparison with MRI findings. *Dis. Colon Rectum* 57: 709–714.

28 Phang, P.T., Gollub, M.J., Loh, B.D. et al. (2012). Accuracy of endorectal ultrasound for measurement of the closest predicted radial mesorectal margin for rectal cancer. *Dis. Colon Rectum* 55: 59–64.

29 Shur, J., Corr, A., Burling, D., and Jenkins, J.T. (2018). SS 2.9 Endorectal ultrasound is accurate for the assessment of anterior resection margin in low rectal cancer. *Insights Imaging* 9: S663.

30 Marusch, F., Ptok, H., Sahm, M. et al. (2011). Endorectal ultrasound in rectal carcinoma – do the literature results really correspond to the realities of routine clinical care? *Endoscopy* 43: 425–431.

31 Balyasnikova, S. and Brown, G. (2016). Optimal imaging strategies for rectal cancer staging and ongoing management. *Curr. Treat. Options Oncol.* 17: 32.

32 von Schulthess, G.K., Steinert, H.C., and Hany, T.F. (2006). Integrated PET/CT: current applications and future directions. *Radiology* 238: 405–422.

33 Suzuki, K., Dozois, R.R., Devine, R.M. et al. (1996). Curative reoperations for locally recurrent rectal cancer. *Dis. Colon Rectum* 39: 730–736.

34 Yamada, K., Ishizawa, T., Niwa, K. et al. (2001). Patterns of pelvic invasion are prognostic in the treatment of locally recurrent rectal cancer. *Br. J. Surg.* 88: 988–993.

35 Wanebo, H.J., Antoniuk, P., Koness, R.J. et al. (1999). Pelvic resection of recurrent rectal cancer: technical considerations and outcomes. *Dis. Colon Rectum* 42: 1438–1448.

36 Moore, H.G., Shoup, M., Riedel, E. et al. (2004). Colorectal cancer pelvic recurrences: determinants of resectability. *Dis. Colon Rectum* 47: 1599–1606.

37 Georgiou, P.A., Tekkis, P.P., Constantinides, V.A. et al. (2013). Diagnostic accuracy and value of magnetic resonance imaging (MRI) in planning exenterative pelvic surgery for advanced colorectal cancer. *Eur. J. Cancer* 49: 72–81.

38 Kim, Y.H., Kim, D.Y., Kim, T.H. et al. (2005). Usefulness of magnetic resonance volumetric evaluation in predicting response to preoperative concurrent chemoradiotherapy in patients with resectable rectal cancer. *Int. J. Radiat. Oncol. Biol. Phys.* 62: 761–768.

39 Hartley, A., Ho, K.F., McConkey, C., and Geh, J.I. (2005). Pathological complete response following pre-operative chemoradiotherapy in rectal cancer: analysis of phase II/III trials. *Br. J. Radiol.* 78: 934–938.

40 Rullier, E. and Sebag-Montefiore, D. (2006). Sphincter saving is the primary objective for local treatment of cancer of the lower rectum. *Lancet Oncol.* 7: 775–777.

41 Ryan, J.E., Warrier, S.K., Lynch, A.C., and Heriot, A.G. (2015). Assessing pathological complete response to neoadjuvant chemoradiotherapy in locally advanced rectal cancer: a systematic review. *Color. Dis.* 17: 849–861.

42 Hoffmann, K.-T., Rau, B., Wust, P. et al. (2002). Restaging of locally advanced carcinoma of the rectum with MR imaging after preoperative radio-chemotherapy plus regional hyperthermia. *Strahlenther. Onkol.* 178: 386–392.

43 Beyond TME Collaborative (2013). Consensus statement on the multidisciplinary management of patients with recurrent and primary rectal cancer beyond total mesorectal excision planes. *Br. J. Surg.* 100: 1009–1014.

44 Barbaro, B., Vitale, R., Leccisotti, L. et al. (2010). Restaging locally advanced rectal cancer with MR imaging after chemoradiation therapy. *Radiographics* 30: 699–716.

45 Dresen, R.C., Beets, G.L., Rutten, H.J. et al. (2009). Locally advanced rectal cancer: MR imaging for restaging after neoadjuvant radiation therapy with concomitant chemotherapy. Part I. Are we able to predict tumor confined to the rectal wall? *Radiology* 252: 71–80.

46 Barbaro, B., Fiorucci, C., Tebala, C. et al. (2009). Locally advanced rectal cancer: MR imaging in prediction of response after preoperative chemotherapy and radiation therapy. *Radiology* 250: 730–739.

47 Jhaveri, K.S. and Hosseini-Nik, H. (2015). MRI of rectal cancer: an overview and update on recent advances. *Am. J. Roentgenol.* 205: W42–W55.

48 Patel, U.B., Blomqvist, L.K., Taylor, F. et al. (2012). MRI after treatment of locally advanced rectal cancer: how to report tumor response – the MERCURY experience. *Am. J. Roentgenol.* 199: W486–W495.

49 Vliegen, R.F., Beets, G.L., Lammering, G. et al. (2008). Mesorectal fascia invasion after neoadjuvant chemotherapy and radiation therapy for locally advanced rectal cancer: accuracy of MR imaging for prediction. *Radiology* 246: 454–462.

50 Chen, C.C., Lee, R.C., Lin, J.K. et al. (2005). How accurate is magnetic resonance imaging in restaging rectal cancer in patients receiving preoperative combined chemoradiotherapy? *Dis. Colon Rectum* 48: 722–728.

51 Kuo, L.J., Chern, M.C., Tsou, M.H. et al. (2005). Interpretation of magnetic resonance imaging for locally advanced rectal carcinoma after preoperative chemoradiation therapy. *Dis. Colon Rectum* 48: 23–28.

52 Muthusamy, V.R. and Chang, K.J. (2007). Optimal methods for staging rectal cancer. *Clin. Cancer Res.* 13: 6877s–6884s.

53 Allen, S.D., Padhani, A.R., Dzik-Jurasz, A.S., and Glynne-Jones, R. (2007). Rectal carcinoma: MRI with histologic correlation before and after chemoradiation therapy. *Am. J. Roentgenol.* 188: 442–451.

54 Maretto, I., Pomerri, F., Pucciarelli, S. et al. (2007). The potential of restaging in the prediction of pathologic response after preoperative chemoradiotherapy for rectal cancer. *Ann. Surg. Oncol.* 14: 455–461.

55 Del Vescovo, R., Trodella, L.E., Sansoni, I. et al. (2012). MR imaging of rectal cancer before and after chemoradiation therapy. *Radiol. Med.* 117: 1125–1138.

56 Gagliardi, G., Hawley, P.R., Hershman, M.J., and Arnott, S.J. (1995). Prognostic factors in surgery for local recurrence of rectal cancer. *Br. J. Surg.* 82: 1401–1405.

57 Potter, K.C., Husband, J.E., Houghton, S.L. et al. (2009). Diagnostic accuracy of serial CT/magnetic resonance imaging review vs. positron emission tomography/CT in colorectal cancer patients with suspected and known recurrence. *Dis. Colon Rectum* 52: 253–259.

58 Sammour, T. and Skibber, J.M. (2018). Evaluation of treatment of locally recurrent rectal cancer. In: *Rectal Cancer: Modern Approaches to Treatment* (ed. G.J. Chang), 231–245. Cham: Springer International Publishing.

59 Watson, A.J., Lolohea, S., Robertson, G.M., and Frizelle, F.A. (2007). The role of positron emission tomography in the management of recurrent colorectal cancer: a review. *Dis. Colon Rectum* 50: 102–114.

60 Selvaggi, F., Fucini, C., Pellino, G. et al. (2015). Outcome and prognostic factors of local recurrent rectal cancer: a pooled analysis of 150 patients. *Tech. Coloproctol.* 19: 135–144.

61 Floriani, I., Torri, V., Rulli, E. et al. (2010). Performance of imaging modalities in

diagnosis of liver metastases from colorectal cancer: a systematic review and meta-analysis. *J. Magn. Reson. Imaging* 31: 19–31.

62 Bellomi, M., Rizzo, S., Travaini, L.L. et al. (2007). Role of multidetector CT and FDG-PET/CT in the diagnosis of local and distant recurrence of resected rectal cancer. *Radiol. Med.* 112: 681–690.

63 Agarwal, A., Marcus, C., Xiao, J. et al. (2014). FDG PET/CT in the management of colorectal and anal cancers. *Am. J. Roentgenol.* 203: 1109–1119.

64 Zhang, C., Chen, Y., Xue, H. et al. (2009). Diagnostic value of FDG-PET in recurrent colorectal carcinoma: a meta-analysis. *Int. J. Cancer* 124: 167–173.

65 Sugarbaker, P.H. and Jablonski, K.A. (1995). Prognostic features of 51 colorectal and 130 appendiceal cancer patients with peritoneal carcinomatosis treated by cytoreductive surgery and intraperitoneal chemotherapy. *Ann. Surg.* 221: 124–132.

66 Portilla, A.G., Sugarbaker, P.H., and Chang, D. (1999). Second-look surgery after cytoreduction and intraperitoneal chemotherapy for peritoneal carcinomatosis from colorectal cancer: analysis of prognostic features. *World J. Surg.* 23: 23–29.

67 Sugarbaker, P.H. (1999). Successful management of microscopic residual disease in large bowel cancer. *Cancer Chemother. Pharmacol.* 43: S15–S25.

68 Elias, D., Blot, F., El Otmany, A. et al. (2001). Curative treatment of peritoneal carcinomatosis arising from colorectal cancer by complete resection and intraperitoneal chemotherapy. *Cancer* 92: 71–76.

69 Glehen, O. and Gilly, F.N. (2003). Quantitative prognostic indicators of peritoneal surface malignancy: carcinomatosis, sarcomatosis, and peritoneal mesothelioma. *Surg. Oncol. Clin. North Am.* 12: 649–671.

70 Tentes, A.A., Tripsiannis, G., Markakidis, S.K. et al. (2003). Peritoneal cancer index: a prognostic indicator of survival in advanced ovarian cancer. *Eur. J. Surg. Oncol.* 29: 69–73.

71 Harmon, R.L. and Sugarbaker, P.H. (2005). Prognostic indicators in peritoneal carcinomatosis from gastrointestinal cancer. *Int. Semin. Surg. Oncol.* 2: 3.

72 Low, R.N., Barone, R.M., and Lucero, J. (2015). Comparison of MRI and CT for predicting the peritoneal cancer index (PCI) preoperatively in patients being considered for cytoreductive surgical procedures. *Ann. Surg. Oncol.* 22: 1708–1715.

73 Koh, J.L., Yan, T.D., Glenn, D., and Morris, D.L. (2009). Evaluation of preoperative computed tomography in estimating peritoneal cancer index in colorectal peritoneal carcinomatosis. *Ann. Surg. Oncol.* 16: 327–333.

74 Chua, T.C., Al-Zahrani, A., Saxena, A. et al. (2011). Determining the association between preoperative computed tomography findings and postoperative outcomes after cytoreductive surgery and perioperative intraperitoneal chemotherapy for pseudomyxoma peritonei. *Ann. Surg. Oncol.* 18: 1582–1589.

75 Fujii, S., Matsusue, E., Kanasaki, Y. et al. (2008). Detection of peritoneal dissemination in gynecological malignancy: evaluation by diffusion-weighted MR imaging. *Eur. Radiol.* 18: 18–23.

4

Neoadjuvant Therapy Options for Advanced Rectal Cancer

Alexandra Zaborowski[1], Paul Kelly[2], and Brian Bird[3]

[1] Department of Surgery, St. Vincent's University Hospital, Dublin, Ireland
[2] Department of Radiation Oncology, Bon Secours, Cork, Ireland
[3] Department of Medical Oncology, Bon Secours, Cork, Ireland

Background

Combined-modality therapy was a paradigm shift in managing locally advanced rectal cancer (LARC) in the latter part of the twentieth century. Neoadjuvant chemoradiotherapy (nCRT; long-course radiotherapy with concomitant fluoropyrimidine-based chemotherapy) then interval total mesorectal excision (TME) is the standard of care for patients with bulky cT3/4 tumors or predicted node-positive disease in most countries. Short-course radiotherapy (five fractions without chemotherapy) is also an evidence-based standard and was pioneered in Scandinavia, the Netherlands, and the UK. Several large studies have demonstrated superior disease-related outcomes with neoadjuvant therapy over surgery alone [1–4]. Following systematically taught TME and widespread adoption of tri-modality therapy, five-year local recurrence rates decreased to 5% or less [5]. However, long-term overall survival (OS) did not improve in parallel and the leading cause of rectal-cancer-related death is now distant disease failure, with approximately 20–30% of patients developing distant metastases despite receiving postoperative chemotherapy in some countries [6]. Increasing emphasis has been placed on optimized systemic therapy to improve long-term OS.

In the USA and some European countries adjuvant chemotherapy has been recommended in the management of LARC. This is largely based on extrapolation from the results of trials in colonic cancer demonstrating improved disease-free survival (DFS) and OS. Oncologists generally estimate that adjuvant fluoropyrimidine-based chemotherapy reduces the relative risk of systemic recurrence of colon cancer by one-third, with oxaliplatin adding another 5–6% benefit [7, 8]. Early trials in rectal cancer observed similar survival advantages; however, these trials were conducted prior to the introduction of neoadjuvant therapy [9, 10]. The role of adjuvant chemotherapy in the modern era of nCRT is less defined. ADORE—a large phase II Korean trial—randomized patients post nCRT to four cycles of adjuvant 5-fluorouracil (5-FU) or FOLFOX (5-FU, leucovorin, and oxaliplatin) and demonstrated improvement in DFS [11]. Four randomized European trials have failed to demonstrate a significant survival benefit [12–15]. Notably, these trials demonstrated that compliance with adjuvant chemotherapy is poor following rectal cancer surgery. In the largest of these studies, the European Organization for Research and Treatment of Cancer (EORTC) 22921 trial, over half of

---

Surgical Management of Advanced Pelvic Cancer, First Edition.
Edited by Michael E. Kelly and Desmond C. Winter.
© 2022 John Wiley & Sons Ltd. Published 2022 by John Wiley & Sons Ltd.

patients did not complete the intended four cycles [15]. Any apparent absence of survival advantage with adjuvant chemotherapy may be related, in part, to poor tolerance of postoperative treatment. Furthermore, a meta-analysis evaluating the impact of time from surgery to adjuvant therapy on survival in colorectal cancers demonstrated that a four-week increase in time was associated with a significant decrease in DFS (hazard ratio [HR] 1.14, 95% confidence interval [CI] 1.10–1.18) [16]. Alternative approaches are required to optimize delivery. Total neoadjuvant therapy (TNT) has emerged as an attractive alternative strategy—systemic chemotherapy given before nCRT (i.e. induction chemotherapy) or after it (consolidation chemotherapy) in the preoperative setting.

Potential Advantages of TNT

1) Targeting of subclinical micrometastases: Early administration of full-dose systemic chemotherapy has the potential of eradicating occult micrometastases, reducing distant disease failure, and prolonging long-term survival.
2) Assessment of tumor biology: TNT provides an opportunity to evaluate the innate biomolecular profile of the tumor. Disease progression during full-dose systemic chemotherapy suggests aggressive tumor biology. Patients with unfavorable treatment-resistant disease may receive little or no benefit from subsequent resection.
3) Increased tumor downstaging: Additional full-dose systemic chemotherapy may improve resectability by inducing tumor downsizing. This may be related to the direct effects of the chemotherapy and/or indirectly due to the prolonged interval to resection. Patients who experience marked tumor regression may become suitable for less radical or sphincter-preserving surgery, although this is controversial. As a general principle, adjacent structures directly invaded by the tumor (including sphincters) should be considered for en-bloc resection unless sure they are not involved. Deviation from the initial planned surgical approach requires excellent imaging, endoscopy, and multidisciplinary input in addition to judicious intraoperative decision-making.
4) Increased pathological complete response (pCR): A pCR represents a strong positive prognostic indicator, associated with improved local control and disease-specific survival [17].
5) Potential for organ preservation: The clinical implication of improved tumor regression is the selective practice of surgery and potential for non-operative management. An expectant "watch and wait" approach may be appropriate in patients who demonstrate a good response to neoadjuvant therapy.
6) Superior compliance: Surgical morbidity and postoperative complications may limit compliance to adjuvant chemotherapy. Delivery in the preoperative period may improve compliance by avoiding such limitations.

Potential Disadvantages of TNT

1) Disease progression: Delay to definitive surgery may allow local disease progression, resulting in more technically challenging resection and increased perioperative morbidity, or even unresectability. However, progression on full-dose chemotherapy indicates an unfavorable disease profile that suggests disease course and outcome would not be altered by surgery.
2) Negative effect on performance status: Full-dose systemic chemotherapy may negatively impact fitness, thereby delaying or preventing surgery. Reduced physiological reserve due to treatment-related toxicity could increase the risk of perioperative morbidity (or even mortality). In practice this should not be the case with reasonable assessment of performance status, comprehensive geriatric assessment, adequate organ function parameters, and general well-being [18]. It is better to wait for full recovery than to compromise outcome for timing.

Short-Term Outcomes

Pathological Response

Neoadjuvant therapy has the potential to eradicate tumors entirely. A pCR, defined as an absence of tumor cells in the resected specimen, represents an important predictor of favorable oncological outcome [15, 19]. In a meta-analysis of 16 studies involving 3363 patients with LARC treated with nCRT, those who achieved a pCR had less local recurrence (odds ratio [OR] 0.25, 95% CI 0.10–0.59, p = 0.002) and better five-year DFS (OR 4.33, 95% CI 2.31–8.09, p < 0.001) [17].

Pathological outcomes following TNT are limited, available data are conflicting, and whether TNT improves pCR rates is unclear. Furthermore, pCR rates are influenced by interval to surgery as radiation-induced tumor necrosis is time-dependent. Several large series and meta-analyses have demonstrated increased pCR rates with intervals of > 6–8 weeks following completion of nCRT [20–22]. The GRECCAR6 phase III multicenter randomized control trial of 265 patients found no significant difference in pCR rates after an interval of 7 weeks compared to 11 weeks between nCRT and surgery, with standard practice now an interval of 8–10 weeks [23]. Whether pathological response observed with TNT is due to the direct effect of chemotherapy or prolonged interval to surgery or both is unclear.

The CONTRE (Complete Neoadjuvant Treatment for Rectal Cancer) study reported a pCR rate of 33% following eight cycles of induction-modified FOLFOX6 [24]. Surgery was performed 6–10 weeks following completion of nCRT. Another North American study reported a rate of up to 38%, with the longest regimen (six cycles of induction FOLFOX with an interval of up to 19 weeks) but only 18% in patients treated with standard nCRT [25]. Interestingly, the Spanish GCR-3 phase II trial reported no significant difference in pCR rate between induction capecitabine plus oxaliplatin (CAPOX) and conventional nCRT (14.3 vs. 13.5%) [26]. In this study, the interval to surgery was considerably shorter (five to six weeks). A large registry-based study of 36 268 patients with clinical stage II or III disease, 3421 of whom received induction chemotherapy, also reported no difference in pCR rates between the TNT and conventional groups [27]. These registry-based data must be interpreted with caution as exact chemotherapeutic regimens are unknown. Furthermore, selection criteria for TNT were unavailable, and thus a significant proportion of the TNT group may have included patients with advanced disease with unfavorable biology (cT4, significant nodal burden, threatened mesorectal margin).

In a systematic review of 10 prospective studies involving 648 patients treated with TNT, the overall pCR rate was 21.8% (range 10–40%) [28]. In the 10 comparative studies included, the overall pCR rate following TNT was 19% and TNT increased the odds of pCR by 39% (OR 1.39, 95% CI 1.08–1.81, p = 0.01). Similar findings were reported in a meta-analysis of 28 studies (retrospective and prospective) of 3579 patients receiving TNT (n = 2688) or conventional nCRT (n = 891) [29]. The pooled pCR rate with TNT was 22.4% (95% CI 19.4–25.7, p < 0.001). Interpretation and application of these data are difficult and hampered by the heterogeneity of systemic agents used, timing of chemotherapy, and interval to surgery.

The Dutch–Swedish RAPIDO trial compared three-year DFS following short-course radiotherapy (5×5 Gy), full-dose preoperative CAPOX and interval TME, with conventional nCRT, TME, and selective adjuvant chemotherapy (CAPOX or FOLFOX) [30]. The RAPIDO trial found that, compared to traditional neoadjuvant CRT and surgery, short-course radiotherapy followed by neoadjuvant chemotherapy prior to surgery reduced distant metastatic events at three years (20% vs. 26.8%). It increased pCR from 14% to 28%, with a putative survival advantage, but without altering quality of life or overall surgical morbidity. The PRODIGE 23 trial, another prospective randomized trial examining TNT, compared induction triplet neoadjuvant chemotherapy (six cycles of modified FOLFIRINOX; 5-FU, leucovorin, irinotecan, and oxaliplatin) followed by neoadjuvant CRT, surgery, and a further three months of chemotherapy (either FOLFOX or capecitabine) with conventional nCRT, surgery, and six months of adjuvant chemotherapy [31]. It found pCR improved from 11.7% to 27.5% and three-year metastasis-free survival from 71.7% to 78.8% with TNT over the control arm. Metastatic disease on restaging prior to surgery was also lower with TNT (1% vs. 4.7%).

Long-Term Oncological Outcomes

The key clinical question is whether delivery of up-front full-dose systemic chemotherapy and increased compliance improves disease-specific outcomes. Long-term survival data following TNT are lacking and predominantly limited to small case series. A systematic review of oncological outcomes following TNT, including seven prospective studies reporting five-year survival data, found similar long-term survival outcomes when compared with standard nCR. The overall weighted mean five-year OS and DFS were 74.4 and 65.4% respectively. Comparative analysis of seven studies by Petrelli et al., however, demonstrated that patients who received TNT had better DFS (HR 0.75, 95% CI 0.52–1.07, $p = 0.11$) and OS (HR 0.73, 95% CI 0.59–0.9, $p = 0.004$) than those who received conventional nCRT only [29]. In a multi-institutional phase II trial, better disease-specific survival was observed with consolidation chemotherapy (two, four, or six cycles of modified FOLFOX) compared with conventional nCRT [32]. After a median follow-up of 59 months, five-year DFS was 81% following consolidation chemotherapy compared to 50% with nCRT ($p = 0.0005$). There were no significant differences in survival among the experimental arms. Notably, the primary endpoint of this trial was pCR and it was not adequately powered to show differences in survival. Similarly, a North American multicenter retrospective analysis of 110 patients with cT3/4 N0–2 disease treated with short-course radiotherapy also observed improved DFS with consolidation FOLFOX [33]. DFS at three years was 85% compared with 68% among patients treated with standard nCRT and adjuvant chemotherapy ($p = 0.032$). A single-arm Chinese study of 96 patients with cT3/4 or node-positive disease treated with consolidation XELOX (capecitabine and oxaliplatin) also reported comparable five-year DFS of 83% [34]. Interestingly, the Polish phase III randomized trial of 515 patients with cT4 or fixed cT3 reported no significant difference in DFS between those receiving short-course radiotherapy with three cycles of consolidation FOLFOX4 compared to traditional CRT [35]. DFS at eight years was 43 vs. 41% respectively.

The most meaningful potential advantage of early full-dose chemotherapy is targeting subclinical micrometastases and reducing distant disease failure. In a systematic review of ten prospective studies, the overall weighted mean distant recurrence rate was 20.6% (range 5–31%). Eight studies reported distant failure rates consistent with the standard treatment paradigm (19–31%). The remaining two studies reported significantly lower rates [36, 37]. This discrepancy may be related to the shorter length of follow-up because of differences in clinical stage, compliance, and/or the use of adjuvant therapy. It will be interesting to see if the three-year metastasis-free survival benefit seen in RAPIDO and PRODIGE 23 is maintained with prolonged follow-up.

Organ Preservation

In addition to event-free survival and local control outcomes, preservation of bowel function and quality of life continue to represent significant challenges in the management of LARC. The prevalence of low anterior resection syndrome (LARS) is 60–90% following low or ultra-low sphincter-sparing surgery for rectal cancer [38]. The syndrome is associated with a significant and sustained reduction in quality of life [39, 40]. A potential advantage of improved tumor regression and downstaging with TNT is the selective practice of non-operative management and avoidance of a stoma. A multinational experience (1009 patients) of conventional nCRT and a "watch and wait" approach found two-year local tumor regrowth was 25% [41].

A retrospective single-center analysis of 628 patients with LARC observed more complete responders at one year with TNT compared with conventional nCRT and adjuvant chemotherapy [42]. This was the subject of a recently presented multicenter, randomized, phase II trial assessing if TNT increases the proportion of patients managed with organ preservation. Patients were randomized to induction or consolidation FOLFOX (before or after long-course chemoradiation), followed by restaging with magnetic resonance imaging (MRI)/endoscopy 8–12 weeks later. Incomplete responders proceeded to TME, while complete clinical responders were managed non-operatively [43]. Three-year disease- and metastasis-free survival rates were similar in the OPRA (organ preservation of rectal adenocarcinoma) trial arms, but the rate of organ preservation was improved by consolidation (58%) rather than induction (43%) chemotherapy.

In patients with early disease (cT1–2N0), the standard of care currently is surgery without neoadjuvant therapy. Systemic therapy with curative intent may be an alternative to surgery if long-term disease-specific outcomes were comparable. Those who achieve a clinical complete response (cCR) may be eligible for organ preservation, with salvage surgery reserved for cases of locoregional recurrence. A retrospective analysis of 81 patients with cT2N0 disease reported an increased likelihood of a cCR and avoidance of definitive surgery at five years with consolidation chemotherapy (six cycles of 5-FU) with high-dose radiotherapy (54 Gy) compared with standard nCRT (67 vs. 30%; $p = 0.001$) [44].

Chemotherapy and Compliance

Chemotherapy for LARC has traditionally been fluoropyrimidine-based. In the postoperative (adjuvant) setting, oxaliplatin improves progression-free and disease-free survival in colonic cancer [7]. The role of oxaliplatin in neoadjuvant treatment has been debated. Apart from the German CAO/ARO/AIO-04 trial [45], several trials and meta-analyses have failed to demonstrate a survival advantage with oxaliplatin added to radiosensitizing fluoropyrimidine nCRT [46–50]. Furthermore, oxaliplatin was associated with significant toxicity including neurotoxicity and increased risk of infection. For TNT, the optimum regimen is unknown (e.g. capecitabine alone, CAPOX, or FOLFOX). Toxicity of treatment regimens is a concern, and poor compliance could be a major challenge if patients do not complete the intended dose-intensity. Encouragingly, several trials evaluating induction and/or consolidation chemotherapy reported favorable compliance rates of over 90% with toxicity profiles comparable to those of standard nCRT [36, 51, 52]. In the Spanish GCR-3 study, 91% of patients completed the study protocol in the induction chemotherapy arm compared with 54% in the nCRT/adjuvant chemotherapy arm ($p < 0.001$) [53]. Garcia-Aguilar et al. reported compliance rates of 77–82% depending on the number of cycles of mFOLFOX given [25]. The two most recent phase 3 TNT trials (RAPIDO and PRODIGE 23) clearly demonstrate that it is safe and efficacious to incorporate oxaliplatin into neoadjuvant chemotherapy regimens. Neither trial included oxaliplatin during radiotherapy.

Novel Chemotherapeutic Agents

Integration of targeted agents in the treatment of LARC has been the focus of several modern early phase trials [54]. Preclinical studies have demonstrated that vascular endothelial growth factor (VEGF) blockade in combination with standard chemoradiotherapy enhances tumor regression. VEGF blockade induces alterations to the vasculature of the tumor microenvironment, increasing tumor perfusion and oxygenation and improving intratumoral drug delivery [55]. A meta-analysis reported a pooled pCR rate of 27% with neoadjuvant therapy including bevacizumab [56]. A small single-institution prospective phase II trial evaluating induction FOLFOX with bevacizumab followed by radiotherapy reported favorable pathological, toxicity, and survival outcomes [57]. Forty-three patients with clinical stage II–III low rectal adenocarcinoma and MRI-defined high-risk features (cT4, cN2, predicted positive lateral nodal involvement, threatened circumferential resection margin [CRM]) were included. The pCR rate was 37.2% and three-year DFS was 86%. Irinotecan has no adjuvant role in colon cancer and can have significant toxicities including colitis and sepsis. It has been successfully incorporated into neoadjuvant, adjuvant, and palliative chemotherapy for pancreatic cancer in the FOLFIRINOX regimen [58]. Several French trials use it as the backbone of a TNT approach in rectal cancer, but there is hesitancy to adopt it elsewhere.

The Italian TRUST trial also observed favorable results with induction FOLFOXIRI (5-FU, leucovorin, irinotecan, and oxaliplatin) and bevacizumab plus nCRT [59]. This phase II single-arm study of 49 patients with predicted node-positive or clinical T3/4 disease reported a pCR rate of 36% and two-year DFS of 80%. The GEMCAD 1402 trial randomized patients to induction mFOLFOX with or without aflibercept (VEGF inhibitor) [60]. In per protocol analysis, a pCR was achieved in 25.2% of the experimental arm and 14.5% of the control group (p= 0.10). In the EXPERT-C trial, patients with MRI-defined high-risk disease were randomized to induction CAPOX with cetuximab (epidermal growth factor receptor [EGFR] inhibitor) or CAPOX alone, followed by standard nCRT [61]. In this study, however, no significant difference in the primary endpoint of pCR was observed among groups. Capecitabine and cetuximab are no longer combined in routine practice as there is unacceptable synergistic skin toxicity. Although the addition of targeted agents has yielded some positive oncological outcomes, concerns exist surrounding their safety profile and associated toxicity. The AVACROSS phase II single-arm study evaluating induction XELOX with bevacizumab reported a high postoperative complication rate (58%), with 24% of patients requiring surgical reintervention [62]. No agent has emerged as superior to oral or intravenous 5-FU as a radiosensitizer. In colon cancer there has been no therapy added to systemic adjuvant therapy since oxaliplatin nearly two decades ago. Bevacizumab does not improve survival, and the monoclonal antibodies cetuximab and panitumumab which target EGFR have no adjuvant role even in *RAS/RAF* wild-type colon cancer. There was considerable enthusiasm for the poly-ADP ribose polymerase (PARP) inhibitor veliparib as a radiosensitizer, but unfortunately this was not confirmed by the NRG-GI002 phase II trial [63].

Immunotherapeutics

The past few decades have witnessed unprecedented advances in the field of cancer immunology. The focus of systemic therapy is developing novel strategies to enhance the ineffective antitumor response of the immune system. Immunotherapy with checkpoint blockade (mainly programed cell death protein 1 [PD-1]) has had limited efficacy in the vast majority of patients with metastatic colorectal cancer. Durable responses have predominantly been observed in patients with microsatellite instability-high (MSI-H) colorectal cancer [64]. The high mutational burden of microsatellite instability (MSI) tumors is thought to provoke a strong intratumoral T-cell response, which can be further enhanced with anti-PD-1 therapy. Pembrolizumab is now accepted as a first-line standard of care for MSI-H stage IV colon cancer based on the KEYNOTE-177 study [65]. There is concern that over one-third of MSI-H patients experience rapid disease progression on immunotherapy even though there is a large sustained survival benefit in the majority. *RAS* mutations and left-sided tumor origin had less benefit from immunotherapy, but *BRAF* mutations did not appear to detract from efficacy. Future characterization of blood and tumoral biomarkers may enable precise selection of patients likely to respond to monotherapy and those who require alternative approaches, potentially facilitating the integration of immunotherapy into the neoadjuvant treatment paradigm. There have been some early reports of dramatic responses to neoadjuvant immunotherapy in MSI-H rectal cancer [66]. While 10–15% of all colon cancer is MSI-H, only 3–5% of rectal cancer is. The holy grail of colon cancer research is a means by which to enable immunotherapy to benefit patients with microsatellite stable (MSS) disease. Can radiotherapy render MSS rectal cancer vulnerable to immunotherapy? The upregulation of programed cell death-ligand 1 (PD-L1) in rectal cancer post-radiotherapy may be associated with improved outcomes [67, 68]. Several early phase trials are exploring the PD-L1 antagonists avelumab (AVANA) and atezolizumab (R-IMMUNE) in combination with preoperative chemoradiotherapy [69–71]. Other studies such as PEMREC combine pembrolizumab with short-course radiation therapy [72]. In stage III non-small cell lung cancer, durvalumab is used following definitive chemoradiation based on the PACIFIC trial [73]. Similar approaches in rectal cancer such as the Dutch TARZAN trial (short-course radiation therapy followed by atezolizumab and bevacizumab) and the Chinese CHINOREC trial (nCRT followed by ipilimumab and nivolumab) are underway. There is no role for immunotherapy in MSS disease outside of clinical trials.

Locally Recurrent Rectal Cancer

The incidence of locally recurrent rectal cancer (LRRC) remains approximately 5%. A negative resection margin, the most important predictor of outcome, may be difficult to achieve due to the anatomical location, involvement of surrounding structures, and the challenges of prior surgery. As a result, upfront chemoradiotherapy may downstage tumors and improve resectability. In patients who have received radiotherapy for treatment of their primary tumor, reirradiation options are limited. Induction chemotherapy has been proposed as a potential means of improving tumor downstaging and clear margin rates. Moreover, it may eradicate occult micrometastases. Development of metastatic disease is common following local recurrence and represents the leading cause of cancer-related death following successful treatment of local recurrence. Preliminary results of a cohort study in the Netherlands demonstrated R0 and pCR rates of 55 and 17% respectively with induction chemotherapy compared to 49 and 4% with CRT alone ($p = 0.506$ and $p = 0.015$ respectively) [57, 74]. Among the induction chemotherapy group, achieving a pCR was strongly associated with improved three-year DFS (both local recurrence and distant metastases). Two European prospective randomized trials, the French GRECCAR15 and the Dutch PelvEx2 Induction Chemotherapy Trial, aim to determine the optimum preoperative management for LRRC (NCT03879109, Dutch Cancer Society no. 12960/2020–1). GRECCAR15 is comparing induction FOLFIRINOX (six cycles) followed by CRT (30.2 Gy with capecitabine) to induction FOLFIRINOX alone. The primary outcome of interest is the R0 resection rate.

Future Developments

Long-term outcome data following induction or consolidation chemotherapy are lacking, and whether the total neoadjuvant approach can improve survival remains to be elucidated. Several prospective randomized trials are currently ongoing to evaluate long-term disease-specific outcomes, including the PROSPECT and TNTCRT trials [75]. The awaited North American PROSPECT trial will show us if some high-risk patients who respond well to induction FOLFOX can omit neoadjuvant radiotherapy. GRECCAR12 (lower-risk patients) is still recruiting and builds on GRECCAR2 comparing neoadjuvant FOLFIRINOX followed by CRT to CRT alone [76, 77]. In both arms, good responders will have local excision of the primary to avoid major surgery. Similarly, the Chinese TNTCRT trial is designed to assess whether induction and consolidation CAPOX, nCRT, and TME improves DFS compared with standard nCRT and TME with adjuvant chemotherapy (NCT03177382). Circulating tumor DNA (ctDNA) is under investigation to guide adjuvant chemotherapy in stage II colon cancer [78, 79]. The DESTINY-CRC01 trial proved that a drug–antibody conjugate (trastuzumab deruxtecan to target the HER2 receptor) is active against metastatic colon cancer that appropriately express the molecular target [80]. A deeper understanding of radiobiology may lead to molecularly targeted radio-sensitizing agents [81, 82]. It may become possible to use immunotherapy in MSS LARC.

Summary Box

- Early delivery of high-dose systemic chemotherapy represents a promising treatment strategy for both LARC and LRRC.
- Favorable short-term outcomes include improved chemotherapy compliance and superior pathological response.
- Long-term survival data are limited and interpretation is hampered by marked heterogeneity among neoadjuvant/adjuvant treatment regimes.
- Prospective randomized trials will determine whether this approach can improve distant disease control and quality of life, and increase the proportion of patients suitable for non-operative management.
- With increasing emphasis on personalized care, the future of rectal cancer management should include risk-adapted strategies incorporating the biomolecular and radiological profile of the tumor.

References

1 Sauer, R., Liersch, T., Merkel, S. et al. (2012). Preoperative versus postoperative chemoradiotherapy for locally advanced rectal cancer: results of the German CAO/ARO/AIO-94 randomized phase III trial after a median follow-up of 11 years. *J. Clin. Oncol.* 30: 1926–1933.

2 Peeters, K.C.M.J., Marijnen, C.A.M., Nagtegaal, I.D. et al. (2007). The TME trial after a median follow-up of 6 years: increased local control but no survival benefit in irradiated patients with resectable rectal carcinoma. *Ann. Surg.* 246: 693–701.

3 Swedish Rectal Cancer Trial, Cedermark, B., Dahlberg, M. et al. (1997). Improved survival with preoperative radiotherapy in resectable rectal cancer. *N. Engl. J. Med.* 336: 980–987.

4 Folkesson, J., Birgisson, H., Pahlman, L. et al. (2005). Swedish Rectal Cancer Trial: long lasting benefits from radiotherapy on survival and local recurrence rate. *J. Clin. Oncol.* 23: 5644–5650.

5 Bosset, J.-F., Collette, L., Calais, G. et al. (2006). Chemotherapy with preoperative radiotherapy in rectal cancer. *N. Engl. J. Med.* 355: 1114–1123.

6 Peacock, O., Waters, P.S., Bressel, M. et al. (2019). Prognostic factors and patterns of failure after surgery for T4 rectal cancer in the beyond total mesorectal excision era. *Br. J. Surg.* 106: 1685–1696.

7 André, T., de Gramont, A., Vernerey, D. et al. (2015). Adjuvant fluorouracil, leucovorin, and oxaliplatin in stage II to III colon cancer: updated 10-year survival and outcomes according to BRAF mutation and mismatch repair status of the MOSAIC study. *J. Clin. Oncol.* 33: 4176–4187.

8 Kuebler, J.P., Wieand, H.S., O'Connell, M.J. et al. (2007). Oxaliplatin combined with weekly bolus fluorouracil and leucovorin as surgical adjuvant chemotherapy for stage II and III colon cancer: results from NSABP C-07 J. *Clin. Oncol.* 25: 2198–2204.

9 Krook, J.E., Moertel, C.G., Gunderson, L.L. et al. (1991). Effective surgical adjuvant therapy for high-risk rectal carcinoma. *N. Engl. J.Med.* 324: 709–715.

10 Petersen, S.H., Harling, H., Kirkeby, L.T. et al. (2012). Postoperative adjuvant chemotherapy in rectal cancer operated for cure. *Cochrane Database Syst. Rev.* 3: CD004078.

11 Hong, Y.S., Nam, B.-H., Kim, K.-P. et al. (2014). Oxaliplatin, fluorouracil, and leucovorin versus fluorouracil and leucovorin as adjuvant chemotherapy for locally advanced rectal cancer after preoperative chemoradiotherapy (ADORE): an open-label, multicentre, phase 2, randomised controlled trial. *Lancet Oncol.* 15: 1245–1253.

12 Sainato, A., Cernusco Luna Nunzia, V., Valentini, V. et al. (2014). No benefit of adjuvant fluorouracil leucovorin chemotherapy after neoadjuvant chemoradiotherapy in locally advanced cancer of the rectum (LARC): long term results of a randomized trial (I-CNR-RT). *Radiother. Oncol. J.* 113: 223–229.

13 Glynne-Jones, R., Counsell, N., Quirke, P. et al. (2014). Chronicle: results of a randomised phase III trial in locally advanced rectal cancer after neoadjuvant chemoradiation randomising postoperative adjuvant capecitabine plus oxaliplatin (XELOX) versus control. *Ann. Oncol.* 25: 1356–1362.

14 Breugom, A.J., van Gijn, W., Muller, E.W. et al. (2015). Adjuvant chemotherapy for rectal cancer patients treated with preoperative (chemo)radiotherapy and total mesorectal excision: a Dutch Colorectal Cancer Group (DCCG) randomized phase III trial. *Ann. Oncol. Off.* 26: 696–701.

15 Bosset, J.-F., Calais, G., Mineur, L. et al. (2014). Fluorouracil-based adjuvant chemotherapy after preoperative chemoradiotherapy in rectal cancer: long-term results of the EORTC 22921 randomised study. *Lancet Oncol.* 15: 184–190.

16 Biagi, J.J., Raphael, M.J., Mackillop, W.J. et al. (2011). Association between time to initiation of adjuvant chemotherapy and survival in colorectal cancer: a systematic review and meta-analysis. *JAMA* 305: 2335–2342.

17 Martin, S.T., Heneghan, H.M., and Winter, D.C. (2012). Systematic review and meta-analysis of outcomes following pathological complete response to neoadjuvant chemoradiotherapy for rectal cancer. *Br. J.Surg.* 99: 918–928.

18 Kenis, C., Decoster, L., Van Puyvelde, K. et al. (2014). Performance of two geriatric screening tools in older patients with cancer. *J. Clin. Oncol.* 32: 19–26.

19 Maas, M., Nelemans, P.J., Valentini, V. et al. (2010). Long-term outcome in patients with a pathological complete response after chemoradiation for rectal cancer: a pooled analysis of individual patient data. *Lancet Oncol.* 11: 835–844.

20 Kalady, M.F., de Campos-Lobato, L.F., Stocchi, L. et al. (2009). Predictive factors of pathologic complete response after neoadjuvant chemoradiation for rectal cancer. *Ann. Surg.* 250: 582–589.

21 Tulchinsky, H., Shmueli, E., Figer, A. et al. (2008). An interval >7 weeks between neoadjuvant therapy and surgery improves pathologic complete response and disease-free survival in patients with locally advanced rectal cancer. *Ann. Surg. Oncol.* 15: 2661–2667.

22 Ryan, É.J., O'Sullivan, D.P., Kelly, M.E. et al. (2019). Meta-analysis of the effect of extending the interval after long-course chemoradiotherapy before surgery in locally advanced rectal cancer. *Br. J. Surg.* 106: 1298–1310.

23 Lefevre, J.H., Mineur, L., Kotti, S. et al. (2016). Effect of interval (7 or 11 weeks) between neoadjuvant radiochemotherapy and surgery on complete pathologic response in rectal cancer: a multicenter, randomized, controlled trial (GRECCAR-6) *J. Clin. Oncol.* 34: 3773–3780.

24 Perez, K., Safran, H., Sikov, W. et al. (2017). Complete neoadjuvant treatment for rectal

cancer: the Brown University Oncology Group CONTRE study. *Am. J. Clin. Oncol.* 40: 283–287.

25 Garcia-Aguilar, J., Chow, O.S., Smith, D.D. et al. (2015). Effect of adding mFOLFOX6 after neoadjuvant chemoradiation in locally advanced rectal cancer: a multicentre, phase 2 trial. *Lancet Oncol.* 16: 957–966.

26 Fernandez-Martos, C., Garcia-Albeniz, X., Pericay, C. et al. (2015). Chemoradiation, surgery and adjuvant chemotherapy versus induction chemotherapy followed by chemoradiation and surgery: long-term results of the Spanish GCR-3 phase II randomized trial. *Ann. Oncol.* 26: 1722–1728.

27 Hardiman, K.M., Antunez, A.G., Kanters, A. et al. (2019). Clinical and pathological outcomes of induction chemotherapy before neoadjuvant radiotherapy in locally-advanced rectal cancer. *J. Surg. Oncol.* 120: 308–315.

28 Zaborowski, A., Stakelum, A., and Winter, D.C. (2019). Systematic review of outcomes after total neoadjuvant therapy for locally advanced rectal cancer. *Br. J. Surg.* 106: 979–987.

29 Petrelli, F., Trevisan, F., Cabiddu, M. et al. (2020). Total neoadjuvant therapy in rectal cancer: a systematic review and meta-analysis of treatment outcomes. *Ann. Surg.* 271: 440–448.

30 Hospers, G., Bahadoer, R.R., Dijkstra, E.A. et al. (2020). Short-course radiotherapy followed by chemotherapy before TME in locally advanced rectal cancer: the randomized RAPIDO trial. *J. Clin. Oncol.* 38: 4006.

31 Conroy, T., Lamfichekh, N., Etienne, P.-L. et al. (2020). Total neoadjuvant therapy with mFOLFIRINOX versus preoperative chemoradiation in patients with locally advanced rectal cancer: final results of PRODIGE 23 phase III trial, a UNICANCER GI trial. *J. Clin. Oncol.* 38: 4007.

32 Marco, M.R., Zhou, L., Patil, S. et al. (2018). Consolidation mFOLFOX6 chemotherapy after chemoradiotherapy improves survival in patients with locally advanced rectal cancer: final results of a multicenter phase II trial. *Dis. Colon Rectum* 61: 1146–1155.

33 Markovina, S., Youssef, F., Roy, A. et al. (2017). Improved metastasis- and disease-free survival with preoperative sequential short-course radiation therapy and FOLFOX chemotherapy for rectal cancer compared with neoadjuvant long-course chemoradiotherapy: results of a matched pair analysis. *Int. J. Radiat. Oncol. Biol. Phys.* 99: 417–426.

34 Zheng, R., Lian, S., Huang, X. et al. (2019). The survival benefit of intensified full-dose XELOX chemotherapy concomitant to radiotherapy and then resting-period consolidation chemotherapy in locally advanced rectal cancer. *J. Cancer* 10: 730–736.

35 Cisel, B., Pietrzak, L., Michalski, W. et al. (2019). Long-course preoperative chemoradiation versus 5 × 5 Gy and consolidation chemotherapy for clinical T4 and fixed clinical T3 rectal cancer: long-term results of the randomized Polish II study. *Ann. Oncol.* 30: 1298–1303.

36 Zampino, M.G., Magni, E., Leonardi, M.C. et al. (2009). Capecitabine initially concomitant to radiotherapy then perioperatively administered in locally advanced rectal cancer. *Int. J. Radiat. Oncol. Biol. Phys.* 75: 421–427.

37 Yu, X., Wang, Q., Xiao, W. et al. (2018). Neoadjuvant oxaliplatin and capecitabine combined with bevacizumab plus radiotherapy for locally advanced rectal cancer: results of a single-institute phase II study. *Cancer Commun.* 38: 24.

38 CLC, B., Lunniss, P.J., Knowles, C.H. et al. (2012). Anterior resection syndrome. *Lancet Oncol.* 13: e403–e408.

39 EHA, P., Palmer, G.J., Juul, T. et al. (2019). Low anterior resection syndrome and quality of life after sphincter-sparing rectal cancer surgery: a long-term longitudinal follow-up. *Dis. Colon Rectum* 62: 14–20.

40 van Heinsbergen, M., Janssen-Heijnen, M.L., Leijtens, J.W. et al. (2018). Bowel dysfunction after sigmoid resection underestimated: multicentre study on quality of life after surgery for carcinoma

of the rectum and sigmoid. *Eur. J. Surg. Oncol.* 44: 1261–1267.

41 van der Valk, M.J.M., Hilling, D.E., Bastiaannet, E. et al. (2018). Long-term outcomes of clinical complete responders after neoadjuvant treatment for rectal cancer in the International Watch & Wait Database (IWWD): an international multicentre registry study. *Lancet* 391: 2537–2545.

42 Cercek, A., CSD, R., Strombom, P. et al. (2018). Adoption of total neoadjuvant therapy for locally advanced rectal cancer. *JAMA Oncol.* 4: e180071.

43 Garcia-Aguilar, J., Patil, S., Kim, J.K. et al. (2020). Preliminary results of the organ preservation of rectal adenocarcinoma (OPRA) trial. *J. Clin. Oncol.* 38: 4008.

44 Smith, J.J., Chow, O.S., Gollub, M.J. et al. (2015). Organ preservation in rectal adenocarcinoma: a phase II randomized controlled trial evaluating 3-year disease-free survival in patients with locally advanced rectal cancer treated with chemoradiation plus induction or consolidation chemotherapy, and total mesorectal excision or nonoperative management. *BMC Cancer* 15: 767.

45 Rödel, C., Graeven, U., Fietkau, R. et al. (2015). Oxaliplatin added to fluorouracil-based preoperative chemoradiotherapy and postoperative chemotherapy of locally advanced rectal cancer (the German CAO/ARO/AIO-04 study): final results of the multicentre, open-label, randomised, phase 3 trial. *Lancet Oncol.* 16: 979–989.

46 Gérard, J.-P., Azria, D., Gourgou-Bourgade, S. et al. (2012). Clinical outcome of the ACCORD 12/0405 PRODIGE 2 randomized trial in rectal cancer. *J. Clin. Oncol. Off.* 30: 4558–4565.

47 Aschele, C., Cionini, L., Lonardi, S. et al. (2011). Primary tumor response to preoperative chemoradiation with or without oxaliplatin in locally advanced rectal cancer: pathologic results of the STAR-01 randomized phase III trial. *J. Clin. Oncol.* 29: 2773–2780.

48 Allegra, C.J., Yothers, G., O'Connell, M.J. et al. (2015). Neoadjuvant 5-FU or capecitabine plus radiation with or without oxaliplatin in rectal cancer patients: a phase III randomized clinical trial. *J. Natl Cancer Inst.* 107.

49 Hüttner, F.J., Probst, P., Kalkum, E. et al. (2019). Addition of platinum derivatives to fluoropyrimidine-based neoadjuvant chemoradiotherapy for stage II/III rectal cancer: systematic review and meta-analysis. *J. Natl Cancer Inst.* 111: 887–902.

50 Fu, X.-L., Fang, Z., Shu, L.-H. et al. (2017). Meta-analysis of oxaliplatin-based versus fluorouracil-based neoadjuvant chemoradiotherapy and adjuvant chemotherapy for locally advanced rectal cancer. *Oncotarget* 8: 34340–34351.

51 Dueland, S., Ree, A.H., Grøholt, K.K. et al. (2016). Oxaliplatin-containing preoperative therapy in locally advanced rectal cancer: local response, toxicity and long-term outcome. *Clin. Oncol. R. Coll. Radiol.* 28: 532–539.

52 Kogler, P., AF, D.V., Eisterer, W. et al. (2018). Intensified preoperative chemoradiation by adding oxaliplatin in locally advanced, primary operable (cT3NxM0) rectal cancer: impact on long-term outcome. Results of the phase II TAKO 05/ABCSG R-02 trial. Strahlenther. *Onkol. Organ Dtsch. Rontgengesellschaft Al* 194: 41–49.

53 Fernández-Martos, C., Pericay, C., Aparicio, J. et al. (2010). Phase II, randomized study of concomitant chemoradiotherapy followed by surgery and adjuvant capecitabine plus oxaliplatin (CAPOX) compared with induction CAPOX followed by concomitant chemoradiotherapy and surgery in magnetic resonance imaging-defined, locally advanced rectal cancer: Grupo Cancer de Recto 3 study. *J. Clin. Oncol.* 28: 859–865.

54 Clifford, R., Govindarajah, N., Parsons, J.L. et al. (2018). Systematic review of treatment intensification using novel agents for chemoradiotherapy in rectal cancer. *Br. J. Surg.* 105: 1553–1572.

55 Willett, C.G., Boucher, Y., di Tomaso, E. et al. (2004). Direct evidence that the VEGF-specific antibody bevacizumab has antivascular effects in human rectal cancer. *Nat. Med.* 10: 145–147.

56 Zhong, X., Wu, Z., Gao, P. et al. (2018). The efficacy of adding targeted agents to neoadjuvant therapy for locally advanced rectal cancer patients: a meta-analysis. *Cancer Med.* 7: 565–582.

57 Konishi, T., Shinozaki, E., Murofushi, K. et al. (2019). Phase II trial of neoadjuvant chemotherapy, chemoradiotherapy, and laparoscopic surgery with selective lateral node dissection for poor-risk low rectal cancer. *Ann. Surg. Oncol.* 26: 2507–2513.

58 Conroy, T., Hammel, P., Hebbar, M. et al. (2018). FOLFIRINOX or gemcitabine as adjuvant therapy for pancreatic cancer. *N. Engl. J. Med.* 379: 2395–2406.

59 Masi, G., Vivaldi, C., Fornaro, L. et al. (2019). Total neoadjuvant approach with FOLFOXIRI plus bevacizumab followed by chemoradiotherapy plus bevacizumab in locally advanced rectal cancer: the TRUST trial. *Eur. J. Cancer Oxf. Engl.* 110: 32–41.

60 Fernández-Martos, C., Pericay, C., Losa, F. et al. (2019). Effect of aflibercept plus modified FOLFOX6 induction chemotherapy before standard chemoradiotherapy and surgery in patients with high-risk rectal adenocarcinoma: the GEMCAD 1402 randomized clinical trial. *JAMA Oncol.* 5 (11): 1566–1573.

61 Dewdney, A., Cunningham, D., Tabernero, J. et al. (2012). Multicenter randomized phase II clinical trial comparing neoadjuvant oxaliplatin, capecitabine, and preoperative radiotherapy with or without cetuximab followed by total mesorectal excision in patients with high-risk rectal cancer (EXPERT-C). *J. Clin. Oncol.* 30: 1620–1627.

62 Nogué, M., Salud, A., Vicente, P. et al. (2011). Addition of bevacizumab to XELOX induction therapy plus concomitant capecitabine-based chemoradiotherapy in magnetic resonance imaging–defined poor-prognosis locally advanced rectal cancer: the AVACROSS study. *The Oncologist* 16: 614–620.

63 George, T.J., Yothers, G., Hong, T.S. et al. (2019). NRG-GI002: a phase II clinical trial platform using total neoadjuvant therapy (TNT) in locally advanced rectal cancer (LARC)—first experimental arm (EA) initial results. *J. Clin. Oncol.* 15: 3505.

64 Le, D.T., Uram, J.N., Wang, H. et al. (2015). PD-1 blockade in tumors with mismatch-repair deficiency. *New Engl. J.Med.* 372: 2509–2520.

65 André, T., Shiu, K.-K., Kim, T.W. et al. (2020). Pembrolizumab in microsatellite-instability–high advanced colorectal cancer. *N. Engl. J. Med.* 383: 2207–2218.

66 Zhang, J., Cai, J., Deng, Y., and Wang, H. (2019). Complete response in patients with locally advanced rectal cancer after neoadjuvant treatment with nivolumab. *Oncoimmunology* 8.

67 Chiang, S.-F., Huang, C.-Y., Ke, T.-W. et al. (2019). Upregulation of tumor PD-L1 by neoadjuvant chemoradiotherapy (neoCRT) confers improved survival in patients with lymph node metastasis of locally advanced rectal cancers. *Cancer Immunol. Immunother.* 68: 283–296.

68 Hecht, M., Büttner-Herold, M., Erlenbach-Wünsch, K. et al. (1990). PD-L1 is upregulated by radiochemotherapy in rectal adenocarcinoma patients and associated with a favourable prognosis. *Eur. J. Cancer Oxf. Engl.* 65: 52–60.

69 Salvatore, L., Bensi, M., Pietrantonio, F. et al. (2019). 662TiP—phase II study of preoperative (PREOP) chemoradiotherapy (CTRT) plus avelumab (AVE) in patients (PTS) with locally advanced rectal cancer (LARC): the AVANA Study. *Ann. Oncol.* 30: v249.

70 Cohen, R., Shi, Q., and André, T. (2020). Immunotherapy for early stage colorectal cancer: a glance into the future. *Cancers* 12.

71 Arnold, C.R., Mangesius, J., Jäger, R., and Ganswindt, U. (2020). Neoadjuvant

chemoradiotherapy in rectal cancer. *Mag. Eur. Med. Oncol.* 13: 329–333.

72 Kössler, T., Buchs, N., Dutoit, V. et al. (2020). P-115 PEMREC: a phase II study to evaluate safety and efficacy of neo-adjuvant pembrolizumab and radiotherapy in localized microsatellite stable rectal cancer. *Ann. Oncol.* 31: S127.

73 Antonia, S.J., Villegas, A., Daniel, D. et al. (2018). Overall survival with durvalumab after chemoradiotherapy in stage III. *N. Engl. J. Med.* 379: 2342–2350.

74 van Zoggel, D.M.G.I., Bosman, S.J., Kusters, M. et al. (2018). Preliminary results of a cohort study of induction chemotherapy-based treatment for locally recurrent rectal cancer. *Br. J. Surg.* 105: 447–452.

75 Bossé, D., Mercer, J., Raissouni, S. et al. (2016). PROSPECT eligibility and clinical outcomes: results from the Pan-Canadian Rectal Cancer Consortium. *Clin. Colorectal Cancer* 15: 243–249.

76 Rullier, E., Rouanet, P., Tuech, J.-J. et al. (2017). Organ preservation for rectal cancer (GRECCAR 2): a prospective, randomised, open-label, multicentre phase 3 trial. *Lancet* 390: 469–479.

77 Rullier, E., Vendrely, V., Asselineau, J. et al. (2020). Organ preservation with chemoradiotherapy plus local excision for rectal cancer: 5-year results of the GRECCAR 2 randomised trial. *Lancet Gastroenterol. Hepatol.* 5: 465–474.

78 Anon. Circulating tumor DNA testing in predicting treatment for patients with stage IIA colon cancer after surgery. 2019. www.ClinicalTrials.gov.

79 Folprecht, G., Reinacher-Schick, A., Tannapfel, A. et al. (2020). Circulating tumor DNA-based decision for adjuvant treatment in colon cancer stage II evaluation: (CIRCULATE-trial) AIO-KRK-0217. *J. Clin. Oncol.* 38: TPS273.

80 Siena, S., di Bartolomeo, M., Raghav, K.P.S. et al. (2020). A phase II, multicenter, open-label study of trastuzumab deruxtecan (T-DXd; DS-8201) in patients (pts) with HER2-expressing metastatic colorectal cancer (mCRC): DESTINY-CRC01. *J. Clin. Oncol.* 38 (15): 4000.

81 Akiyoshi, T., Tanaka, N., Kiyotani, K. et al. (2019). Immunogenomic profiles associated with response to neoadjuvant chemoradiotherapy in patients with rectal cancer. *Br. J. Surg.* 106: 1381–1392.

82 Koyama, F.C., Ramos, C.M.L., Ledesma, F. et al. (2018). Effect of Akt activation and experimental pharmacological inhibition on responses to neoadjuvant chemoradiotherapy in rectal cancer. *Br. J. Surg.* 105: e192–e203.

5

Preoperative Optimization Prior to Exenteration

Marta Climent[1] and Miguel Pera[2]

[1] *Department of Surgery, Bellvitge University Hospital, Barcelona, Spain*
[2] *Hospital del Mar Universidad Autónoma de Barcelona, Spain*

Background

A patient's general physical condition is the most important determinant of postoperative complications. Pelvic exenteration is a major multivisceral resection with significant morbidity, and therefore patients need to be carefully selected and counseled. Full clinical history, evaluation of comorbidities, and regular medication are paramount for assessing suitability for a pelvic exenteration. Some comorbidities might require further investigations or assessment by other specialists in an attempt to optimize the patient before the surgery. Conditions like pre-existing neurological symptoms or other functional issues are important, especially as most patients will have one or two stomas [1].

Clinical Examination

Digital rectal examination provides vital information relating to the localization of the tumor, its diameter, and its involvement of the sphincter complex. A bimanual recto-vaginal and abdominal examination is mandatory to confirm the presence of a central pelvic recurrence, which ideally should be mobile and not fixed to the pelvic sidewall. If necessary, examination under anesthesia, with cystoscopy or colonoscopy often provides useful information [1].

Laboratory Tests

As part of the preoperative assessment, any detected anemia should be corrected [2]. If the patient has diabetes, optimization of glycemic control is essential [3]. In addition, electrolyte or renal impairments should be checked. Nutritional risk assessment should be performed routinely, with full screening including checking plasma albumin [4], prealbumin, total cholesterol, and total protein [5]. C-reactive protein (CRP) has been shown to be a good independent prognostic marker in patients [6].

Risk Assessment of Morbidity and Mortality

Current approaches to predict postoperative outcomes include scores such as the American Society of Anesthesiologists (ASA) classification and the Physiological and Operative Severity Score for the enumeration of Mortality and Morbidity (POSSUM) [7]. Ihemelandu

Surgical Management of Advanced Pelvic Cancer, First Edition.
Edited by Michael E. Kelly and Desmond C. Winter.
© 2022 John Wiley & Sons Ltd. Published 2022 by John Wiley & Sons Ltd.

et al. noted that the Eastern Cooperative Oncology Group (ECOG) performance status and Health-Related Quality of Life (HRQoL) measured by Functional Assessment of Cancer Therapy (FACT-C) questionnaire are valuable predictors of postoperative morbidity in patients undergoing major surgery [8]. ECOG status has been described as well as a useful tool in the preoperative assessment of patients undergoing pelvic exenteration [9]. Preoperative physical fitness has also been identified as an independent predictor of surgical outcome. For this reason, assessment of functional capacity before a major surgery is paramount. Cardiopulmonary exercise testing (CPET) is probably the most reliable, objective, and precise means of evaluating presurgical physical fitness and the physiologic reserve. This is a dynamic and non-invasive assessment of the cardiorespiratory system at rest and under stress, integrating expired oxygen and carbon dioxide concentrations with the measurement of ventilatory flow, thus deriving oxygen consumption (V_{O2}) and carbon dioxide production (V_{CO2}) under conditions of varying physiologic stress imposed by a range of defined external workloads. Heart rate, oxygen saturations, blood pressure, and electrocardiogram are monitored simultaneously [10]. The most frequent mode of exercise used is cycle ergometry. CPET is the gold standard method of measuring aerobic capacity, predicting postoperative outcomes, and identifying high-risk patients [11, 12]. Several studies and systematic reviews have demonstrated that CPET is a useful tool for preoperative risk stratification in patients undergoing cardiac and non-cardiac surgery. Studies observe that lower V_{O2} peak and aerobic threshold (AT) indicate patients at increased risk of postoperative morbidity [13]. Alternative tests are six-minute walk tests, shuttle walking, and stair climbing.

Preoperative Optimization

Identification and correction of modifiable risk factors, like malnourishment or anemia, in the preoperative assessment can improve surgical outcomes. All these factors in addition to poor preoperative physical performance correlate with increased complications and mortality risk after major surgery [2, 3, 12]. Figure 5.1 shows a preoperative algorithm, including some of the risk factors that should be evaluated. Assessment of preoperative functional capacity should be performed with CPET, if available, not only to identify those patients who may benefit from preoperative exercise training but also to prescribe the intensity of the program [14]. To get a good adherence to the exercise program, preferences and needs of patients have to be considered and led by a specialized physiotherapist. Some patients would require supervision in hospital rather than a home-based program [2, 12]. Neoadjuvant therapies provide the opportunity to train patients before major cancer operations [10]. A recent systematic review supports the role of exercise training in patients undergoing neoadjuvant treatment [15]. Adherence rates were acceptable (66–96%), but the overall impact on HRQoL is still not known.

Anemia Management

Preoperative anemia in patients with cancer is multifactorial, with one-third of patients having iron deficiency at presentation [3, 16]. The negative impact of preoperative anemia on surgical outcomes is well known. A multivariate analysis of 39 309 patients undergoing major surgery showed that severe anemia was associated with higher in-hospital mortality (odds ratio (OR) 2.82, 95% confidence interval (CI) 2.06–3.85) and postoperative admission to intensive care ($p < 0.001$) [17]. A systematic review and meta-analysis reported increased acute kidney injury and infection in patients with preoperative anemia [18]. On the other hand, allogenic red cell transfusion, which occurs at a higher rate among anemic patients, is also associated with increased mortality and morbidity [3, 18]. Therefore, in order to reduce the risk of postoperative complications, it is necessary to correct anemia before surgery. Oral iron replacement is not always effective in

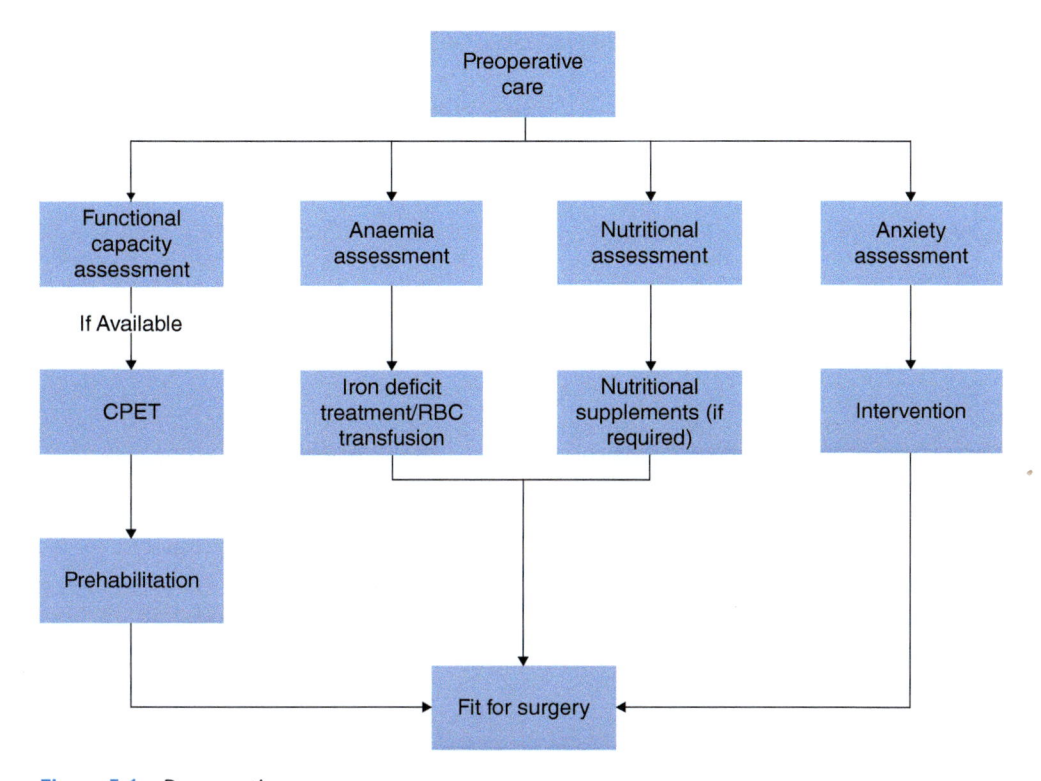

Figure 5.1 Preoperative care.

patients with cancer because of the time required for its efficacy and because its action is limited by the inflammation. Therefore the intravenous (IV) treatment option is the most indicated. A single dose of IV ferric carboxymaltose (15 mg/kg body weight) in patients with ferritin < 300 mcg/l, transferrin saturation < 25%, and Hb < 12.0 g/dl for women and Hb < 13.0 g/dl for men has been shown to reduce the need of transfusion during major abdominal surgery in 60% of patients [16].

Optimization of Nutritional Status

Cancer-related malnutrition is multifactorial, including anorexia, nausea, vomiting, and metabolic disorders. It is not uncommon in patients undergoing major abdominal surgery. Although there is a lack of a standardized definition, it is well known that malnutrition is a significant risk factor of postoperative complications. Nutritional status can be measured using several tools. The gold standard for the American Society for Parenteral and Enteral Nutrition (ASPEN) is the Subjective Global Assessment (SGA), based on performance status and physical examination. It is widely used, but the main disadvantage is the high interobserver variability [19]. In 2003, the European Society of Parenteral and Enteral Nutrition (ESPEN) adopted Nutritional Risk Screening 2002 (NRS-2002) to screen patients for malnutrition in the hospital. NRS-2002 is based on oral food intake, weight loss, patient's age, body mass index (BMI), and severity of underlying disease (Table 5.1) [4].

According to the ESPEN guidelines, a minimum of seven days of preoperative nutritional support that provides at least 10 kcal/kg/day is considered adequate for patients who are nutritionally at risk (NRS score at least 3) [4]. Oral nutrition support with a standard whole protein formula enriched with immune modulating substrates (arginine, ω-3 fatty acids, and

Table 5.1 Nutritional Risk Screening (based on NRS-2002) [4].

	Impaired nutritional status	Severity of disease	
Absent – Score 0	Normal nutritional status	Absent – Score 0	Normal nutritional requirements
Mild – Score 1	Weight loss > 5% in three months or food intake below 50–75% of normal requirement in preceding week	Mild – Score 1	Chronic patients, in particular with acute complications: cirrhosis, chronic obstructive pulmonary disease (COPD), chronic hemodialysis, diabetes, oncology
Moderate – Score 2	Weight loss > 5% in two months or BMI 18.5–20.5 plus impaired general condition or food intake 25–60% of normal requirement in preceding week	Moderate – Score 2	Major abdominal surgery, severe pneumonia, hematologic malignancy
Severe – Score 3	Weight loss > 5% in one month (> 15% in three months) or BMI < 18.5 plus impaired general condition or food intake 0–25% of normal requirement in preceding week	Severe – Score 3	Intensive care patients (APACHE > 10)
Age	If ≥ 70 years: add 1 to total score above	= Age-adjusted total score	

Score ≥ 3: the patient is nutritionally at-risk and a nutritional care plan is initiated

Score < 3: weekly rescreening of the patient. If the patient, for instance, is scheduled for a major operation, a preventive nutritional care plan is considered to avoid the associated risk status

nucleotides) is strongly recommended [20]. Whenever feasible, enteral feeding should be preferred to parenteral nutrition [21]. Combination with parenteral nutrition may be considered in patients in whom 60% of caloric requirement cannot be achieved with the enteral route.

Mechanical Bowel Preparation and Oral Antibiotic Prophylaxis

Mechanical bowel preparation (MBP) with concurrent oral antibiotics has recently been the subject of many trials. In North America this has been integrated into patient pathways [22]. A recent survey (2017) by the European Society of Coloproctology observed that only 16.8% of the European surgeons used oral antibiotics with MBP prior to rectal resection [23]. This was largely attributable to the fact that most enhanced recovery protocols recommend avoiding MBP [24].

However, a French Research Group of Rectal Cancer Surgery (GRECCAR) multicenter trial noted that patients undergoing elective rectal cancer surgery without MBP (retrograde enema and oral laxatives) had a higher risk of infectious complications (34% vs. 16%, p = 0.005) [25]. A meta-analysis of 38 randomized clinical trials including 8458 patients compared four preoperative management strategies (MBP with oral antibiotics, oral antibiotics only, MBP only, or no preparation). The cohort of patients receiving only oral antibiotics had the lowest rate of surgical site infection [26]. Several other studies have reported conflicting results [23, 27], and there remains several further prospective trials in progress.

Thromboprophylaxis

Cancer patients undergoing a surgical procedure have twice the risk of postoperative venous thromboembolism (VTE) and threefold risk of pulmonary embolism (PE) [28]. Therefore the use of prophylaxis is vital in reducing VTE events. Among pharmacological methods, low molecular weight heparin (LMWH) has some advantages to unfractionated heparin (UFH), including the ease of administration and a lower risk of hemorrhage. For these reasons, LMWH is considered the first choice [28, 29]. In addition, the use of mechanical thromboprophylactic modalities such as compression stockings or intermittent pneumatic compression devices is advocated [28].

The enoxaparin and cancer (ENOXACAN) II multicenter trial observed a 60% reduction of VTE in cancer patients who received LMWH for extended duration (four weeks) compared to those only getting it for one week, without increased risk of bleeding [29]. The cancer, bemiparin, and surgery evaluation (CANBESURE) trial also demonstrated a considerable relative risk reduction (82.4%) of major VTE in having extended prophylaxis [30]. As a result, the use of extended prophylaxis is becoming protocolized in many institutions.

Stoma Education

Preoperative education helps reduce stoma-related complications including peristomal skin irritation and pouch leakage, and overall improves quality of life [31]. Ultimately, it provides an opportunity to prepare patients for a stoma, helping acceptance of new body image and promoting self-care [31–36]. Person et al. evaluated the impact of preoperative stoma site marking on patients' quality of life, independence, and complication rates in a series of 105 patients (60 permanent and 45 temporary stomas). The quality of life of patients whose stoma sites were educated preoperatively was significantly better [32]. Several trials and systematic reviews have demonstrated the positive impact of a structured stoma education program regarding length of hospital stay, psychosocial health, and overall healthcare expenditure [34–36].

Summary Box

- A patient's general physical condition is the most important determinant of postoperative complications.
- CPET is a reliable preoperative indicator, highlighting those at risk of surgical stress.
- Preoperative optimization involves a multidisciplinary team of surgeons, anesthesiologists, physiotherapists, stoma therapists, and dieticians.
- A minimum of seven days of preoperative nutritional support providing at least 10 kcal/kg/day is considered adequate for patients who are nutritionally at risk.
- Preoperative stoma education, correction of anemia, and psychological support have a positive impact on postoperative quality of life.
- Patients undergoing pelvic exenteration should receive extended VTE prophylaxis.

References

1 Salom, E. and Penalver, M. (2003). Pelvic exenteration and reconstruction. *Cancer J.* 9: 415–424.

2 Carli, F., Gillis, C., and Scheede-Bergdahl, C. (2017). Promoting a culture of prehabilitation for the surgical cancer patient. *Acta Oncol.* 56: 128–133.

3 Ripollés-Melchor, J., Carli, F., Coca-Martínez, M. et al. (2018). Committed to be fit. The value of preoperative care in the perioperative medicine era. *Minerva Anestesiol.* 84: 1–11.

4 Kondrup, J., Allison, S.P., Elia, M. et al. (2003). ESPEN guidelines for nutrition screening 2002. *Clin. Nutr.* 22: 415–421.

5 Zhang, Z., Pereira, S.L., Luo, M., and Matheson, E.M. (2017). Evaluation of blood biomarkers associated with risk of malnutrition in older adults: a systematic review and meta-analysis. *Nutrients* 9: 829–849.

6 McMillan, D.C. (2013). The systemic inflammation-based Glasgow Prognostic Score: a decade of experience in patients with cancer. *Cancer Treat. Rev.* 39: 534–540.

7 West, M.A., Parry, M.G., Lythgoe, D. et al. (2014). Cardiopulmonary exercise testing for the prediction of morbidity risk after rectal cancer surgery. *Br. J. Surg.* 101: 1166–1172.

8 Ihemelandu, C.U., McQuellon, R., Shen, P. et al. (2013). Predicting postoperative morbidity following cytoreductive surgery with hyperthermic intraperitoneal chemotherapy (CS+HIPEC) with preoperative FACT-C (functional assessment of cancer therapy) and patient-rated performance status. *Ann. Surg. Oncol.* 20: 3519–3526.

9 Chew, M.H., Yeh, Y.-T., Toh, E.-L. et al. (2017). Critical evaluation of contemporary management in a new pelvic exenteration unit: the first 25 consecutive cases. *World J. Gastrointest. Oncol.* 15: 218–227.

10 Levett, D.Z.H. and Grocott, M.P.W. (2015). Cardiopulmonary exercise testing, prehabilitation, and Enhanced Recovery After Surgery (ERAS). *Can. J. Anesth.* 62: 131–142.

11 West, M.A., Loughney, L., Lythgoe, D. et al. (2015). Effect of prehabilitation on objectively measured physical fitness after neoadjuvant treatment in preoperative rectal cancer patients: a blinded interventional pilot study. *Br. J. Anaesth.* 114: 244–251.

12 Wilson, R.J.T., Davies, S., Yates, D. et al. (2010). Impaired functional capacity is associated with all-cause mortality after major elective intra-abdominal surgery. *Br. J. Anaesth.* 105: 297–303.

13 Hennis, P.J., Meale, P.M., and Grocott, M.P.W. (2011). Cardiopulmonary exercise testing for the evaluation of perioperative risk in non-cardiopulmonary surgery. *Postgrad. Med. J.* 87: 550–557.

14 Mayo, N.E., Feldman, L., Scott, S. et al. (2011). Impact of preoperative change in physical function on postoperative recovery: argument supporting prehabilitation for colorectal surgery. *Surgery* 150: 505–514.

15 Loughney, L., West, M.A., Kemp, G.J. et al. (2016). Exercise intervention in people with cancer undergoing neoadjuvant cancer treatment and surgery: a systematic review. *Eur. J. Surg. Oncol.* 42: 28–38.

16 Froessler, B., Palm, P., Weber, I. et al. (2016). The important role for intravenous iron in perioperative patient blood management in major abdominal surgery. *Ann. Surg.* 264: 41–46.

17 Baron, D.M., Hochrieser, H., Posch, M. et al. (2014). Preoperative anaemia is associated with poor clinical outcome in non-cardiac surgery patients. *Br. J. Anaesth.* 113: 416–423.

18 Fowler AJ, Ahmad T, Phull MK, Allard S, Gillies MA, Pearse RM (2015). Meta-analysis of the association between preoperative anaemia and mortality after surgery. *Br J Surg.* Oct;102(11):1314–24.

19 Schiesser, M., Müller, S., Kirchhoff, P. et al. (2008). Assessment of a novel screening score for nutritional risk in predicting

complications in gastro-intestinal surgery. *Clin. Nutr.* 27: 565–570.

20 Weimann, A., Braga, M., Harsanyi, L. et al. (2006). ESPEN guidelines on enteral nutrition: surgery including organ transplantation. *Clin. Nutr.* 25: 224–244.

21 Arends, J., Bachmann, P., Baracos, V. et al. (2017). ESPEN guidelines on nutrition in cancer patients. *Clin. Nutr.* 36: 11–48.

22 Scarborough, J.E., Mantyh, C.R., Sun, Z., and Migaly, J. (2015). Combined mechanical and oral antibiotic bowel preparation reduces incisional surgical site infection and anastomotic leak rates after elective colorectal resection: an analysis of colectomy-targeted ACS NSQIP. *Ann. Surg.* 262: 331–337.

23 Glasbey, J.C., Blanco-Colino, R., Kelly, M. et al. (2018). Association of mechanical bowel preparation with oral antibiotics and anastomotic leak following left sided colorectal resection: an international, multi-centre, prospective audit. *Colorectal Dis.* 20: 15–32.

24 McSorley, S.T., Steele, C.W., and McMahon, A.J. (2018). Meta-analysis of oral antibiotics, in combination with preoperative intravenous antibiotics and mechanical bowel preparation the day before surgery, compared with intravenous antibiotics and mechanical bowel preparation alone to reduce surgical-site infections in elective colorectal surgery. *Br. J. Surg.* 2: 185–194.

25 Bretagnol, F., Panis, Y., Rullier, E. et al. (2010). Rectal cancer surgery with or without bowel preparation: the French GRECCAR III multicenter single-blinded randomized trial. *Ann. Surg.* 252: 863–868.

26 Toh, J.W.T., Phan, K., Hitos, K. et al. (2018). Association of mechanical bowel preparation and oral antibiotics before elective colorectal surgery with surgical site infection: a network meta-analysis. *JAMA* 1: 1–20.

27 Koskenvuo, L., Lehtonen, T., Koskensalo, S. et al. (2019). Mechanical and oral antibiotic bowel preparation versus no bowel preparation for elective colectomy (MOBILE): a multicentre, randomised, parallel, single-blinded trial. *Lancet* 394: 840–848.

28 Mandala, M., Falanga, A., and Roila, F. (2011). Management of venous thromboembolism (VTE) in cancer patients: ESMO Clinical Practice Guidelines. *Ann. Oncol.* 22: 85–92.

29 Bergqvist, D., Agnelli, G., Cohen, A.T. et al. (2002). Duration of prophylaxis against venous thromboembolism with enoxaparin after surgery for cancer. *N. Engl. J. Med.* 13: 975–980.

30 Kakkar, V.V., Balibrea, J.L., Martínez-González, J., and Prandoni, P. (2010). Extended prophylaxis with bemiparin for the prevention of venous thromboembolism after abdominal or pelvic surgery for cancer: the CANBESURE randomized study. *J. Thromb. Haemost.* 8: 1223–1229.

31 McKenna, L.S., Taggart, E., Stoelting, J., and Kirkbride, Forbes, G., G.B. (2016). The impact of preoperative stoma marking on health-related quality of life. A comparison cohort study. *J. Wound Ostomy Cont. Nurs.* 43: 57–61.

32 Person, B., Ifargan, R., Lachter, J. et al. (2012). The impact of preoperative stoma site marking on the incidence of complications, quality of life, and patient's independence. *Dis. Colon Rectum* 55: 783–787.

33 Maydick, D. (2016). A descriptive study assessing quality of life for adults with a permanent ostomy and the influence of preoperative stoma site marking. *Ostomy Manag.* 62: 14–24.

34 Faury, S., Koleck, M., Foucaud, J. et al. (2017). Patient education interventions for colorectal cancer patients with stoma: a systematic review. *Patient Educ. Couns.* 100: 1807–1819.

35 Chaudhri, S., Brown, L., Hassan, I., and Horgan, A.F. (2005). Preoperative intensive, community-based vs. traditional stoma education: a randomized, controlled trial. *Dis. Colon Rectum* 48: 504–509.

36 Danielsen, A.K., Burcharth, J., and Rosenberg, J. (2013). Patient education has a positive effect in patients with a stoma: a systematic review. *Colorectal Dis.* 15: 276–283.

6

Patient Positioning and Surgical Technology

Ben Creavin, Michael E. Kelly, and Desmond C. Winter

Department of Colorectal Surgery, St. Vincent's University Hospital, Dublin, Ireland

Background

The role and techniques involved in pelvic exenteration have evolved significantly since first being reported. There is increased emphasis on perioperative risk and patient safety management [1–4]. A surgical procedure begins prior to the patient entering the operating room. Setup of both the equipment and layout of the operating room are key components in the process of performing an operation and it should not be overlooked. The position of the patient is fundamental to ensuring a safe procedure is performed and should be done correctly prior to commencing the surgery. Patient positioning is extremely important as it impacts on operative access and anesthetic needs, and can reduce potential complications for the patient. Ultimate responsibility of patient position lies with the principal operator, although all surgical staff are responsible for ensuring that the position and safety of the patient is maintained throughout the procedure.

Minimally invasive surgery has led to significant advancements in surgical technology. Robotic surgery has improved the dexterity of minimally invasive instruments, reducing shearing injury to tissues. Hand-held laparoscopic instruments have been reassessed in light of the robotic era and have forced manufacturers to redesign standard instruments. Traditional methods of suture ligating a vessel are challenging in deep pelvic surgery and have been aided by the use of energy devices, clips, and stapling devices.

This chapter examines the core aspects that ensure a safe and efficient pelvic exenteration. It highlights aspects of operative room setup to enhance workflow, and describes in detail the positioning of patients for this procedure and the potential pitfalls associated with them, along with the necessary surgical technology needed to ensure the procedure can be performed effectively.

Operating Room Setup

Setup of the operating room is an important component in any surgical procedure and should be discussed with all members of the surgical team prior to commencing the operation. Ideally, operating rooms should be organized in a systematic manner to ensure efficiency and enhance workflow, both of which will contribute to the overall success of the operation while reducing the total operative time [5, 6]. Complex pelvic surgery requires multiple surgical teams with specific equipment, which

---

Surgical Management of Advanced Pelvic Cancer, First Edition.
Edited by Michael E. Kelly and Desmond C. Winter.
© 2022 John Wiley & Sons Ltd. Published 2022 by John Wiley & Sons Ltd.

need to be accommodated in the operating room. Preoperative assessment of this equipment is essential to ensure correct calibration and functionality [6]. If a minimally invasive approach is the goal of exenterative surgery, provisions for backup equipment along with instruments for a quick conversion to an open operation need to be available. For these reasons, planning and highlighting potential issues with all the surgical team is advised prior to commencing surgery.

General Room Setup

Although the majority of pelvic exenterations are performed in an open setting with dual surgical teams, minimally invasive exenterations are becoming more feasible due to improvements of preoperative management and planning [7]. Sufficient space is needed to accommodate the patient on the operating table, anesthetic machines, adjuncts for performing laparoscopic surgery, and circulating theater staff. Ideally, having a single boom with insufflation, generators, and digital recording and printing devices would declutter the operative field and allow free flow around the surgical table [8]. If feasible, carbon dioxide mains in theater prevent the need for changing individual gas canisters. Light cables, carbon dioxide tubing, and camera cords need to be secured to the bed and should be directed off the head of the bed in an organized fashion to avoid entanglement. Operative lights should be mounted to the ceiling and be positioned above the surgical field to provide adequate visualization for the surgeon [5]. A head light can be utilized in open pelvic exenteration, especially when dissecting deep in the pelvis.

The location and size of individual monitors is of extreme importance as it helps with the ergonomics of the procedure. If possible, ceiling-mounted monitors relaying feedback of the assistant's camera along with any pre- or intraoperative imaging obtained would again improve the movement of the surgical team around the patient. Exenterative surgery requires significant dissection, which influences the surgeon's position at the table. Locating the monitors in minimally invasive pelvic exenteration opposite the principal surgeon improves the ergonomics and reduces the strain on the surgeon. Monitor visualization for the assistant is also important so that the operative field can be kept focused and in view at all times [5, 8].

The position of the surgeon during pelvic exenteration is dynamic and requires constant repositioning of the surgical team, especially the scrub nurse. It is important to place the scrub nurse, instrument table, and mayo stand at the end of the table, either to the right or left foot [6]. Elevated mayo stands can be utilized and positioned over the patient to aid in instrument selection and provide extra space during the procedure. During the abdominal approach the scrub nurse can be positioned either at the foot of the bed or in between the patient's legs to allow space for the surgeon and assistant to perform the operation. However, with both an abdominal and perineal approach being implemented at the same time, two scrub nurses with independent instrument tables are needed [6, 9].

Adjuncts to Operating Room Setup

Urological stenting along with other intraoperative imaging may be required during pelvic exenteration. Adequate space for a mobile C-arm and monitors to display the images needs to be integrated into the operating room setup. The advent of the "hybrid" operating theater has eased the integration of both surgical and interventional procedures in pelvic exenteration. While mobile C-arms are the mainstay in operating theaters currently, there is a need for more advanced and definitive imaging (computed tomography (CT) and magnetic resonance imaging (MRI)) in the operating theater, especially in advanced pelvic surgery. Hybrid theaters combine surgical, radiological, and interventional capabilities, allowing intra- and postoperative on table imaging and intervention, further streamlining patient care [10].

Hybrid theaters facilitate orthopedic, urological, and vascular colleagues in the one theater, significantly improving the efficiency of the operation. However, in order to facilitate a hybrid-operating theater, special consideration for radiation safety, audio visual systems, imagining technology, costs, and sterility issues need to be addressed early [10]. Hybrid theaters also accommodate the use of intraoperative radiation therapy. This concept has been explored in the area of pelvic exenteration, with only a few centers implementing this approach. While results are conflicting, accommodation of this intervention may be needed in operating theaters in the future [11–13].

Robotic Room Setup

Robotic approaches to colorectal surgery have gained recognition in recent years and have recently extended into the field of pelvic exenteration. Operating room setup is more complicated for robotic surgery and requires complex and expensive equipment. There are a number of core principles in setting up and positioning a patient in robotic surgery compared to open or laparoscopic approaches. Again, it is important to discuss all aspects of the procedure prior to commencing the setup of a robotic surgery. A dedicated robotic team is extremely important as they will have a clear understanding of the setup process and will be able to identify and alleviate any technical problems encountered [14]. Well-trained staff in equipment setup, patient positioning, docking, and technical malfunctions will increase the efficiency of the operation and reduce anesthetic times [15].

A standard robotic system consists of four main components: (i) the patient cart, (ii) surgeon console, (iii) vision cart, and (iv) instrumentation [16]. The patient cart consists of remote manipulator arms which are controlled by the surgeon console. It mimics the surgeon's movements and is capable of performing tasks such as cutting, grasping, suturing, and electrocautery [14, 16]. The patient console is draped in a sterile fashion and is united with the sterile field of the patient for the operation. A large operating theater is needed in order to drape the patient console without running the risk of contamination. The surgeon console is where the instruments are controlled and allow the surgeon to visualize the operation and communicate with the surgical team. The surgeon console is located outside the sterile field; however, the principal operator must be able to see the operating table at all times [16]. Dual console systems are available on newer robotic models. Operating theater rooms with adequate space are a must and provisions should be drawn up for this. The visualization cart allows a direct view of the surgical field in a 3D fashion [14]. It is again positioned outside the surgical sterile field but needs to be easily seen by the first assistant and scrub nurse. The instruments make up the last core component of the robotic system. Instruments have been adapted from laparoscopic equipment and provide the surgeon with a full range of motion and dexterity to perform the operation.

The setup of the robotic system is challenging and time consuming; however, improvement in setup times is seen with increased case numbers and trained staff. Prior to the patient entering the operating room and docking, the robotic system needs to be calibrated. Systematic placement of each component of the robotic system in the operating room is extremely important in performing this operation. The patient console should be positioned in a dedicated spot that allows easy and short access to the operating table in order to decrease the risk of robotic damage and contamination during docking [14]. Docking for pelvic exenteration usually occurs over the right hip, but the newer version of the robot (Si) allows for repositioning without the need to undock. Care must be taken when docking the robot to ensure no harm is done to the patient, especially when the patient's legs are in stirrups [14, 17]. Correct port placement is vital to limit external and internal collisions of the instruments. Furthermore, provisions should be made for an emergency undocking and conversion to laparotomy [15]. Following the completion of the robotic phase of the operation, undocking in a safe manner is also highly important. Instruments should be removed under direct vision with the robotic arms undocked systematically. Care must be taken when removing the robot from the patient to prevent damage to the robot and contamination, as redocking may be needed by the surgeon at a later point in the operation [14, 16].

Patient Positioning

The position of the patient is fundamental to ensuring a safe procedure is performed and should be undertaken correctly prior to commencing surgery. Patient positioning impacts on operative access and visualization, anesthetic needs, and potential comfort and complications for the patient. This is especially true in pelvic exenteration when dual surgical teams are performing the operation. Ultimate responsibility of patient position lies with the principal operator, although all surgical staff are responsible for ensuring that the position and safety of the patient is maintained throughout the procedure.

Modified Lloyd-Davies

A modified Lloyd-Davies (lithotomy–Trendelenburg position) approach is the most common position encountered in pelvic exenterative surgery [2, 11]. Patients are placed in a supine position, with provisions being made for sacrectomy. The patient's coccyx should hang just off the bed with either a rolled-up towel/padding or a 2-l bag of saline underneath the patient's lumbar spine to elevate the distal sacrum [11]. The hips are extended and knees flexed to 45° and slightly abducted with supporting equipment for the calves [18]. Ideally, Allen stirrups are used where the lower limbs are placed in a casing protected by soft material and adjustable strapping. These stirrups aid in repositioning during surgery, support the base of the foot, are more physiological, and reduce the possibility of complications associated with other forms of leg supports. It is imperative that padding is used in these stirrups to provide support and comfort to the patient while preventing complications. Pneumatic compression stockings providing intermittent compression to the legs are important to prevent venous stasis and thrombosis when the legs are elevated [6]. The ankle, knee, and shoulder should all be aligned in the final positioning of the patient. Arms should be tucked in all cases either against the body or in abduction [5]. Padding should be used to protect pressure points, with careful attention to the degree of abduction to prevent overextension of the brachial plexus. Consultation with the anesthetics team is important to prevent issues with access to intravenous (IV) lines and monitoring [18].

To aid in surgical dissection and visualization of the pelvis, patients can be tilted into a Trendelenburg position or laterally during the procedure. To ensure that patients do not move or slide on the table, straps and specific securing mats can be used to ensure patient safety. Straps across the chest along with shoulder supports may be utilized to prevent cephalic and lateral movement of patients. Careful placement of these devices with padding is important to avoid compressing neurovascular structures [5, 6, 9, 18, 19]. Furthermore, they should not interfere with bear-hugger equipment keeping the patient warm during the procedure. Newer forms of securing the patient to the bed have been developed more recently. Gel mats placed under the patient prevent the patient from sliding and have the added advantage of being doubled up and placed at the lumbar region to elevate the sacrum. Bean-bag-type mats have also become available [2, 6]. A suction device hardens these mats which molds it around the patient's body, preventing sliding and injury to the patient.

When the patient is fully positioned on the table and after induction of anesthesia, an orogastric or nasogastric tube can be placed to decompress the stomach, while a Foley urinary catheter with/without a temperature probe should be placed to monitor urinary output and prevent inadvertent damage to the bladder intraoperatively [6].

Jackknife Prone

The challenging issue in positioning patients for pelvic exenteration occurs when the sacrum is involved in the disease process. Sacrectomy is usually performed in the jackknife prone position following the completion of the abdominal and perineal phase [20, 21]. While this position allows excellent access to the sacrum, it is time consuming transferring the patient intraoperatively and loss of vascular control in the abdomen can occur [22].

Controlling the patient's neck and airway is extremely important in transferring the patient into this position. Pillows are placed on the table for positioning under the patient prior to transferring them: one under the chest should be small enough to prevent respiratory compromise and one under the pelvis below the hips should expose the perineal region [18]. The table is split, with the patient's legs pointing toward the floor, again to provide better exposure to the perineal region. Taping of the buttocks improves visualization during the procedure. A pillow can also be placed under the ankles to prevent compression and flexion of the feet. The head is positioned lower than the heart and can be either positioned to one side or placed in a ring to relieve pressure and ensure adequate ventilation is being delivered. Care is needed to ensure accidental extubation does not occur. The arms can be tucked in against the body or put in extension around the head [18].

Solomon et al. recently described an alternative approach to a prone sacrectomy, especially when the lower sacrum is involved (S3 and below). Patients are positioned in the preferred modified Lloyd-Davies position as previously described with elevation and floating of the sacrum off the bed. Sacrectomy is then performed through an abdominal and perineal approach, with excellent results being seen [22]. This approach allows better access to the lateral compartment of the pelvis, which will aid in vessel control, identification, and dissection of important structures, especially the sciatic nerve. Furthermore, this approach will help the reconstructive phase of the perineum and avoid the anesthetic challenges associated with a prone approach [22].

Complications Associated with Patient Positioning

Patient position and physiological aspects of the procedure can cause unwanted complications in pelvic exenterative surgery. Identifying risks factors early may prevent complications or reduce the impact these complications have on patients.

Compartment syndrome is a feared and significant complication in pelvic surgery. Increased hydrostatic pressure in the central compartments in the lower limbs leads to accumulation of edema in the tissue, resulting in increased capillary pressure, changes in vascular permeability, and altered venous return and arterial flow. Ultimately this leads to muscle ischemia and secondary necrosis of the tissue [18, 23]. Numerous factors have been attributed to its development, including positioning of the legs, the type of leg support used, epidural analgesia, and the duration of surgery [23, 24]. Patient factors play a role too, with a raised body mass index (BMI), gender, age, and previous arterial disease contributing to its development [18]. Patients experiencing increased pain, weakness, and sensory issues in the lower limbs should be suspected of having compartment syndrome. A fasciotomy in the early phase of disease progression can save the patient from an amputation. Correct positioning of the patient is extremely important in order to prevent the development of compartment syndrome. In a Trendelenberg position, placing the calves lower than the right atrium without extreme angulation of the hips is helpful, along with avoiding hypotension intraoperatively, ensuring nothing is resting on the legs, and letting the legs out of the supports in prolonged procedures can help reduce the incidence of this complication [23].

Nerve injuries are seen in up to 2% of pelvic surgeries; however, the majority tend to resolve [25]. Both compressive and stretching injuries occur in varying degrees and can be prevented by having patients in a neutral position, ensuring adequate padding is applied to pressure points and avoiding long surgeries [26, 27]. Compression of the common peroneal nerve (lateral to the head of the fibula) while the patient's legs are in stirrups can lead to foot drop and club foot in patients [18]. Compression and extension of the sciatic nerve leads to weakness or paralysis of the muscles below the knee, while abducting the hip > 30° can damage the obturator nerve. Simultaneous flexion of the hips while positioning the patient may help in reducing these injuries. The femoral nerve can be damaged by retraction or flexion of the hip and compression of the nerve in the inguinal region. This will lead to decreased sensation in the anterior and medial side of the thigh and weakness of the quadriceps muscle. Injuries to the brachial plexus and ulnar nerve are uncommon in pelvic surgery and tend to resolve soon after the injury is encountered [18, 25].

Venous thromboembolisms are commonly encountered following pelvic surgery. Patient position, pneumoperitoneum in laparoscopic surgery, and disease factors all contribute to developing venous thromboembolism (VTE) in pelvic surgery [28, 29]. Pneumoperitoneum and a Trendelenberg position increase preload and intra-abdominal pressure which put increased pressure on the respiratory system and myocardial oxygen requirements [18, 30]. Reverting to a supine position when possible and reducing intra-abdominal pressure can resolve these issues gradually. Furthermore, the use of pneumatic compression stockings will increase venous return in the legs, reducing the incidence of VTE [31].

Surgical Equipment and Energy Devices

Numerous devices exist currently to ensure safe dissection, hemostasis, and reconstruction in surgery. All members of the exenterative process should understand the basic function of each device used during the procedure. To aid in wound protection and visualization in the abdominal phase, an Alexis™ (Applied Medical) wound retractor can be used in open exenterations, while a Lone Star™ (Cooper Surgical) retractor can help with visualization in the perineal phase [32]. Stapling devices, both linear and circular, can aid in transection of the bowel and anastomosis, while providing vessel ligation in certain instances. This too is true for clip applicators that provide quick hemostasis for small vessels. Osteotomes should be on hand in cases where sacrectomy is being performed [2, 11, 22].

Visualization in pelvic surgery can be difficult and is aided by adequate hemostasis and maintaining the embryological planes of dissection. The rapid developments of monopolar, bipolar, and ultrasonic energy devices have overtaken traditional methods of hemostasis by suture ligation.

Monopolar devices require an electrode pad to be placed on a patient in order to facilitate a closed electrical circuit for dissection. Monopolar devices such as hand or hook diathermy achieve dissection and hemostasis in a cutting or coagulation process [33]. While monopolar devices provide rapid hemostasis, a complete and intact energy circuit is required to ensure it functions properly. Understanding the relationship between current density and tissue heating is important as tissues can be heated far from where the current is applied. Lateral thermal spread should be considered when applying the energy settings to the generator to ensure that critical structures adjacent to the point of dissection are not compromised [34, 35]. Caution should be taken in patients with implanted defibrillators and pacemakers to prevent tissue damage in unwanted regions, especially if the implant creates an alternative electrical circuit [36].

Bipolar devices rely on electrodes in close proximity, and thus the effect on the patient's tissue is local and requires less power to affect tissues compared to monopolar devices. Grasping tissues between the teeth of the device provides a current between the tissue and the electrodes to provide local dissection [33]. Furthermore, bipolar devices have the added advantage of sealing vessels up to 7 mm in diameter (LigaSure™, Covidien; and Enseal™, Ethicon) [19]. By grasping the tissue and applying an energy source, both physical pressure and electrothermal energy are delivered to the tissue. Ultimately, denaturing of the elastin and collagen of the vessels occurs, ensuring a sealing effect. A feedback mechanism is installed on the device to measure the density of the tissue and provide adequate electrothermal energy. A built-in cutting device is used to transect the planes once the vessel is sealed and the blunt tip to the device facilitates blunt dissection of tissues [34]. Compared with monopolar devices, bipolar electrosurgery devices have been shown to be faster at tissue dissection, to be better at vessel sealing, encounter less blood loss, and are more cost-effective [33].

Ultrasonic energy devices such as the Harmonic™ (Ethicon) and SonSurg™ (Olympus) use low-frequency mechanical vibrations (ultrasonic energy 20–60 kHz) to perform tissue cutting and coagulation [37]. Piezoelectric transducers located in the device convert electrical energy to mechanical vibration which is transferred to the blades of the device [33]. Ultimately, this induces protein denaturation by breaking down hydrogen bonds in the tissue [38]. The cutting effect of ultrasonic devices is achieved based on the protein density of the tissues. High-protein-dense tissues rely on mechanical stretching of the tissue beyond its elastic capacity, whereas low-density proteins rely on cell rupture from vaporization of intracellular water [33]. A mist is produced due to cavitation effect; however, no smoke is produced and no active energy is transmitted into the tissue, which gives it an advantage over alternative energy sources [33]. Ultrasonic devices have an active blade that can be rotated and an area approved for sealing vessels up to 7 mm; however, studies have questioned their reliability at sealing large vessels [39]. Built-in mechanisms including power settings at the generator, degree of activation at the device (minimum or maximum), and degree of tension on tissues will determine the spectrum of coagulation or cutting the device will achieve. Compared to electrosurgical devices, ultrasonic devices are slower at coagulating tissues and produce higher temperatures, which can cause damage to tissues that come into contact with the blades after dissection is performed [33].

More recently, the Thunderbeat™ device has been introduced to the market as a single multifunctional device providing dual ultrasonic and bipolar energy [40]. This dual device has the added advantages of both providing the dissection aspects of ultrasound and benefiting from the sealing vessels up to 7 mm. This device has been shown to improve dissection and vessel sealing time, while reducing lateral thermal spread, reducing its impact on adjacent tissues [40].

Summary Box

- Pelvic exenterative surgery is complex. Operative room setup and patient positioning is the ultimate responsibility of the principal operator.
- Minimally invasive pelvic exenteration is becoming more popular. Monitor and boom setup are extremely important to facilitate good ergonomics and enhance workflow, all of which will contribute to the overall success of the operation while reducing the total operative time.
- A modified Lloyd-Davies (lithotomy–Trendelenburg position) approach is the most common position encountered in pelvic exenterative surgery, with sacrectomy being feasible through an abdominal and pelvic approach.
- Patient position and physiological aspects of the procedure can cause unwanted complications in pelvic exenterative surgery. Identifying risk factors early may prevent complications or reduce the impact these complications have on patients.
- Visualization in pelvic surgery can be difficult and is aided by adequate hemostasis and maintaining the embryological planes of dissection. The rapid developments of monopolar, bipolar, and ultrasonic energy devices have overtaken traditional methods of hemostasis by suture ligation.

References

1 Brunschwig, A. (1948). Complete excision of pelvic viscera for advanced carcinoma; a one-stage abdominoperineal operation with end colostomy and bilateral ureteral implantation into the colon above the colostomy. *Cancer* 1: 177–183.

2 Koh, C.E., Solomon, M.J., Brown, K.G. et al. (2017). The evolution of pelvic exenteration practice at a single center: lessons learned from over 500 cases. *Dis. Colon Rectum* 60: 627–635. Fundamental paper for all surgeons performing pelvic exenterative surgery. Gives an honest account of their experience and tips on how to improve your practice.

3 Brown, K.G.M., Solomon, M.J., and Koh, C.E. (2017). Pelvic exenteration surgery: the evolution of radical surgical techniques for advanced and recurrent pelvic malignancy. *Dis. Colon Rectum* 60: 745–754.

4 Pawlik, T.M., Skibber, J.M., and Rodriguez-Bigas, M.A. (2006). Pelvic exenteration for advanced pelvic malignancies. *Ann. Surg. Oncol.* 13: 612–623.

5 Sharp, N. and Papaconstantinou, H. (2017). Room setup, equipment and patient positioning. In: Operative Techniques in Single Incision Laparoscopic Colorectal Surgery (eds. D. Geisler, D. Keller and E. Haas), 19–24. Boston: Springer.

6 Nakajima, K., Milsom, J.W., and Böhm, B. (2006). Patient preparation and operating room setup. In: Laparoscopic Colorectal Surgery (eds. J.W. Milsom, B. Böhm and K. Nakajima), 48–52. New York: Springer.

7 Srinivasaiah, N., Shekleton, F., and Kelly, M.E. (2018). Minimally invasive surgery techniques in pelvic exenteration: a systematic and meta-analysis review. *Surg. Endosc.* 32: 4707–4715.

8 Delaney, C., Neary, P., Heriot, A., and Senagore, A. (2007). Instrumentation and setup. In: Operative Techniques in Laparoscopic Colorectal Surgery, Chapter 3. Philadelphia: Lippincott Williams & Wilkins. Excellent summary of operative room and equipment setup. Provides some tips and tricks to improve ergonomics and workflow.

9 Young-Fadok, T.M. (2006). Colorectal resections: patient positioning and operating room setup. In: The SAGES Manual (eds. R.L. Whelan, J.W. Fleshman and D.L. Fowler), 150–162. New York: Springer.

10 Siddharth, V., Kant, S., Chandrashekhar, R., and Gupta, S. (2014). Planning premises and design considerations for hybrid operating room. *Int. J. Res. Foundation Hosp. Healthc. Adm.* 2: 50–56.

11 Warrier, S.K., Heriot, A.G., and Lynch, A.C. (2016). Surgery for locally recurrent rectal cancer: tips, tricks, and pitfalls. *Clin. Colon Rectal Surg.* 29: 114–122.

12 Tan, J., Heriot, A.G., Mackay, J. et al. (2013). Prospective single-arm study of intraoperative radiotherapy for locally advanced or recurrent rectal cancer. *J. Med. Imaging Radiat. Oncol.* 57: 617–625.

13 Mirnezami, R., Chang, G.J., Das, P. et al. (2013). Intraoperative radiotherapy in colorectal cancer: systematic review and meta-analysis of techniques, long-term outcomes, and complications. *Surg. Oncol.* 22: 22–35.

14 Oh, S.Y., Harnsberger, C.R., and Ramamoorthy, S.L. (2015). Operating room setup and general techniques for robotic surgery. In: Advanced Techniques in Minimally Invasive and Robotic Colorectal Surgery (ed. O. Bardakcioglu), 25–33. Boston: Springer.

15 Agcaoglu, O., Aliyev, S., Taskin, H.E. et al. (2012). Malfunction and failure of robotic systems during general surgical procedures. *Surg. Endosc.* 26: 3580–3583.

16 Bhama, A.R. and Cleary, R.K. (2016). Setup and positioning in robotic colorectal surgery. *Semin. Colon Rectal Surg.* 27: 130–133.

17 Ramamoorthy, S. and Obias, V. (2013). Unique complications of robotic colorectal surgery. *Surg. Clin. North Am.* 93: 273–286.

18 Roig-Vila, J.V., García-Armengol, J., Bruna-Esteban, M. et al. (2009). Operating position in colorectal surgery. The importance of the basics. *Cirugía Española (English Edition)* 86: 204–212.

19 Jafari, M.D., Stamos, M.J., and Mills, S. (2015). Patient positioning, instrumentation, and trocar placement. In: Minimally Invasive Approaches to Colon and Rectal Disease: Technique and Best Practices (eds. H.M. Ross, S. Lee, M.G. Mutch, et al.), 15–24. New York: Springer.

20 Dozois, E.J., Privitera, A., Holubar, S.D. et al. (2011). High sacrectomy for locally recurrent rectal cancer: can long-term survival be achieved? *J. Surg. Oncol.* 103: 105–109.

21 Melton, G.B., Paty, P.B., Boland, P.J. et al. (2006). Sacral resection for recurrent rectal cancer: analysis of morbidity and treatment results. *Dis. Colon Rectum* 49: 1099–1107.

22 Solomon, M.J., Tan, K.K., Bromilow, R.G. et al. (2014). Sacrectomy via the abdominal approach during pelvic exenteration. *Dis. Colon Rectum* 57: 272–277.

23 Beraldo, S. and Dodds, S.R. (2006). Lower limb acute compartment syndrome after colorectal surgery in prolonged lithotomy position. *Dis. Colon Rectum* 49: 1772–1780.

24 Schofield, P.F. and Grace, R.H. (2004). Acute compartment syndrome of the legs after colorectal surgery. *Colorectal Dis.* 6: 285–287.

25 Cardosi, R.J., Cox, C.S., and Hoffman, M.S. (2002). Postoperative neuropathies after major pelvic surgery. *Obstet. Gynecol.* 100: 240–244.

26 Kroll, D.A., Caplan, R.A., Posner, K. et al. (1990). Nerve injury associated with anesthesia. *Anesthesiology* 73: 202–207.

27 Winfree, C.J. and Kline, D.G. (2005). Intraoperative positioning nerve injuries. *Surg. Neurol.* 63: 5–18; discussion 18.

28 Stahl, T.J., Gregorcyk, S.G., Hyman, N.H., and Buie, W.D. (2000). Practice parameters for the prevention of venous thrombosis. The Standards Practice Task Force of the American Society of Colon and Rectal Surgeons. *Dis. Colon & Rectum* 43: 1037–1047.

29 Bergqvist, D. (2006). Venous thromboembolism: a review of risk and prevention in colorectal surgery patients. *Dis. Colon & Rectum* 49: 1620–1628.

30 Rist, M., Hemmerling, T.M., Rauh, R. et al. (2001). Influence of pneumoperitoneum and patient positioning on preload and splanchnic blood volume in laparoscopic surgery of the lower abdomen. *J. Clin. Anesth.* 13: 244–249.

31 Feng, J.-P., Xiong, Y.-T., Fan, Z.-Q. et al. (2016). Efficacy of intermittent pneumatic compression for venous thromboembolism prophylaxis in patients undergoing gynecologic surgery: a systematic review and meta-analysis. *Oncotarget* 8: 20371–20379.

32 Zhang, L., Elsolh, B., and Patel, S.V. (2018). Wound protectors in reducing surgical site infections in lower gastrointestinal surgery: an updated meta-analysis. *Surg. Endosc.* 32: 1111–1122.

33 Sankaranarayanan, G., Resapu, R.R., Jones, D.B. et al. (2013). Common uses and cited complications of energy in surgery. *Surg. Endosc.* 27: 3056–3072.

34 Bohm, B., Milsom, J., and Nakajima, K. (2006). Surgical energy devices. In: Laparoscopic Colorectal Surgery (eds. B. Bohm, J. Milsom and K. Nakakima), 30–47. New York: Springer.

35 Sutton, P.A., Awad, S., Perkins, A.C., and Lobo, D.N. (2010). Comparison of lateral thermal spread using monopolar and bipolar diathermy, the harmonic scalpel and the Ligasure. *Br. J. Surg.* 97: 428–433.

36 Govekar, H.R., Robinson, T.N., Varosy, P.D. et al. (2012). Effect of monopolar radiofrequency energy on pacemaker function. *Surg. Endosc.* 26: 2784–2788.

37 O'Daly, B.J., Morris, E., Gavin, G.P. et al. (2008). High-power low-frequency

ultrasound: a review of tissue dissection and ablation in medicine and surgery. *J. Mater. Process. Technol.* 200: 38–58.

38 Lee, S.J. and Park, K.H. (1999). Ultrasonic energy in endoscopic surgery. *Yonsei Med. J.* 40: 545–549.

39 Phillips, C.K., Hruby, G.W., Durak, E. et al. (2008). Tissue response to surgical energy devices. *Urology* 71: 744–748.

40 Devassy, R., Hanif, S., Krentel, H. et al. (2019). Laparoscopic ultrasonic dissectors: technology update by a review of literature. *Med. Devices (Auckl.)* 12: 1–7.

7

Intraoperative Assessment of Resectability and Operative Strategy

Rory Kokelaar, Dean Harris, and Martyn Evans

Department of Surgery, Morriston Hospital, Swansea, Wales, UK

Background

Despite improved preoperative staging and neoadjuvant therapies, the final assessment of operability of advanced pelvic neoplasms is made at the time of surgery. Unexpected intraoperative findings occur, and the exenterative surgeon must have a clear strategy for dealing with these. Even when staging is accurate, the challenge of exenterative surgery requires surgeons to think strategically when performing multivisceral resections in situations where the pelvis has had prior surgery or radiation. Additionally, non-tumor-related factors may limit or affect the technical resectability of an advanced pelvic malignancy. A failure to proceed, a suboptimal excision, or an irretrievable situation can rapidly occur if insufficient planning or hasty decisions at time of surgery are made. Therefore an appropriate and methodical approach to intraoperative assessment of resectability and surgical strategy are required.

The Preoperative Phase

Planning

Multidisciplinary Team
Successful management of advanced pelvic malignancy begins with the multidisciplinary team (MDT). Most non-specialist MDTs discuss a relatively low volume of patients with locally advanced primary or recurrent pelvic cancer and collaborative groups have recommended that all advanced pelvic malignancies should be discussed in a superspecialized MDT [1, 2]. This MDT needs to include specialists from a broad spectrum, drawing upon expertise on a case-by-case basis for multivisceral or radical resections. An MDT undertaking pelvic exenterative surgery should bring together colorectal surgeons and oncologists with colleagues in urology, gynecologic oncology, and plastic-reconstructive, vascular, and orthopedic surgery; a practice now well established in most centres dealing with complex cases.

The aim of the superspecialist MDT is to provide expertise in managing these particularly challenging cases, fostering a high-volume and high-quality, evidence-based service [3]. Currently, much of the published evidence supporting exenterative approaches is limited to single-center experiences, and consensus across the community of MDTs is lacking. Even standard definitions of what constitutes exenterative surgery are poorly defined, undermining the evidence base. Overcoming this challenge is one of the key objectives of the PelvEx Collaborative [4, 5].

Surgical Management of Advanced Pelvic Cancer, First Edition.
Edited by Michael E. Kelly and Desmond C. Winter.
© 2022 John Wiley & Sons Ltd. Published 2022 by John Wiley & Sons Ltd.

Operating Environment

Pelvic exenterative surgery is frequently arduous and complex, and with significant intraoperative risk [6, 7]. Operative time typically exceeds six hours and can involve personnel changes in operating teams, anesthetists, and theater nursing staff. Specialist services such as cell salvage, intraoperative radiography and fluoroscopy, intraoperative radiotherapy (IORT), and frozen section all need to be orchestrated in order to facilitate the efficient running of the operation. There are two critical elements to ensuring the smooth running of such a complex operation: planning and leadership.

Adequate foresight of what may be required during surgery for advanced pelvic malignancy allows specialists from a range of services to be available for planned, or on occasion unexpected elements of a complex procedure. Anticipating the challenges of a bespoke patient-specific approach to advanced pelvic disease must include strategies for overcoming them. The requirement for turning the patient prone or supine during the procedure, exposure for flap harvesting, or gaining vascular access for bypass must all be anticipated in advance of beginning such a procedure. On-the-fly adjustments will lead to increased operating times and significant avoidable intraoperative duress, if not operative compromises and suboptimal oncological outcomes [8]. Expertise in deploying medical technologies is crucial in the planning stage, ranging from ensuring the correct number, size, and type of abdominal wall meshes or vascular grafts are available, through to the application of laparoscopic (and increasingly robotic) platforms. Each of these considerations can be facilitated by the organizational behavior of the unit in which the MDT is embedded, and the subsequent governance of and integration of MDT practices to care [9].

The orchestration of complex exenterative procedures should be led by the clinician responsible for the patient's care acting as the hub within a web of professionals centered upon the patient and their procedure. It is no longer appropriate that this surgeon is a stand-alone operator who should perform every element of the procedure, although the overarching responsibility remains with them and they should have intimate working knowledge and experience of every component.

Personnel

A broad pool of expertise is required to optimally perform exenterative surgery. When considering intraoperative decision-making and operative strategy there are three tiers of service required for delivery of an effective service: the core teams, regular participants, and occasional contributors. The personnel required to execute a procedure for advanced pelvic malignancy will depend on the nature and extent of the disease, the planned procedure, and to a certain degree the expertise available at a particular center. The primary principle of this statement is that if a center does not have the expertise required to perform a particular element of the planned procedure (remembering that the core principle of exenterative surgery is achieving an R0 resection) then it should not be undertaking it. The exceptions to this principle are where expertise may be brought in on a case-by-case basis to facilitate a procedure, during the development of a superspecialist center where there is limited previous experience and a learning curve is to be anticipated (and mitigated), or during development of novel approaches where there is no prior expertise [10]. Additionally, there will unfortunately always be cases where additional expertise will be required due to an unintended complication, or an unexpected scenario, although these should be limited by adequate planning and anticipation.

Core Teams

The core operating teams required to undertake exenterative surgery are tripartite – surgical, anesthetic, and theater – led by the triumvirate of consultant surgeon, consultant anesthetist, and theater nursing lead. Each team should then comprise individuals with expertise in surgery for advanced pelvic malignancy. The constituents of teams described here are not absolute requirements but designed as a guide to what is required to undertake this demanding surgery, and to serve as a framework to consider if sufficient expertise is available to proceed [11].

As a minimum, the core operating team should comprise the consultant surgeon with a specialist practice in exenterative surgery and assistants, a senior anesthetist, and an experienced theater scrub team. Developing expertise in each of these teams is important in delivering an effective and safe service. To this end, the importance of regular and reliable rostering of staff to participate in this surgery cannot be emphasized enough, as is the role of specialist education and fellowship programs.

Regular Participants

Beyond the core teams, additional services should be available either as planned contributors or as failsafes for managing the unexpected. Those teams who are frequently required to deliver care for patients undergoing exenteration may be considered as regular participants and are integral to service delivery. The main constituent specialities in this category are urology, gynecology, plastic-reconstructive surgery, and intensive care. In planning procedures utilizing teams from this category, it is important that they are available throughout the procedure and have been involved with the MDT decision-making preoperatively. Although essential to the operation, regular participants commonly will only be required for portions of the procedure.

Advanced pelvic malignancies by definition involve structures beyond the classical system-specific planes of excision, involving adjacent organ systems and structures of the pelvis. Most frequently, the reproductive and genitourinary systems are involved, depending on tumor origin and biology, gender of the patient, and previous surgeries, and thus system-specific surgical expertise should be available to facilitate exenteration or to aid in managing composite resections. The completion of a cystectomy and construction of ileal conduit, for example, should be performed by specialist urologists, as should en-bloc prostatectomy and reconstruction [12, 13]. Similarly, radical total abdominal hysterectomy with or without bilateral salpingo-oophorectomy (TAHBSO) should be performed by or under the guidance of a gynecologist, especially when considering the care of women of childbearing age [14, 15]. Although minor excisions of adjacent structures are commonly employed by non-specialist surgeons to achieve a complete excision of locally advanced tumors (such as taking portions of the posterior wall of the vagina or dome of the bladder), this practice should not be considered where specialist expertise is not available should difficulties be encountered, or for surgeons not commonly managing locally advanced disease.

The use of plastic-reconstructive techniques to facilitate radical excisions is the accepted standard of care, and the availability of plastic surgeons with expertise to provide planned soft-tissue reconstruction, particularly of the perineum, should be considered for every patient undergoing surgery for advanced pelvic malignancy [16–18]. Not every patient will require reconstruction, but the availability of expertise is essential in adequate planning or in the uncommon events of delayed reconstruction due to failed primary closure [19, 20].

A requirement to undertaking exenterative surgery is the availability of intensive care or high-dependency care input. Generally speaking, few patients require level III care following uncomplicated exenterative surgery, although a significant proportion require step-down care on a level II or equivalent unit for the immediate 24–48 hours post surgery [21]. A small number of units electively admit intubated and ventilated patients to level III care overnight as part of a two-stage procedure, but this is not widespread practice.

Occasional Contributors

The technical limitations of surgery for advanced pelvic malignancy are constantly under review as both the techniques and evidence base for increasingly radical resections grow. However, an increasing number of procedures intervening on the bony pelvis and major neurovascular structures are being performed in highly specialized centers. This drive to operate into "higher and wider" planes naturally should bring in the expertise of surgeons not commonly involved in surgery for pelvic malignancy on a limited case-by-case basis, namely vascular and orthopedic surgery [22]. This group of surgeons may be considered as the occasional contributors, as (currently) the indications for and patients suitable for these interventions are limited. Additionally, there will be unforeseen circumstances where input from these specialities will be required.

The role of vascular surgeons in surgery for advanced pelvic malignancy has traditionally been to stop unexpected or uncontrollable bleeding. However, with wider and more radical resections there is a role for elective reconstruction of major infra-aortic vessels following resection of advanced tumors of the pelvic sidewall (addressed in Chapter 12) [23, 24]. There is also an occasional role for vascular surgeons in approaches to the retroperitoneum for isolated or oligometastatic disease of the para-aortic nodes, although the evidence base for this is as yet inconclusive [25].

The potential contribution to pelvic exenterative surgery of orthopedic surgeons and bone-specific techniques may be underestimated. Resections of the low sacrum and coccyx form an integral part of surgery for locally advanced or recurrent rectal cancers and are frequently performed routinely by colorectal surgeons. As planes of excision have extended, increasingly adventurous bony excisions have been undertaken in a small number of centers with success [26, 27]. However, within the sphere of pelvic bony sarcoma surgery, increasingly complex, radical, and successful resections are being undertaken (see Chapters 11, 12, and 13) [3]. Whether these can be translated into viable options for pelvic exenterative surgery for non-sarcoma pathology is as yet unproven, although increasingly specialist orthopedic surgeons should be considered part of the wider MDT [28].

The Intraoperative Stage

Once the patient has reached the operating table the final assessment of operability and operative strategy must be decided based upon the intraoperative findings. This element of decision-making is grounded in the preoperative assessments, planning, and consent process, and should always refer back to these preceding steps [29]. The assessment can be broken-down into three stages: external examination, general laparotomy, and the pelvis. Each stage presents an opportunity to reconsider the operative strategy, or halt an attempted resection before an unrecoverable scenario unfolds. It may be beneficial to consider a checklist of criteria that would alter your decision-making (Table 7.1). Ultimately, the goal of exenterative surgery is to achieve R0 resection whilst preserving as much function as possible, and every decision must be taken with this in mind.

Table 7.1 Checkpoints for proceeding at the intraoperative stage.

- Metastatic disease (peritoneal/omental/liver/para-aortic disease)
- Extent of small bowel involvement (short bowel syndrome)
- Height of sacral involvement (unstable pelvis/hemorrhage)
- Sidewall fixity (hemorrhage and neurological deficit)
- At point of causing tumor or adjacent organ ischemia (mesenteric vessel division)
- At point of potential massive hemorrhage
- Presacral veins
- Iliac vein/artery trunk/branches
- Prostatic dorsal venous complex

External Examination

Initial assessment begins with an abdominal examination with the patient asleep and paralyzed. The presence of an unexpected mass or ascites suggesting tumor progression or metastasis presents an opportunity to consider the likelihood of complete resection. At this point an assessment should also be made of the abdominal wall, such as the presence of previous scars or stoma sites. This step is essential in planning the optimal incision and in decision-making regarding the harvesting of flaps for reconstruction. Inappropriate incisions risk limiting pelvic access, damaging tissues/abdominal wall blood supply that may otherwise have been suitable for reconstruction, or complicating stoma siting, or result in abdominal wall failure and hernia formation.

A rectal and/or vaginal (bimanual) examination should then be performed. These examinations are primarily focused on assessing local tumor fixity, indicating direct invasion, and the likelihood of adjacent organ involvement [30]. Examination under anesthesia also gives the surgeon a 3D mental image of the disease and anticipated required surgical resection. The examination may need to be augmented with flexible cystoscopy or sigmoidoscopy. Fixity to bony landmarks such as the pubis, sacrum/coccyx, and sidewalls indicates bony infiltration, or at least involvement of the periosteum, and should raise the question of technical resectability, whether orthopedic input is required, or whether the patient is willing to accept the potential morbidity of a bony resection. If sacral resection is planned, which approach should be undertake first and the orchestration of turning the patient during the procedure should be considered.

Staging laparoscopy is not currently routinely undertaken in the context of advanced pelvic tumors of colorectal origin due to the infrequency of peritoneal spread, and lack of evidence that it changes management, but some centers do perform this step.

General Laparotomy

If a vertical rectus abdomino-myocutaneous flap is planned then consideration should be given to a fascia-preserving incision to facilitate subsequent abdominal closure after flap harvest. Once the patient's abdomen is open it is important to systematically examine each compartment of the abdomen, beginning away from the pelvis. During this examination the presence of distant disease relating to the primary cancer should be detected, as well as coinciding unrelated disease. Particular attention should be paid to disease factors that would preclude or significantly modify the operative strategy. The presence of metastatic disease, particularly if there is widespread peritoneal and/or omental involvement, would normally present an absolute contraindication to proceeding (see Chapter 14 for further detail) [31–33]. The presence of unexpected multiple liver metastasis is also normally considered an absolute contraindication to proceeding, although, ultimately, if the patient is suitable for chemotherapy, these may themselves become operable and thus the pelvic tumor also potentially operable [34, 35]. There are of course a limited number of patients with locally advanced or locally recurrent cancers who have known isolated or oligometastatic liver disease who will undergo simultaneous or delayed liver metastasectomy/formal liver resection.

Another frequent consideration when assessing the operability of an advanced pelvic malignancy, especially in cases of recurrent disease and an empty pelvis, is the involvement of small bowel. Although not a common site for metastasis, small bowel frequently becomes locally infiltrated by pelvic disease requiring en-bloc resection. Often a decision to resect, a small bowel loop adherent to a pelvic mass is needed as one of the first steps in pelvic dissection. Vascular division of the small bowel mesentery in this setting is a relative point of no return and therefore should only be performed when the surgical team is comfortable that there is a reasonable chance of performing an R0 resection of the pelvic disease. Frequently it is a terminal ileal loop that is tethered in the pelvis; in this scenario, if urinary diversion with an ileal conduit is planned, the conduit can be harvested from the small bowel adjacent to the resection. This approach affords the benefit of a single small bowel anastomosis.

Figure 7.1 demonstrates an example of small bowel adherent to a recurrent pelvic tumor. Small bowel stuck onto the pelvic mass can also complicate neoadjuvant radiotherapy or re-irradiation of recurrence [36, 37]. Evidence of radiation ileitis should be noted during laparotomy, although the decision to alter operative management due to its presence would only be required by the most severe of cases.

Intraoperative assessment of operability in the pelvis is highly dependent on the location and local infiltration of the tumor, although the overriding principle is that there is no advantage to anything other than an R0 resection. The surgeon faced with a patient who has received neoadjuvant chemoradiotherapy or a history of previous pelvic surgery will frequently encounter hardened tissue in the conventional surgical tissue planes. At present, it is impossible to determine if the hardened tissue represents fibrosis or viable tumor. In this scenario the correct oncological principle is to widen the surgical resection, if technically feasible, rather than risk an R1/2 resection. Any decision to proceed should be measured against the likelihood of achieving complete excision and the morbidity associated with extending the plane of excision, remembering that technical limits may be beyond the limits acceptable to the patient. The limits to operability broadly fall into three overlapping fields: inoperability due to unacceptable loss of function, inoperability due to loss of pelvic stability, and inoperability due to risk of life-threatening hemorrhage. The challenges of unexpected tumor extension are summarized in Table 7.2, with potential strategies for overcoming them.

Technical limits regarding infiltration of the bony pelvis and periosteum are currently under review. Fortunately, high-resolution magnetic resonance imaging (MRI) is usually highly sensitive to involvement of the bony pelvis, and thus a management strategy can be planned preoperatively. Where the unexpected is encountered, the accepted practice is that a surgeon may safely amputate the sacrum at the S2/3 level to excise a posteriorly invading tumor, given appropriate consent [38, 39]. This

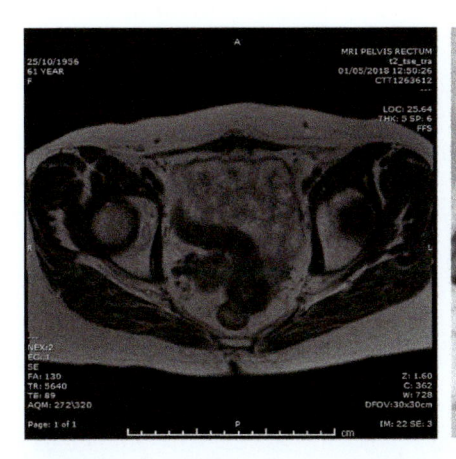

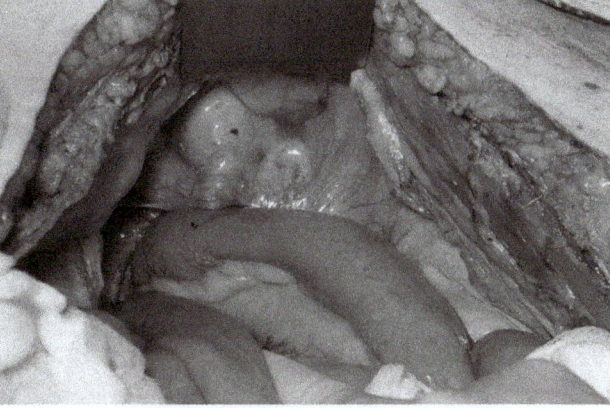

Figure 7.1 T2-turbo spin echo (TSE) MRI and corresponding photograph demonstrating lateral pelvic recurrence with adherent small bowel loops. If the recurrent mass is deemed inoperable then dividing the small bowel mesenteric vessels for access will devascularize the adherent loops. Excision of these alone will result in open tumor. *Source:* Rory Kokelaar, Dean Harris, and Martyn Evans.

Table 7.2 Planes of unexpected tumor extension and potential strategies for management.

Plane of unexpected tumor extension and structures at risk	Potentially curative surgical solution	Comorbidity	Surgical expertise
Anterior – male pelvis Seminal vesicles Prostate and dorsal venous complex Bladder	En-bloc prostatectomy with cysto-urethral reconstruction Partial cystectomy Total pelvic exenteration	Urine leak Major hemorrhage Impaired bladder function Urostomy	Urologist
Anterior – female pelvis Vagina Uterus and reproductive system Bladder Pubic symphysis	En-bloc total/partial vagenectomy En-bloc hysterectomy +/− oophrectomy Total pelvic exenteration Resection of anterior pelvis	Urine leak Infertility Impaired sexual function Pelvic instability	Gynecologist/reproductive health Urologist Plastic-reconstructive (expertise in vaginal reconstruction) Orthopedic surgeon
Lateral sidewall Iliac vessels and branches Sciatic and obturator nerves Ureters Bony pelvic sidewall	Extended lateral sidewall excision (without reconstruction) Arterial and venous reconstruction Nerve graft Ureteric re-implantation/reconstruction IORT	Major hemorrhage Neurologic deficit and disability Urine leak	Vascular surgeon Plastic-reconstructive surgeon (expertise in nerve grafting) Urologist Clinical oncologist
Posterior sacrum and sacroiliac joints Lower lumbar vertebrae Lumbar and sacral nerve roots Presacral veins	Anterior table sacrectomy Sacral division (below S2) Lateral sacrectomy High sacrectomy (+/− L5) with reconstruction IORT	Major hemorrhage Neurologic deficit and disability Pelvic instability	Orthopedic surgeon Clinical oncologist
Pelvic floor Muscular pelvic floor Vulva Root of penis and scrotum	Anterior or posterior triangle of pelvic floor excision with reconstruction Radical pelvic floor excision	Additional ostomies Pelvic floor hernia Impaired sexual function	Plastic-reconstructive surgeon Urologist

procedure typically involves a prone phase to the operation which must be planned in advance but may be completed prior to or following the abdominal component. Above the S2/S3 level, concerns regarding instability of the pelvis have typically been regarded as a contraindication and outside the specialist practice of a small number of sarcoma centers and units with expertise in bony reconstruction [40, 41]. At the S2 level and above, serious consideration has to be made of the potentially significant morbidity associated with damage to the nerve roots, adding reduced mobility to the sexual and continence morbidity associated with neurological injury. As a compromise, more limited excisions of the high

Figure 7.2 T2 MRI demonstrating an anteriorly based rectal tumor invading the seminal vesicles post long course chemoradiotherapy (LCCRT). The plane of excision was fibrosed due to radiotherapy and it was impossible to tell intraoperatively whether viable tumor would involve the resection margin, which was also threatening the prostatic dorsal venous complex. An intraoperative decision was made to progress to total pelvic exenteration (TPE) rather than abdomino-perineal excision resection (APER) with en-bloc excision of seminal vesicles. *Source:* Rory Kokelaar, Dean Harris, and Martyn Evans.

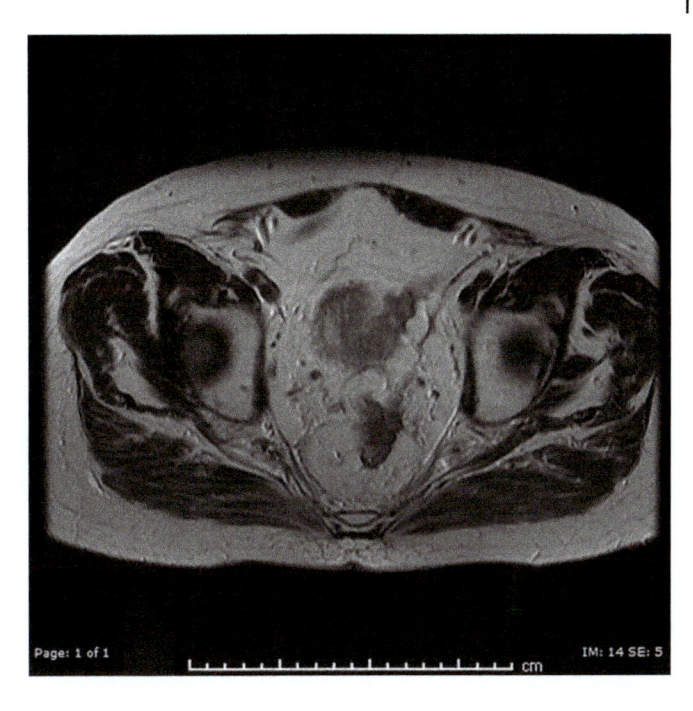

sacrum, such as anterior table sacrectomy, have been employed by a small number of units; although the data underpinning this practice are small, early R0 outcomes are promising [3]. Due to the evolving status of the approach to the high sacrum, if unexpected advanced disease is encountered, it would not be advisable to automatically defer to a palliative scenario.

The risk of life-threatening hemorrhage should not be underestimated in exenterative surgery. Approaches to the lateral pelvic sidewall and its major vessels, the presacral veins, and the prostatic dorsal venous complex all present a significant risk of severe bleeding, especially in a pre-irradiated pelvis or when tumor is invading or encasing these structures. Figure 7.2 demonstrates an anteriorly based rectal tumor invading seminal vesicles. Bleeding is also to be expected during any resection of the bony pelvis. If safe dissection cannot be progressed into a highly vascularized area due to fibrosis or limited access it should be ceased until adequate proximal control is established, either by slinging the major vessels or by ligating and excising the structures en bloc [23, 42]. This practice is not uncommon for tumors invading the lateral pelvic sidewall where the internal iliac artery and vein are at risk. These may be safely ligated by an experienced pelvic oncology surgeon, although ischemia to other pelvic organs and buttock claudication must be considered. Ligation of the common or external iliac vessels is rarely performed but is technically feasible, although it relies on the expertise of a vascular surgeon to perform reconstruction and it should be possible to predict this situation preoperatively [43]. Usually the tumor doesn't involve the vessel directly and a plane can be developed to leave the major vessel intact without fear of a positive margin. Provided that vascular expertise is available in an unexpected major vessel involvement it should be possible to excise and revascularize without the need to abandon surgery.

> **Summary Box**
>
> - The management of advanced pelvic malignancies should be led by an experienced MDT in a specialized center to ensure a high-volume, high-quality service.
> - A bespoke operative strategy should be planned for each individual case and led by the consultant surgeon, drawing on expertise from other surgical disciplines as dictated by the case. Specialist anesthetic and nursing care is also crucial.
> - Assessment of intraoperative resectability should be made at safe threshold points during surgery to prevent adverse outcomes such as critical devascularization, bony pelvic instability, catastrophic hemorrhage, or suboptimal resection, lest an irrecoverable situation inadvertently be encountered.
> - Beyond total mesorectal excision (TME), tumor extension can be managed according to the affected adjacent organ systems and pelvic compartment, given appropriate expertise. Solutions in the anterior pelvis and pelvic floor are gender-dependent, but lateral and posterior extension may be standardized dependent on the structures involved.

References

1 Beyond TME Collaborative (2013). Consensus statement on the multidisciplinary management of patients with recurrent and primary rectal cancer beyond total mesorectal excision planes. *Br. J. Surg.* 100 (8): 1009–1014.

2 Kokelaar, R.F., Evans, M.D., Davies, M. et al. (2016). Locally advanced rectal cancer: management challenges. *Onco. Targets Ther.* 9: 6265–6272.

3 Sineshaw, H.M., Jemal, A., Thomas, C.R. Jr., and Mitin, T. (2016). Changes in treatment patterns for patients with locally advanced rectal cancer in the United States over the past decade: an analysis from the National Cancer Data Base. *Cancer* 122 (13): 1996–2003.

4 PelvEx Collaborative (2018). Factors affecting outcomes following pelvic exenteration for locally recurrent rectal cancer. *Br. J. Surg.* 105 (6): 650–657.

5 PelvEx Collaborative. Surgical and Survival Outcomes Following Pelvic Exenteration for Locally Advanced Primary Rectal Cancer: Results From an International Collaboration. Ann Surg. 2019 Feb;269(2):315-321. doi: 10.1097/SLA.0000000000002528. PMID: 28938268

6 Radwan, R.W., Jones, H.G., Rawat, N. et al. (2015). Determinants of survival following pelvic exenteration for primary rectal cancer. *Br. J. Surg.* 102 (10): 1278–1284.

7 Speicher, P.J., Turley, R.S., Sloane, J.L. et al. (2014). Pelvic exenteration for the treatment of locally advanced colorectal and bladder malignancies in the modern era. *J. Gastrointest. Surg.* 18 (4): 782–788.

8 Koh, C.E., Solomon, M.J., Brown, K.G. et al. (2017). The evolution of pelvic exenteration practice at a single center: lessons learned from over 500 cases. *Dis. Colon Rectum* 60 (6): 627–635.

9 Augestad, K.M., Lindsetmo, R.O., Stulberg, J.J. et al. (2012). System-based factors influencing intraoperative decision-making in rectal cancer by surgeons: an international assessment. *Colorectal Dis.* 14 (10): e679–e688.

10 Brown, K.G.M., Solomon, M.J., and Koh, C.E. (2017). Pelvic exenteration surgery: the evolution of radical surgical techniques for advanced and recurrent pelvic malignancy. *Dis. Colon Rectum* 60 (7): 745–754.

11 Weldon, S.M., Korkiakangas, T., Bezemer, J., and Kneebone, R. (2013). Communication in

the operating theatre. *Br. J. Surg.* 100 (13): 1677–1688.

12 Hautmann, R.E., Abol-Enein, H., Lee, C.T. et al. (2015). Urinary diversion: how experts divert. *Urology* 85 (1): 233–238.

13 Lee, R.K., Abol-Enein, H., Artibani, W. et al. (2014). Urinary diversion after radical cystectomy for bladder cancer: options, patient selection, and outcomes. *BJU Int.* 113 (1): 11–23.

14 Kavallaris, A., Zygouris, D., Dafopoulos, A. et al. (2015). Nerve sparing radical hysterectomy in early stage cervical cancer. Latest developments and review of the literature. *Eur. J. Gynaecol. Oncol.* 36 (1): 5–9.

15 Orozco, L.J., Tristan, M., Vreugdenhil, M.M., and Salazar, A. (2014). Hysterectomy versus hysterectomy plus oophorectomy for premenopausal women. *Cochrane Database Syst. Rev* Jul 28 (7): CD005638.

16 Salom, E.M. and Penalver, M.A. (2003). Pelvic exenteration and reconstruction. *Cancer J.* 9 (5): 415–424.

17 Brodbeck, R., Horch, R.E., Arkudas, A., and Beier, J.P. (2015). Plastic and reconstructive surgery in the treatment of oncological perineal and genital defects. *Frontiers Oncol.* 5: 212.

18 Devulapalli, C., Jia Wei, A.T., DiBiagio, J.R. et al. (2016). Primary versus flap closure of perineal defects following oncologic resection: a systematic review and meta-analysis. *Plast. Reconstr. Surg.* 137 (5): 1602–1613.

19 McArdle, A., Bischof, D.A., Davidge, K. et al. (2012). Vaginal reconstruction following radical surgery for colorectal malignancies: a systematic review of the literature. *Ann. Surg. Oncol.* 19 (12): 3933–3942.

20 Chae, M.P., Rozen, W.M., Whitaker, I.S. et al. (2015). Current evidence for postoperative monitoring of microvascular free flaps: a systematic review. *Ann. Plast. Surg.* 74 (5): 621–632.

21 Mirhashemi, R., Janicek, M.F., and Schoell, W.M. (1999). Critical care issues in cervical cancer management. *Semin. Surg. Oncol.* 16 (3): 267–274.

22 Harji, D.P., Griffiths, B., McArthur, D.R., and Sagar, P.M. (2013). Surgery for recurrent rectal cancer: higher and wider? *Colorectal Disease* 15 (2): 139–145.

23 Austin, K.K. and Solomon, M.J. (2009). Pelvic exenteration with en bloc iliac vessel resection for lateral pelvic wall involvement. *Dis. Colon Rectum* 52 (7): 1223–1233.

24 McKay, A., Motamedi, M., Temple, W. et al. (2007). Vascular reconstruction with the superficial femoral vein following major oncologic resection. *J. Surg. Oncol.* 96 (2): 151–159.

25 Gagniere, J., Dupre, A., Chabaud, S. et al. (2015). Retroperitoneal nodal metastases from colorectal cancer: curable metastases with radical retroperitoneal lymphadenectomy in selected patients. *Eur. J. Surg. Oncol.* 41 (6): 731–737.

26 Milne, T., Solomon, M.J., Lee, P. et al. (2013). Assessing the impact of a sacral resection on morbidity and survival after extended radical surgery for locally recurrent rectal cancer. *Annals of Surgery* 258 (6): 1007–1013.

27 Milne, T., Solomon, M.J., Lee, P. et al. (2014). Sacral resection with pelvic exenteration for advanced primary and recurrent pelvic cancer: a single-institution experience of 100 sacrectomies. *Dis. Colon Rectum* 57 (10): 1153–1161.

28 Kawada, K., Hasegawa, S., Okada, T. et al. (2017). Stereotactic navigation during laparoscopic surgery for locally recurrent rectal cancer. *Techniques in Coloproctology* 21 (12): 977–978.

29 Chew, M.H., Brown, W.E., Masya, L. et al. (2013). Clinical, MRI, and PET-CT criteria used by surgeons to determine suitability for pelvic exenteration surgery for recurrent rectal cancers: a Delphi study. *Dis. Colon Rectum* 56 (6): 717–725.

30 Asoglu, O., Karanlik, H., Muslumanoglu, M. et al. (2007). Prognostic and predictive factors after surgical treatment for locally

recurrent rectal cancer: a single institute experience. *Eur. J. Surg. Oncol.* 33 (10): 1199–1206.
31 Hall, B., Padussis, J., and Foster, J.M. (2017). Cytoreduction and hyperthermic intraperitoneal chemotherapy in the management of colorectal peritoneal metastasis. *Surg. Clin. North Am.* 97 (3): 671–682.
32 Mirnezami, R., Mehta, A.M., Chandrakumaran, K. et al. (2014). Cytoreductive surgery in combination with hyperthermic intraperitoneal chemotherapy improves survival in patients with colorectal peritoneal metastases compared with systemic chemotherapy alone. *Br. J. Cancer* 111 (8): 1500–1508.
33 Solomon, M.J., Egan, M., Roberts, R.A. et al. (1997). Incidence of free colorectal cancer cells on the peritoneal surface. *Dis. Colon Rectum* 40 (11): 1294–1298.
34 Hoch, G., Croise-Laurent, V., Germain, A. et al. (2015). Is intraoperative ultrasound still useful for the detection of colorectal cancer liver metastases? *HPB (Oxford)* 17 (6): 514–519.
35 Peloso, A., Franchi, E., Canepa, M.C. et al. (2013). Combined use of intraoperative ultrasound and indocyanine green fluorescence imaging to detect liver metastases from colorectal cancer. *HPB (Oxford)* 15 (12): 928–934.
36 Reis, T., Khazzaka, E., Welzel, G. et al. (2015). Acute small-bowel toxicity during neoadjuvant combined radiochemotherapy in locally advanced rectal cancer: determination of optimal dose-volume cut-off value predicting grade 2–3 diarrhoea. *Radiat. Oncol.* 10: 30.
37 Xu, B., Guo, Y., Chen, Y. et al. (2015). Is the irradiated small bowel volume still a predictor for acute lower gastrointestinal toxicity during preoperative concurrent chemo-radiotherapy for rectal cancer when using intensity-modulated radiation therapy? *Radiat. Oncol.* 10: 257.
38 Kido, A., Koyama, F., Akahane, M. et al. (2011). Extent and contraindications for sacral amputation in patients with recurrent rectal cancer: a systematic literature review. *J. Orthopaed. Sci.* 16 (3): 286–290.
39 Sasikumar, A., Bhan, C., Jenkins, J.T. et al. (2017). Systematic review of pelvic exenteration with en bloc sacrectomy for recurrent rectal adenocarcinoma: R0 resection predicts disease-free survival. *Dis. Colon Rectum* 60 (3): 346–352.
40 Brown, K.G., Solomon, M.J., Austin, K.K. et al. (2016). Posterior high sacral segmental disconnection prior to anterior en bloc exenteration for recurrent rectal cancer. *Tech. Coloproctol.* 20 (6): 401–404.
41 Dozois, E.J., Privitera, A., Holubar, S.D. et al. (2011). High sacrectomy for locally recurrent rectal cancer: can long-term survival be achieved? *Journal of Surgical Oncology* 103 (2): 105–109.
42 Shaikh, I., Aston, W., Hellawell, G. et al. (2014). Extended lateral pelvic sidewall excision (ELSiE): an approach to optimize complete resection rates in locally advanced or recurrent anorectal cancer involving the pelvic sidewall. *Tech. Coloproctol.* 18 (12): 1161–1168.
43 Brown, K.G., Koh, C.E., Solomon, M.J. et al. (2015). Outcomes after en bloc iliac vessel excision and reconstruction during pelvic Exenteration. *Dis. Colon Rectum* 58 (9): 850–856.

8

Anterior Pelvic Exenteration

Jan W.A. Hagemans[1], Jan M. van Rees[1], Joost Rothbarth[1], Cornelis Verhoef[1], and Jacobus W.A. Burger[2]

[1] *Department of Surgery, Erasmus MC, Rotterdam, The Netherlands*
[2] *Department of Surgery, Catharina Hospital Eindhoven, The Netherlands*

Background

In women, an anterior pelvic exenteration refers to removal of the bladder, uterus, and ovaries, leaving the rectum in situ; posterior pelvic exenteration refers to removal of the rectum, uterus, ovaries, and posterior vaginal wall. In men, an anterior exenteration means removal of the bladder, vesicles, and prostate, but this procedure is more commonly referred to as a cystoprostatectomy. A total pelvic exenteration includes complete excision of all pelvic organs including the bladder (+/− prostate/seminal vesicles) and rectum, and in women the uterus/ovaries and posterior vaginal wall (Figure 8.1). For selective resections of organs or structures that do not result in a formal anterior, posterior, or total pelvic exenteration, we use the term "modified exenteration."

Diagnostics Specific to Anterior Pelvic Exenteration

Before performing any extensive surgical procedures in the anterior pelvic area, diagnostic workup is imperative, both for surgical planning and eligibility. After diagnosis of the malignant disease, local status and distant metastasis need to be evaluated.

One diagnostic modality that is eminently useful in patients with tumors in the anterior pelvic area is magnetic resonance imaging (MRI) with diffusion-weighted images. As it depicts tumor invasion in adjacent structures very accurately, feasibility of a successful complete resection can be evaluated.

As urinary tract involvement is common in anterior pelvic malignancies, ureter obstruction and kidney function have to be evaluated carefully. The radioisotope renography, also known as the MAG3 scan, is especially helpful to detect any dysfunction in one of the kidneys. If one of the kidneys is not functioning properly, we usually choose to either ligate the ureter or remove the affected kidney. Re-anastomosing a kidney that has a little function may cause unnecessary complications such as anastomotic leakage and pyelonephritis.

Surgical Procedure

Traditionally, an anterior pelvic exenteration implies removal of the bladder, lower ureters, reproductive organs, draining lymph nodes,

---

Surgical Management of Advanced Pelvic Cancer, First Edition.
Edited by Michael E. Kelly and Desmond C. Winter.
© 2022 John Wiley & Sons Ltd. Published 2022 by John Wiley & Sons Ltd.

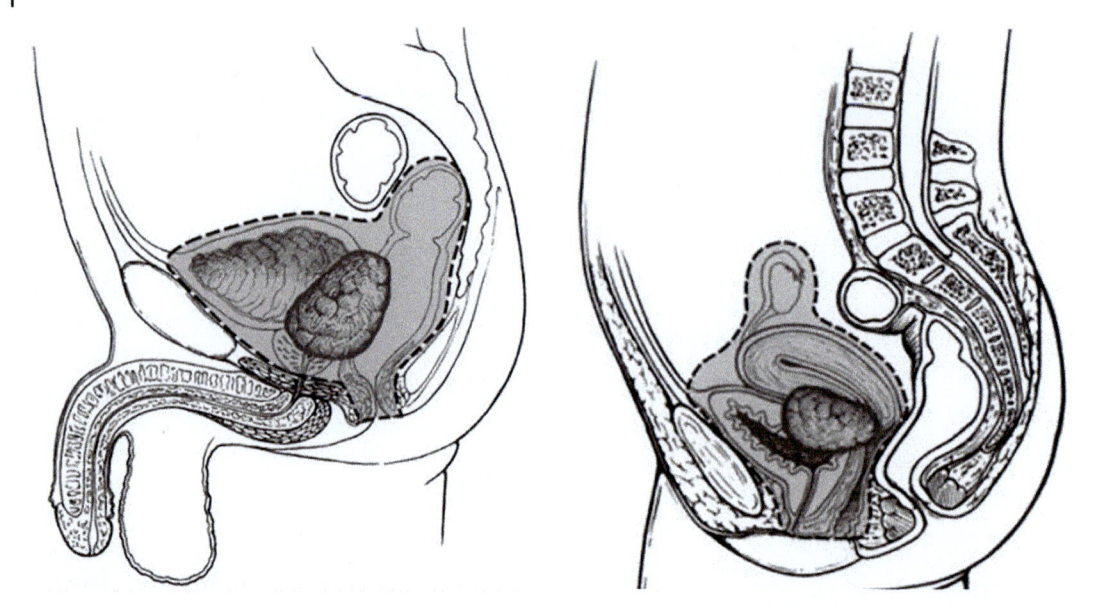

Figure 8.1 Sagital view of a total pelvic exenteration in the male (left) and anterior pelvic exenteration in the female (right) [23]. Source: Jan W.A. Hagemans, Jan M. van Rees, Joost Rothbarth, Cornelis Verhoef, and Jacobus W.A. Burger.

and pelvic peritoneum [1]. However, in clinical practice, the surgical procedure depends on the nature and the extent of the tumor. Anterior pelvic exenterations are performed by surgeon oncologists, gynecologists, and urologists. In case of limited ingrowth in other organs, a selective resection is sufficient. Resections of the ureter, uterus, and part of the bladder are examples of selective procedures that are routinely performed in specialized centers. More extensive tumors and locally recurrent malignancies often require formal anterior, posterior, or total pelvic exenterations. In this chapter, the different approaches for gynecological, urological, and rectal malignancies in the anterior pelvic area are described briefly. In addition, surgical procedures per involved organ in the anterior pelvic area are specified.

Anesthesia and Starting the Procedure

Patients undergoing anterior pelvic exenterations are under general anesthesia and usually receive epidural anesthesia and are placed in the lithotomy position. Patients with advanced or recurrent pelvic cancer are generally not considered candidates for minimally invasive techniques, because tactile feedback is essential in achieving a radical resection. The procedure starts with a midline laparotomy. In our center, we routinely perform an omentoplasty, and therefore the midline incision may be advanced cranially further than strictly necessary for pelvic surgery. Since both locally advanced and locally recurrent pelvic cancer is associated with a high incidence of systemic and peritoneal metastases, careful inspection of the whole abdomen is mandatory before continuing the procedure.

Urological Approach

Anterior pelvic exenteration in urological cancers is often referred to as radical cystoprostectomy and is performed for muscle invasive bladder cancer and T4 prostate cancer. In men, the first step in this procedure is to mobilize and transect the distal ureters as described below. The space between the anterior rectum and posterior prostate may be entered by opening Denonvillier's fascia. The superior and inferior vesical artery are then identified and ligated respectively. To mobilize the bladder, seminal vesicles, and prostate, all tissue laterally from these structures has to be divided. The endopelvic fascia needs to be opened and the puboprostatic ligaments released. After ligation of the dorsal venous complex, the urethra is clipped and transected. By dividing the recto-urethralis muscles, the bladder, seminal vesicles, and prostate can be removed en bloc.

Gynecological Approach

In gynecological cancers, anterior pelvic exenteration includes removing the bladder, urethra, uterus, adnexa, and anterior vaginal wall. The posterior vaginal wall and rectum remain in situ. This procedure is mostly performed for malignancies of the cervix and anterior upper vagina. Anterior pelvic exenteration should only be performed if there is no tumor involvement in the space between the posterior vaginal wall and rectum. After mobilizing the bowel and entering the retroperitoneal space the distal ureters are transected. An incision in the pouch of Douglas is made to dissect the vaginal wall from the rectum. The broad and round ligaments and ovarian vessels are ligated and divided. The superior and inferior vesical arteries are identified and ligated, as are the uterine arteries and veins. The anterior and posterior vaginal wall may then be transected at the desired level. A more detailed description of the resection of the ureter, bladder, and vaginal wall is discussed below.

Rectal Cancer

Locally advanced rectal cancer may invade the anterior pelvic organs such as the bladder and reproductive organs, especially in the case of locally recurrent rectal cancer in the pelvic area. In these cases, a total pelvic exenteration is performed, which is discussed in Chapter 10.

Ureter Dissection

The ureter is identified just above the level of the promontory and dissected in a cranial and caudal direction, while preventing damage to the vasculature of the ureter itself. This is achieved by leaving the ureteral adventitia in place, rather than dissecting the ureter clean.

Fibrosis and tumor are often difficult to differentiate during surgery and any fibrous tissue is considered tumor when performing radical resections. Transection of the ureter opens up the lateral compartment of the pelvis and facilitates radical resection of disease in this compartment. Further resection of all tissues involved is performed, as identified by palpation and macroscopy, and guided by preoperative MRI. When the bladder is not involved, the distal ureter may be cut and ligated, although leaving the ureter open rarely causes leakage from the bladder, because of the uretero-vesical valve. The ureter may be reinserted in the bladder using the so-called psoas-hitch technique. The bladder is mobilized on the contralateral and anterolateral side of the bladder. Ligation of the vesical artery and vein is usually not necessary. The bladder is incised transversely and fixed to the psoas muscle fascia just above the level of the anticipated anastomosis between the ureter and bladder. The ureter is then inserted in the bladder through a small incision, spatulated, and fixed with resorbable sutures. The transverse incision in the bladder is closed longitudinally, and the single J catheter is led out through the bladder wall, abdominal wall, and skin. The single J stent is removed 10 days after surgery when no signs of anastomotic leakage are present on cystogram.

Lateral Compartment

In case of involvement of the pelvic side wall, which occurs frequently in locally advanced and recurrent cancer, the internal iliac artery and vein may also be transected to facilitate more extensive resections up to the acetabulum.

Reconstruction of the internal iliac artery and vein is generally not needed because of sufficient collateral blood supply. In seldom cases in which the external or common iliac vessels are involved, radical resection can sometimes be achieved by complete resection of the external or common iliac vessels.

In case of persistent lymph node metastases in the lateral compartment, a formal lymph node dissection of this area can be performed. The goal of lateral lymph node dissection is to resect all nodes in the pelvic sidewall lateral from the internal iliac vessels after ligating these vessels while preserving the obturator nerve and sacral plexus. In some cases en-bloc resection with these structures is necessary for full clearance of all suspect lateral lymph nodes [2–4]. This procedure is associated with increased urinary and sexual dysfunction, prolonged operation time, and possible increased blood loss [5, 6]. However, in urological cancer, extensive pelvic lymph node dissection is recommended not only to provide accurate staging and prognostic information, but also to possibly identify patients eligible for adjuvant chemotherapy [7–9]. In rectal cancer a recent meta-analysis showed no cancer-specific advantages of extended lymphadenectomy, but there is evidence suggesting that patients with persistent lateral lymph nodes after neoadjuvant (chemo)radiotherapy may benefit from mesorectal excision with lateral lymph node dissection [5, 10–12].

Partial Cystectomy

Successful partial bladder resections are usually performed for radical resection of T4 sigmoid cancer, because these tumors may involve the more cranial aspect of the bladder. It is important to identify the orifices of both ureters to prevent obstruction of the ureter while closing the defect. It is also important to consider whether the size of the remaining bladder, combined with the anticipated function after neoadjuvant therapy, may result in a malfunctioning bladder. A urologist is often required to assist in decision-making. When a small bladder remnant is unlikely to ever function properly, a bladder resection and urinary diversion may be preferable. When partial resection is possible, we open the bladder cranially and choose the dissection planes on palpation and sight. We close the bladder with two layers of 3–0 slowly resorbable sutures. Lower tumors often involve the neck of the bladder and the orifices. Therefore even small bladder wall resections at this level often result in a bladder remnant that is impossible to reconstruct in such a manner that both ureters can be reinserted into a functional remnant. Again, we advise to involve the urologist–oncologist in decision-making. When partial resection is not feasible, a total pelvic exenteration is indicated (see Chapter 10).

Partial Prostatectomy

In case of limited involvement of the prostate, without involvement of the urethra, a partial resection of the prostate may be attempted. It should be noted that the urethra is close to the posterior capsule of the prostate. We insert a large-diameter silicone urinary catheter to palpate the urethra. Softer catheters are palpated less easily. Dissection of the capsule of the prostate should be performed through a perineal approach, usually as part of an abdomino-perineal excision (APE) of the rectum. After performing the usual steps of an APE, we leave the anterior dissection as long as possible. We then identify the urethra by palpation of the silicone catheter and approach the capsule of the prostate caudally and laterally after lateral transection of the pelvic floor. The surgeon may now open the capsule of the prostate and include a layer of prostate in the resection specimen. Continuous palpation may clarify whether the tumor is resected completely and the surgeon can then return to the normal plane with or without including the seminal vesicles in the specimen. When complete removal of the seminal vesicles is performed, the surgeon should be aware that he is approaching the distal ureters from below. It is noteworthy that this type of resection often results in R2 resections, because the extra amount of tissue that can be resected is limited, palpation is difficult, especially in case of extensive fibrosis, and most surgeons are not accustomed to this dissection plane. Ideally, referral of these patients to a specialist center where conversion to a total pelvic exenteration can be performed as needed is advised.

If prostate-conserving surgery cannot be performed, which is common in the case of more advanced tumors invading the prostate or locally recurrent disease in men, a prostatectomy is advised. In some cases, the urethra cannot be re-anastomosed, as patients may have received high-dose radiotherapy and this impairs proper healing of a vesico-urethral anastomosis. Therefore total pelvic exenteration is indicated in these cases.

Uterus and Vaginal Wall

Whereas in men advanced malignancies may extend into the bladder and prostate, in women the uterus and posterior vaginal wall are the first to become involved in tumor extension. Tumor ingrowth into the body of the uterus is relatively rare, as the peritoneal reflection is located lower, at the level of the cervix. Tumor ingrowth at this level can easily be solved by en-bloc resection of the uterus and adnexa, as is performed in gynecological cancer. The ovarian vessels and ligaments are ligated and the uterus mobilized. This can be done by opening the peritoneum and dissecting the bladder from the anterior aspect of the uterus. The vaginal wall is identified and cleared to the caudal aspect of the cervix. The ureters are identified up to their insertion into the bladder or at least up to the point that they are no longer at risk. We then identify the vasculature at the level of the cervix, and isolate and ligate it. When cutting of the many venous branches results in blood loss, it is imperative to be cautious with clamps, diathermy, and energy devices, considering the proximity of the ureter. The vagina is opened anteriorly, below the palpated level of the cervix, using diathermy. The placement of clamps on the vaginal wall and lifting these facilitates separation of the vagina and rectum. The rectum may be cut at the level desired. The vaginal wall may be closed with slowly absorbable sutures, taking care to not include the distal ureter.

Involvement of the cervix and posterior vaginal wall is more common. Findings on the preoperative MRI also guide decision-making. The posterior wall is transected and the vaginal wall freed from the rectum. The lateral wall may be transected with diathermy or an energy device. The defect in the vaginal wall may be large, and when closed primarily, the remnant of the vagina may be small. This may be solved by performing some type of flap reconstruction (e.g. vertical rectus abdominis myocutaneous (VRAM) flap), in which case either skin, fascia, or peritoneum may be used to replace the vaginal wall resected [9]. The alternative is to close the vagina primarily and refer the patient to the gynecologist for dilatation at an early stage. There are no data showing one technique is superior to the other. In the case that the urethra is involved, total pelvic exenteration is indicated. In such cases, near-complete removal of the vagina (colpectomy) is often unavoidable.

Urinary Diversion (Ileal Conduit)

In anterior pelvic exenteration, the gold standard for urinary diversion is the ileal conduit. Although many variances exist, the best-known technique is a Bricker deviation [13–15]. In this procedure, a segment of the terminal ileum with a length of 12–18 cm is isolated at 10 cm from the valve of Bauhin on its mesentery. Usually, a hand-sewed or stapled side-to-side anastomosis is performed to preserve continuation of the digestive tract. The mesentery window is closed with 3–0 absorbable sutures. The distal anastomosis of the ileum is then opened and the ileo-ureteral anastomosis can be constructed. The type of anastomosis performed (e.g. Bricker, Wallace) should be selected by the operating surgeon. The distal ileal loop is usually exteriorized through the lower right quadrant of the abdomen after bluntly dissecting the abdominal muscles and a circular excision in the skin is made.

Urinary Diversion (Colon Conduit)

In some patients, the operator performs a colon conduit as urinary diversion, and this is especially useful when the descending colon or sigmoid is transected during the procedure. The distal colon is cut, leaving a segment of approximately 15–20 cm with an arterial pedicle. This may be the mesenteric inferior artery, the left colonic artery, or in some cases the left branch of the middle colic artery. After mobilization, both ureters may be anastomosed in exactly the same way as in Bricker diversion. The urinary stoma often needs to be placed on the left side of the abdomen, and after mobilization of the transverse colon, the stoma for stool is then placed on the right side of the abdomen. The advantage of this approach is that Bricker diversion results in an extra ileo-ileostomy with a risk of complications such as leakage, whereas diversion with a colon conduit does not require an extra anastomosis.

When performing an ileal or colon conduit, small stents are placed in the ureters to ensure sufficient flow after surgery. The stents are fixed to the bowel wall with 4–0 quickly absorbable braided sutures and led out through the ostomy. If no complications occur, the stent is removed at day 9 and day 10 after surgery under antibiotic prophylaxis.

Morbidity and Mortality

Anterior pelvic exenteration is a comprehensive surgical procedure with a high risk of complications, reinterventions, and postoperative mortality [16–20]. However, due to improved surgical techniques, perioperative care, and patient selection, there have been remarkable improvements in mortality and morbidity in the past decades [18, 21, 22].

Morbidity

The overall morbidity rate after pelvic exenterative surgery is described within a range of 32–84%. The most important risk factor for perioperative morbidity is preoperative pelvic irradiation [17, 20, 23]. Patients often experience general surgical complications such as (intraoperative) bleeding, wound infection, pneumonia, and (pelvic or intra-abdominal) abscesses [24]. Perineal wound problems after exenterative surgery are also common: besides wound infection and abscesses in the short term, perineal hernia or fistulas can occur in the long term [23, 25]. Muscle flap reconstructions may improve perineal wound outcome and pelvic floor dysfunction, but failure of perineal reconstructions often results in catastrophic wound problems [26, 27].

Mortality

Perioperative 30-day mortality after pelvic exenteration is reported within a range of 0–25% [25, 28–31]. A recent population-based study described a mortality rate of 1.9% in women undergoing pelvic exenteration for gynecologic malignancies [31]. Perioperative mortality after radical cystectomy for bladder cancer is reported at between 1.2% and 3.2% [32]. For rectal cancer, a multicenter retrospective study reported day mortality rates of 1.5 and 1.7% for locally advanced and locally recurrent rectal cancer respectively [22].

Complications

Due to the more complex surgery that is performed in total pelvic exenterations, patients undergoing anterior pelvic exenteration may experience fewer complications [33]. However, involvement of the urinary tract and the use of urinary diversions in anterior pelvic exenterations can lead to major problems [34, 35]. Short-term complications of urinary diversion are leakage and obstruction of the urinary enteric anastomosis. Long-term complications include urinary stenosis, fistula, stomal- and peristomal complications, and upper urinary tract deterioration [13]. These complications can sometimes be managed conservatively but more often require re-intervention by prolonged drainage, nephrostomy catheters, or ureter re-implantation [34–36]. Other adverse events such as wound problems and gastrointestinal complications frequently occur in patients undergoing anterior pelvic exenteration [17, 20, 23]. Complications after anterior pelvic exenterations are listed in Table 8.1.

Survival

Prognostic outcomes after pelvic exenteration depend on the origin of the tumor [16]. For bladder cancer, five-year survival rates after radical cystoprostatectomy have been reported between 60 and 67%. Main risk factors for recurrence and reduced bladder-cancer-specific survival are high tumor stage, lymphovascular invasion, and lymph node metastases [37–40]. In advanced and recurrent gynecological malignancies, the five-year overall survival rate after pelvic exenteration is around 50% [41, 42]. Five-year survival after pelvic exenteration for locally advanced recurrent rectal cancer is usually somewhere between 22 and 66%. For locally recurrent rectal cancer, five-year survival after pelvic exenteration is as low as 0–37% [29, 43–45].

Achievement of a clear resection margin is the most important predictive factor for survival in urological, gynecological, and rectal cancers [16, 25, 28].

Quality of Life Following Anterior Pelvic Exenteration

Patients undergoing anterior pelvic exenteration are submitted to a major operation with a high complication rate, prolonged hospital stay, and an extensive rehabilitation process. This can have a huge impact on their quality of life. Patients often receive a permanent urostomy,

Table 8.1 Complications after anterior pelvic exenteration.

General
Hemorrhage
Wound infection
Intra-abdominal abscess
Presacral abscess
Muscle flap necrosis
Pulmonary
Cerebrovascular
Cardiac
Delirium
Venous thrombosis
Urinary diversion related
Urinoma
Urosepsis
Metabolic acidosis
Anastomotic stricture
Obstruction
Fistula
Urinary tract infection
Acute renal failure
Hydronephrosis
Stomal and peristomal problems
Gastrointestinal
Ileus
Small bowel obstruction
Enterocutaneous fistula

colostomy, or both, which can be disabling in various ways [46–48]. However, patient-reported outcomes on quality of life usually improve after exenteration surgery and might even be comparable with those in the general population of disease-free patients [49, 50].

Sexual Dysfunction

Especially in younger women, anterior pelvic exenteration can greatly affect sexual function. Lubrication disorder and dyspareunia are common, especially when parts of the vaginal wall are resected [51, 52]. Due to this, women often experience a lack of sexual desire after pelvic surgery and only a small number of women are sexually active in the postoperative period [51].

Men may experience erectile or ejaculatory dysfunction due to resection of the prostate and vesicles or due to damage to the neurovascular bundle supplying the genitalia [53]. A small number of men who were sexually active before cystoprostatectomy are still potent after surgery. Higher chances of remaining potency after surgery can be achieved when a nerve-sparing operation is performed [38, 53, 54]. It is important to discuss expectations about sexual function after surgery with patients preoperatively [55].

Besides organic sexual dysfunction, both men and women report deterioration in body image and loss in sexual interest [51–53]. It is advisable to offer appropriate psychosexual counseling to patients and it is particularly important in patients who are sexually active [56, 57].

Urinary Dysfunction

As in anterior pelvic exenteration where the bladder is resected, most patients end up with either an ileal or a colon conduit or an orthotopic bladder [13]. Stoma-related problems such as urinary leakage, odor, stomal and peristomal complications, and altered body image are considerable factors affecting patients' quality of life [48]. There is no stoma involvement in an orthotopic bladder and this might have less effect on physical image compared to urinary conduits. However, patients with an orthotopic bladder frequently experience nocturnal incontinence, and postoperative bladder retraining is needed [58]. For patients who receive previous irradiation of the pelvic area, an orthotopic bladder might not be the best option. An ileal or colon conduit might then be preferred. Studies have shown that the quality of life of patients with an ileal conduit and orthotopic bladder is indifferent. Shared decision-making and patient education seem to be the most important factors for postoperative satisfaction [47, 59, 60].

General and Mental Health

General health is often affected, as patients experience greater fatigue, anxiety, and even depression, especially directly after surgery [56, 57]. Numerous other health problems such as pain, abdominal bloating, flatulence, and voiding issues are common [51]. Some patients do not have the ability to return to their profession or occupation after surgery and have difficulties proceeding in their social and leisure activities [48].

Despite these changes and impairments, quality of life usually returns to baseline within a year. Therefore patients should not be denied exenterative surgery based on perceived poor quality of life [50, 61, 62].

Summary Box
• Anterior pelvic exenteration is a complex surgical procedure with considerable perioperative morbidity and mortality rates, but it can be beneficial in a select group of patients. • Urinary diversion complications such as urinary fistula and pyelonephritis are frequent in anterior pelvic exenterations and can be life-threatening.	• Achievement of a clear resection margin is the most important prognostic factor for overall survival. • Anterior pelvic exenteration has a major impact on physical and mental health. Adequate counseling is therefore recommended. • Quality of life is decreased after surgery but rapidly improves in the long term.

References

1. Rodriguez-Bigas, M.A. and Petrelli, N.J. (1996). Pelvic exenteration and its modifications. *Am. J. Surg.* 171 (2): 293–301.
2. Moriya, Y., Sugihara, K., Akasu, T., and Fujita, S. (1997). Importance of extended lymphadenectomy with lateral node dissection for advanced lower rectal cancer. *World J. Surg.* 21 (7): 728–732.
3. Takahashi, T., Ueno, M., Azekura, K., and Ohta, H. (2000). Lateral node dissection and total mesorectal excision for rectal cancer. *Dis. Colon Rectum* 43 (10 Suppl): S59–S68.
4. Moriya, Y., Hojo, K., Sawada, T., and Koyama, Y. (1989). Significance of lateral node dissection for advanced rectal carcinoma at or below the peritoneal reflection. *Dis. Colon Rectum* 32 (4): 307–315.
5. Georgiou, P.A., Mohammed Ali, S., Brown, G. et al. (2017). Extended lymphadenectomy for locally advanced and recurrent rectal cancer. *Int. J. Color. Dis.* 32 (3): 333–340.
6. Fujita, S., Akasu, T., Mizusawa, J. et al. (2012). Postoperative morbidity and mortality after mesorectal excision with and without lateral lymph node dissection for clinical stage II or stage III lower rectal cancer (JCOG0212): results from a multicentre, randomised controlled, non-inferiority trial. *Lancet Oncol.* 13 (6): 616–621.
7. Steven, K. and Poulsen, A.L. (2007). Radical cystectomy and extended pelvic lymphadenectomy: survival of patients with lymph node metastasis above the bifurcation of the common iliac vessels treated with surgery only. *J. Urol.* 178 (4 Pt 1): 1218–1223; discussion 23-4.
8. Herr, H.W., Bochner, B.H., Dalbagni, G. et al. (2002). Impact of the number of lymph nodes retrieved on outcome in patients with muscle invasive bladder cancer. *J. Urol.* 167 (3): 1295–1298.
9. Leissner, J., Ghoneim, M.A., Abol-Enein, H. et al. (2004). Extended radical lymphadenectomy in patients with urothelial bladder cancer: results of a prospective multicenter study. *J. Urol.* 171 (1): 139–144.
10. Fujita, S., Mizusawa, J., Kanemitsu, Y. et al. (2016). A randomized trial comparing mesorectal excision with or without lateral lymph node dissection for clinical stage II, III lower rectal cancer: primary endpoint analysis of Japan clinical oncology group study JCOG0212. *J. Clin. Oncol* 34 (15 Suppl): 3508.
11. Kusters, M., Uehara, K., Velde, C., and Moriya, Y. (2017). Is there any reason to still consider lateral lymph node dissection in rectal cancer? rationale and technique. *Clin. Colon Rectal Surg.* 30 (5): 346–356.
12. Kusters, M., Slater, A., Muirhead, R. et al. (2017). What to do with lateral nodal disease in low locally advanced rectal cancer? A call for further reflection and research. *Dis. Colon Rectum* 60 (6): 577–585.
13. Hautmann, R.E., Abol-Enein, H., Hafez, K. et al. (2007). Urinary diversion. *Urology* 69 (1 Suppl): 17–49.
14. Colombo, R. and Naspro, R. (2010). Ileal conduit as the standard for urinary diversion after radical cystectomy for bladder cancer. *Eur. Urol. Suppl.* 9 (10): 736–744.
15. Bricker, E.M. (1950). Bladder substitution after pelvic evisceration. *Surg. Clin. North Am.* 30 (5): 1511–1521.
16. PelvEx Collaborative (2019). Pelvic exenteration for advanced nonrectal pelvic malignancy. *Ann. Surg.* 270 (5): 899–905.
17. Jakowatz, J.G., Porudominsky, D., Riihimaki, D.U. et al. (1985). Complications of pelvic exenteration. *Arch. Surg.* 120 (11): 1261–1265.
18. Goldberg, J.M., Piver, M.S., Hempling, R.E. et al. (1998). Improvements in pelvic exenteration: factors responsible for reducing morbidity and mortality. *Ann. Surg. Oncol.* 5 (5): 399–406.
19. Shabsigh, A., Korets, R., Vora, K.C. et al. (2009). Defining early morbidity of radical cystectomy for patients with bladder cancer using a standardized reporting methodology. *Eur. Urol.* 55 (1): 164–174.

20 Stimson, C.J., Chang, S.S., Barocas, D.A. et al. (2010). Early and late perioperative outcomes following radical cystectomy: 90-day readmissions, morbidity and mortality in a contemporary series. *J. Urol.* 184 (4): 1296–1300.

21 Brown, K.G.M., Solomon, M.J., and Koh, C.E. (2017). Pelvic exenteration surgery: the evolution of radical surgical techniques for advanced and recurrent pelvic malignancy. *Dis. Colon Rectum* 60 (7): 745–754.

22 PelvEx Collaborative (2019). Changing outcomes following pelvic exenteration for locally advanced and recurrent rectal cancer. *BJS Open* 3 (4): 516–520.

23 Pawlik, T.M., Skibber, J.M., and Rodriguez-Bigas, M.A. (2006). Pelvic exenteration for advanced pelvic malignancies. *Ann. Surg. Oncol.* 13 (5): 612–623.

24 Ferenschild, F.T., Vermaas, M., Verhoef, C. et al. (2009). Total pelvic exenteration for primary and recurrent malignancies. *World J. Surg.* 33 (7): 1502–1508.

25 PelvEx Collaborative (2019;269(2):315–21). Surgical and survival outcomes following pelvic exenteration for locally advanced primary rectal cancer: results from an international collaboration. *Ann. Surg.*

26 Tobin, G.R. and Day, T.G. (1988). Vaginal and pelvic reconstruction with distally based rectus abdominis myocutaneous flaps. *Plast. Reconstr. Surg.* 81 (1): 62–73.

27 Chessin, D.B., Hartley, J., Cohen, A.M. et al. (2005). Rectus flap reconstruction decreases perineal wound complications after pelvic chemoradiation and surgery: a cohort study. *Ann. Surg. Oncol.* 12 (2): 104–110.

28 PelvEx Collaborative (2018). Factors affecting outcomes following pelvic exenteration for locally recurrent rectal cancer. *Br. J. Surg.* 105 (6): 650–657.

29 Yang, T.X., Morris, D.L., and Chua, T.C. (2013). Pelvic exenteration for rectal cancer: a systematic review. *Dis. Colon Rectum* 56 (4): 519–531.

30 Isbarn, H., Jeldres, C., Zini, L. et al. (2009). A population based assessment of perioperative mortality after cystectomy for bladder cancer. *J. Urol.* 182 (1): 70–77.

31 Matsuo, K., Mandelbaum, R.S., Adams, C.L. et al. (2019). Performance and outcome of pelvic exenteration for gynecologic malignancies: a population-based study. *Gynecol. Oncol.* 153 (2): 368–375.

32 Alfred Witjes, J., Lebret, T., Compérat, E.M. et al. (2017). Updated 2016 EAU guidelines on muscle-invasive and metastatic bladder cancer. *Eur. Urol.* 71 (3): 462–475.

33 Petruzziello, A., Kondo, W., Hatschback, S.B. et al. (2014). Surgical results of pelvic exenteration in the treatment of gynecologic cancer. *World J. Surg. Oncol.* 12: 279.

34 Bladou, F., Houvenaeghel, G., Delpero, J.R., and Guerinel, G. (1995). Incidence and management of major urinary complications after pelvic exenteration for gynecological malignancies. *J. Surg. Oncol.* 58 (2): 91–96.

35 Ramirez, P.T., Modesitt, S.C., Morris, M. et al. (2002). Functional outcomes and complications of continent urinary diversions in patients with gynecologic malignancies. *Gynecol. Oncol.* 85 (2): 285–291.

36 Teixeira, S.C., Ferenschild, F.T., Solomon, M.J. et al. (2012). Urological leaks after pelvic exenterations comparing formation of colonic and ileal conduits. *Eur. J. Surg. Oncol.* 38 (4): 361–366.

37 John, P.S., Gary, L., Richard, C. et al. (2001). Radical cystectomy in the treatment of invasive bladder cancer: long-term results in 1,054 patients. *J. Clin. Oncol.* 19 (3): 666–675.

38 Schoenberg, M.P., Walsh, P.C., Breazeale, D.R. et al. (1996). Local recurrence and survival following nerve sparing radical cystoprostatectomy for bladder cancer: 10-year followup. *J. Urol.* 155 (2): 490–494.

39 Madersbacher, S., Hochreiter, W., Burkhard, F. et al. (2003). Radical cystectomy for bladder cancer today – a homogeneous series without neoadjuvant therapy. *J. Clin. Oncol.* 21 (4): 690–696.

40 Shariat, S.F., Karakiewicz, P.I., Palapattu, G.S. et al. (2006). Outcomes of radical cystectomy for transitional cell carcinoma of the bladder: a contemporary series from the bladder cancer research consortium. *J. Urol.* 176 (6 Pt 1): 2414–2422; discussion 22.

41 Park, J.Y., Choi, H.J., Jeong, S.Y. et al. (2007). The role of pelvic exenteration and reconstruction for treatment of advanced or recurrent gynecologic malignancies: analysis of risk factors predicting recurrence and survival. *J. Surg. Oncol.* 96 (7): 560–568.

42 Berek, J.S., Howe, C., Lagasse, L.D., and Hacker, N.F. (2005). Pelvic exenteration for recurrent gynecologic malignancy: survival and morbidity analysis of the 45-year experience at UCLA. *Gynecol. Oncol.* 99 (1): 153–159.

43 Harris, C.A., Solomon, M.J., Heriot, A.G. et al. (2016). The outcomes and patterns of treatment failure after surgery for locally recurrent rectal cancer. *Ann. Surg.* 264 (2): 323–329.

44 Vermaas, M., Ferenschild, F.T., Verhoef, C. et al. (2007). Total pelvic exenteration for primary locally advanced and locally recurrent rectal cancer. *Eur. J. Surg. Oncol.* 33 (4): 452–458.

45 Bhangu, A., Ali, S.M., Brown, G. et al. (2014). Indications and outcome of pelvic exenteration for locally advanced primary and recurrent rectal cancer. *Ann. Surg.* 259 (2): 315–322.

46 Marquis, P., Marrel, A., and Jambon, B. (2003). Quality of life in patients with stomas: the Montreux study. *Ostomy Wound Manage* 49 (2): 48–55.

47 Yang, L.S., Shan, B.L., Shan, L.L. et al. (2016). A systematic review and meta-analysis of quality of life outcomes after radical cystectomy for bladder cancer. *Surg. Oncol.* 25 (3): 281–297.

48 Månsson, Å. and Månsson, W. (1999). When the bladder is gone: quality of life following different types of urinary diversion. *World J. Urol.* 17 (4): 211–218.

49 Guren, M.G., Wiig, J.N., Dueland, S. et al. (2001). Quality of life in patients with urinary diversion after operation for locally advanced rectal cancer. *Eur. J. Surg. Oncol.* 27 (7): 645–651.

50 Young, J.M., Badgery-Parker, T., Masya, L.M. et al. (2014). Quality of life and other patient-reported outcomes following exenteration for pelvic malignancy. *Br. J. Surg.* 101 (3): 277–287.

51 Harji, D.P., Griffiths, B., Velikova, G. et al. (2016). Systematic review of health-related quality of life in patients undergoing pelvic exenteration. *Eur. J. Surg. Oncol.* 42 (8): 1132–1145.

52 Rausa, E., Kelly, M.E., Bonavina, L. et al. (2017). A systematic review examining quality of life following pelvic exenteration for locally advanced and recurrent rectal cancer. *Colorectal Dis.* 19 (5): 430–436.

53 Modh, R.A., Mulhall, J.P., and Gilbert, S.M. (2014). Sexual dysfunction after cystectomy and urinary diversion. *Nat. Rev. Urol.* 11 (8): 445–453.

54 Zippe, C.D., Raina, R., Massanyi, E.Z. et al. (2004). Sexual function after male radical cystectomy in a sexually active population. *Urology* 64 (4): 682–685; discussion 5–6.

55 Hart, S., Skinner, E.C., Meyerowitz, B.E. et al. (1999). Quality of life after radical cystectomy for bladder cancer in patients with an ileal conduit, cutaneous or urethral Kock pouch. *J. Urol.* 162 (1): 77–81.

56 Roos, E.J., de Graeff, A., van Eijkeren, M.A. et al. (2004). Quality of life after pelvic exenteration. *Gynecol. Oncol.* 93 (3): 610–614.

57 Corney, R.H., Crowther, M.E., Everett, H. et al. (1993). Psychosexual dysfunction in women with gynaecological cancer following radical pelvic surgery. *BJOG Int. J. Obstet. Gynaecol.* 100 (1): 73–78.

58 Chang, D.T. and Lawrentschuk, N. (2015). Orthotopic neobladder reconstruction. *Urol. Ann.* 7 (1): 1–7.

59 Autorino, R., Quarto, G., Di Lorenzo, G. et al. (2009). Health related quality of life after radical cystectomy: comparison of ileal

conduit to continent orthotopic neobladder. *Eur. J. Surg. Oncol.* 35 (8): 858–864.

60 Hara, I., Miyake, H., Hara, S. et al. (2002). Health-related quality of life after radical cystectomy for bladder cancer: a comparison of ileal conduit and orthotopic bladder replacement. *BJU Int.* 89 (1): 10–13.

61 Rezk, Y.A., Hurley, K.E., Carter, J. et al. (2013). A prospective study of quality of life in patients undergoing pelvic exenteration: interim results. *Gynecol. Oncol.* 128 (2): 191–197.

62 Vera, M.I. (1981). Quality of life following pelvic exenteration. *Gynecol. Oncol.* 12 (3): 355–366.

9

Posterior Pelvic Exenteration

Werner Hohenberger, Maximilian Brunner, and Susanne Merkel

Department of Surgery, University Hospital Erlangen, Friedrich-Alexander-Universität Erlangen-Nürnberg, Erlangen, Germany

Background

Up to 10% of solid malignant tumors in the pelvis require multivisceral resection [1–3]. Extended surgery necessitating total pelvic exenteration occurs in 20% of cases [4–6]. Approximately three-quarters of advanced primary tumors need a posterior pelvic exenteration to achieve clear margins. However, in cases of recurrent cancer, more than 50% need a total pelvic exenteration.

Posterior pelvic exenteration involves removal of the rectum, the uterus including eventually the posterior part of the vagina, and/or the adnexa, and rarely the sacrum. The main principles to be followed strictly in these cases are to perform en-bloc resections always and to achieve clear margins. Although in almost half of the patients there is no true tumor invasion but cancer-associated inflammation, the circumferential margin may be challenged.

In selected cases of limited peritoneal seedings, in addition to pelvic exenteration, hyperthermic intraperitoneal chemotherapy (HIPEC) may be discussed [7, 8]. However, without obstruction, fistulizing disease, or sealed perforation, in case of peritoneal metastasis, neoadjuvant chemotherapy may be performed first and definitive surgery postponed. In addition, in patients with distant metastases of the liver and lung, neoadjuvant chemotherapy could be considered [9, 10].

Preoperative Assessment

This is discussed extensively elsewhere. But important to posterior exenteration is the need to perform a good gynecological examination to assess vaginal involvement. Special attention has to be payed to any invasion of unresectable structures such as the sciatic nerve or the sacrum above the S3 level. Any threatened marginal [11] suggests that some form or combination of neoadjuvant therapy is better suited initially [12].

Intraoperative Decision-Making

Good preoperative examination and radiology assessment ensure that posterior pelvic exenteration should suffice to clear all neoplasm microscopically. Nevertheless, one should always be aware that intraoperatively a decision to perform a total pelvic exenteration might be necessary. Therefore many surgeons do not really decide in advance to what extent pelvic exenteration will be needed. It is rather more important for the patient to get adequate information about the possible sequelae.

Surgical Management of Advanced Pelvic Cancer, First Edition.
Edited by Michael E. Kelly and Desmond C. Winter.
© 2022 John Wiley & Sons Ltd. Published 2022 by John Wiley & Sons Ltd.

Table 9.1 Pelvic and abdominal organs to be removed during posterior pelvic exenteration for primary rectal cancer (n = 119).

Organ	n	Percentage
Uterus	119	100
Vagina	32	26.9
Adnexa	13	10.9
Bladder segment	8	6.7
Small intestine	10	8.4
Additional colon segment	1	0.8
Kidney	1	0.8
Liver metastases	4	3.4
Peritoneal metastases	4	3.4

Most frequently, a patient just needing a posterior pelvic exenteration will be a woman with a rectosigmoid cancer invading the uterus or with a low rectal cancer infiltrating the vagina. In these cases, the decision for a rectal excision is always determined by an eventual invasion of the rectal sphincter muscles. If the tumor is invading the base of the bladder, the prostate, or the urethra, generally a total pelvic exenteration will be needed. A summary of the pelvic and abdominal organs removed during posterior pelvic exenteration for primary rectal cancer in 119 woman in our surgical department is presented in Table 9.1.

Surgical Technique

At surgery, a diagnostic assessment should be performed. Some advocate the routine use of staging laparoscopy. Then the field/tissue planes around the tumor (not involved) should be approached. Mobilization of the proximal colon along the embryologic planes, starting with the distal descending colon and the sigmoid, is followed by complete mobilization of the splenic flexure, if needed. Early, the ureters must be identified and placed in vascular slings. The gonadal vessels are divided, usually cranially and close to the common and external iliac artery. The next steps are the posterior mobilization of the rectum and the isolation of the uterus from the bladder, anteriorly. Finally, the vagina is transected.

Mobilization of Left Colon and Upper Rectum

Typically, dissection of the pelvis starts with the isolation of the sigmoid colon by incising the peritoneum lateral to the proximal sigmoid, following then the interface between the mesocolic and the parietal fascia. Usually the dissection can be continued all along the posterior mesorectal fascia down to the lower rectal third and laterally on both sides, as is common practice with any low anterior resection, with care to preserve the autonomous nerves. However, with severe fibrosis or if the internal iliac artery has to be dissected, the inferior hypogastric plexus cannot always be identified, or may need to be sacrificed.

This extent of dissection is recommended as a first step, because it allows bringing the tumor block forward under complete control. If a tumor is fixed to the sacrum or laterally to the pelvic sidewall, modification of the procedure is required.

Isolation of Ureters The ureters run behind the parietal fascia and will be easily identified. This allows for safe sigmoid mobilization. They are isolated before they cross the iliac vessels, where they are medial to the gonadal vessels. They too should be placed in vascular slings and dissected down to the entrance into the bladder.

Mobilization of Uterus Including Adnexa

A salpingo-oophorectomy is frequently part of a posterior exenteration. Commonly, the ovarian vessels are divided at the level of the iliac vessels, followed by the mobilization of the adnexa down to the fundus of the uterus. They are covered by a thin layer, which is part of the parietal plane and the broad ligament. It is divided, close to the uterus. The round ligaments are divided and the vesico-uterine pouch is incised. The adhesions of the uterus to the urinary bladder are now separated. They may be marked and need sharp transection. Laterally to both sides, a convolute of veins requires adequate measures to control bleeding. A sponge is placed into the vagina to identify its anterior wall. If the posterior wall of the vagina is invaded by tumor, the incision may be extended as far as needed, to achieve clear margins. If the anal sphincter is infiltrated, an en-bloc rectal excision with resection of the perineum will be necessary. In these cases, for reconstruction of the posterior wall of the vagina and the perineum itself, a flap is essential.

Dissection of Internal Iliac Artery

In bulky tumors or diffuse fibrous infiltration of the pelvis, a safe dissection of the anatomical structures is mandatory to avoid bleeding and an R1 resection. This requires full exposure of the internal iliac artery and vein, and a central ligation of the originating vessels. It is imperative to dissect the veins even more carefully than the arteries and to avoid any tears. Following this rule, placing a vascular sling around the internal iliac artery is helpful. In these cases, the inferior hypogastric plexus usually has to be sacrificed completely because it can no longer be identified within the scar tissue.

Dissection of Obturator Foramen and Anterior Approach to Sciatic Nerve

Advanced tumors can extend into the obturator foramen. Lateral lymph node metastases may also necessitate dissection at this site. The obturator nerve crosses this area longitudinally. It can almost always be preserved. The obturator vessels, however, must always be divided.

Sometimes, continuous growth of a tumor to the lateroposterior sidewall of the pelvis can be resected only after anterior exposure of the sciatic nerve. Its isolation will usually need a central tie of all proximal branches of the internal iliac artery apart from the superior and inferior gluteal arteries with resection of the coccygeal muscle.

Postoperative Outcome and Prognosis

One-third of the 119 patients had postoperative complications (Table 9.2). Urological complications were the most frequent with 18.5%. Surgery of local recurrences represents a particularly challenging task (Figure 9.1). In summary, survival was mainly influenced by the presence of distant metastases and whether curative resection (R0) could be achieved (Table 9.3; Figure 9.2).

Table 9.2 Postoperative complications after posterior pelvic exenteration (n = 119).

Postoperative complication	n	Percentage
Postoperative morbidity	39	32.8
Anastomotic leak (patients with anastomosis)	6/85	7
Urological complications	22	18.5
Bleeding	3	2.5
Wound infection	5	4.2
Septic multiorgan failure	2	1.7
Pulmonary complications	6	5.0
Cardiovascular complications	3	2.5
Other complications	5	4.2

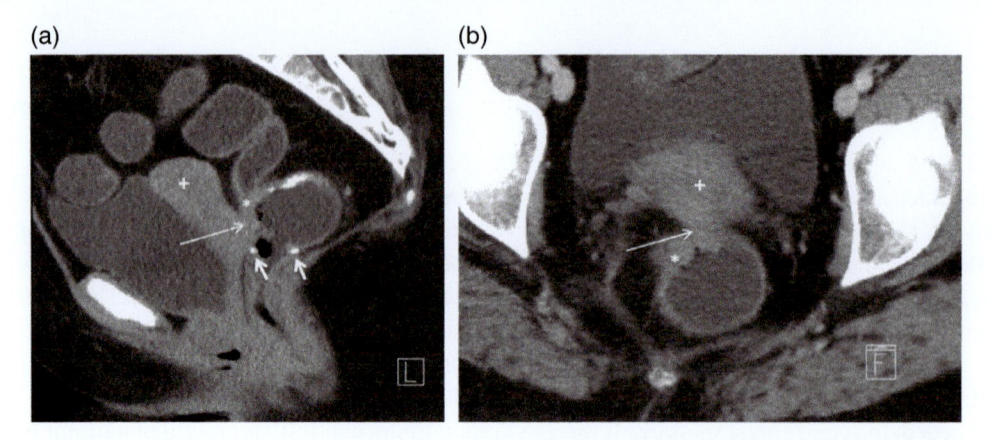

Figure 9.1 Local recurrence of a rectal cancer with infiltration of the uterus, which will be probably resectable by a posterior pelvic exenteration with preservation of the anal sphincter. A: Sagittal; B: transversal. + Uterus; * local recurrence of rectal cancer; long thin arrow, infiltration of the uterus; short thick arrows; staple line after previous rectal resection. *Source:* Werner Hohenberger, Maximilian Brunner, and Susanne Merkel.

Table 9.3 Prognosis after posterior pelvic exenteration.

	n	Median overall survival (months)	Two-year overall survival (95% CI)	Five-year overall survival (95% CI)	p
All	119	36	59.7 (50.9–68.5)	35.9 (27.3–44.5)	
R0	91	52	71.4 (62.2–80.6)	44.0 33.8–54.2)	
R1, 2, X	28	7	21.4 (6.1–36.7)	10.7 (0–22.1)	< 0.001
M0	90	51	71.1 (61.7–80.5)	45.6 (35.4–55.8)	
M1	29	12	24.1 (8.6–39.6)	4.3 (0–12.3)	< 0.001
Rectum	85	35	61.2 (50.8–71.6)	32.5 (22.5–42.5)	
Sigmoid	34	39	55.9 (39.2–72.6)	44.1 (27.4–60.8)	0.191
Rectum M0 R0	56	50	73.2 (61.6–84.8)	42.9 (30.0–55.8)	
Sigmoid M0 R0	25	98	76.0 (59.3–92.7)	60.0 (40.8–79.2)	0.083
1978–1994	76	35	59.2 (48.2–70.2)	34.2 (23.6–44.8)	
1995–2015	43	36	60.5 (46.8–74.2)	38.9 (24.2–53.6)	0.523

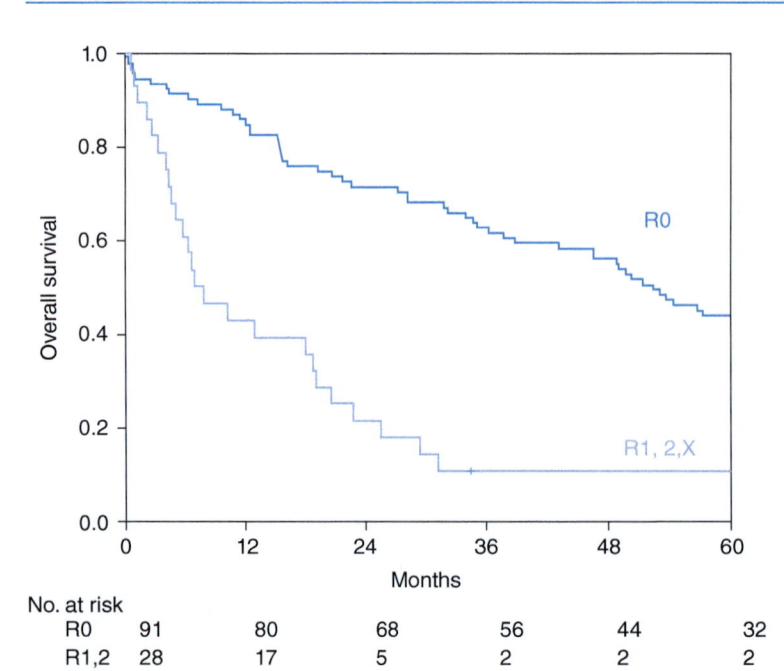

Figure 9.2 Overall survival after curative (R0) and non-curative (R1, 2, X) posterior pelvic resection. *Source:* Werner Hohenberger, Maximilian Brunner, and Susanne Merkel.

No. at risk
R0   91   80   68   56   44   32
R1,2 28   17   5   2   2   2

> **Summary Box**
>
> - Posterior pelvic exenteration is needed in less than 5% of primary tumors of pelvic organs, and more frequently, however, with recurrent malignancies.
> - Even if a true tumor invasion is not confirmed (adhesion/inflammation), multivisceral resection including any involved organ has to be performed, to avoid risk of positive margin.
> - Long-term prognosis is mainly influenced by the presence of distant metastases and whether curative resection is possible.

References

1 Smith, J.D., Nash, G.M., Weiser, M.R. et al. (2012). Multivisceral resections for rectal cancer. *Br. J. Surg.* 99 (8): 1137–1143.

2 Crawshaw, B.P., Augestad, K.M., Keller, D.S. et al. (2015). Multivisceral resection for advanced rectal cancer: outcomes and experience at a single institution. *Am. J. Surg.* 209 (3): 526–531.

3 Hohenberger, W., Thom, N., Hermanek, P. Sr., and Gall, F.P. (1992). Pelvic multivisceral resection from the viewpoint of surgery. *Langenbecks Arch. Chir. Suppl. Kongressbd*: 83–88.

4 Bhangu, A., Ali, S.M., Darzi, A. et al. (2012). Meta-analysis of survival based on resection margin status following surgery for recurrent rectal cancer. *Colorectal Dis.* 14 (12): 1457–1466.

5 Rahbari, N.N., Ulrich, A.B., Bruckner, T. et al. (2011). Surgery for locally recurrent rectal cancer in the era of total mesorectal excision: is there still a chance for cure? *Ann. Surg.* 253 (3): 522–533.

6 Heriot, A.G., Byrne, C.M., Lee, P. et al. (2008). Extended radical resection: the choice for locally recurrent rectal cancer. *Dis. Colon Rectum* 51 (3): 284–291.

7 Votanopoulos, K.I., Swett, K., Blackham, A.U. et al. (2013). Cytoreductive surgery with hyperthermic intraperitoneal chemotherapy in peritoneal carcinomatosis from rectal cancer. *Ann. Surg. Oncol.* 20 (4): 1088–1092.

8 Verwaal, V.J., Bruin, S., Boot, H. et al. (2008). 8-year followup of randomized trial: cyto reduction and hyperthermic intraperitoneal chemotherapy versus systemic chemotherapy in patients with peritoneal carcinomatosis of colorectal cancer. *Ann. Surg. Oncol.* 15: 2426–2432.

9 Fernandez-Martos, C., Garcia-Albeniz, X., Pericay, C. et al. (2015). Chemoradiation, surgery and adjuvant chemotherapy versus induction chemotherapy followed by chemoradiation and surgery: long-term results of the Spanish GCR-3 phase II randomized trial. *Ann. Oncol.* 26: 1722–1728.

10 Schou, J.V., Larsen, F.O., Rasch, L. et al. (2012). Induction chemotherapy with capecitabine and oxaliplatin followed by chemoradiotherapy before total mesorectal excision in patients with locally advanced rectal cancer. *Ann. Oncol.* 23: 2627–2633.

11 Georgiou, P.A., Tekkis, P.P., Constantinides, V.A. et al. (2013). Diagnostic accuracy and value of magnetic resonance imaging (MRI) in planning exenterative pelvic surgery for advanced colorectal cancer. *Eur. J. Cancer* 49 (1): 72–81.

12 Sauer, R., Becker, H., Hohenberger, W. et al. (2004). Preoperative versus postoperative chemoradiotherapy for rectal cancer. *N. Engl. J. Med.* 351 (17): 1731–1740.

10

Total Pelvic Exenteration

Satish K. Warrier, Andrew C. Lynch, and Alexander G. Heriot

Department of Surgical Oncology, Peter MacCallum Cancer Centre, Melbourne, Australia

Background

Total pelvic exenteration (TPE) was first described by Brunschwig [1] in 1948 as a palliative operation for cervical cancer. However, since the late 1990s, pelvic exenteration has become a standard procedure for the management of advanced and recurrent pelvic malignancy [2]. TPE involves the en-bloc removal of all the pelvic organs, namely the rectum, prostate, and bladder in male patients, and the rectum, uterus and ovaries, vagina, and bladder in female patients. This may be combined with bone resection or pelvic sidewall vessel resection; however, these aspects are considered in detail in other chapters and will not be addressed further in this chapter. This form of surgery is required for locally advanced or recurrent tumors which have extended locally beyond the confines of their organ of origin to involve other surrounding organs [3]. The reason for the extended resection is to attain resection margins that are microscopically free from tumor, or an R0 resection margin, which has frequently been identified as the major predicting factor to minimize the risk of local recurrence and maximize the likelihood of cure [5]. Given the inherent nature of the surgery itself, pelvic exenteration surgery has been seen as a morbid procedure, traditionally associated with both high morbidity and perioperative mortality rates, reports from the literature ranging from 27 to 86% [5, 6]. With recent advances in anesthetics, intensive care, and perioperative medicine, these rates have decreased substantially since the late 1990s.

Indications

Pelvic exenteration has evolved over time from a procedure that would only be considered in very selective circumstances to one that is considered to be a standard procedure in tertiary and quaternary surgical centers. It has been demonstrated that the procedure can be undertaken with acceptable morbidity and mortality but requires careful planning and a multidisciplinary approach [7–9]. Colorectal cancer is the most common indication for TPE, with 12% of rectal cancers extending beyond the fascia propria [10] and requiring "Beyond TME" surgery [3]. TPE is more common in male patients as compared to female in the case of rectal cancer, as frequently a more limited exenteration involving the rectum, uterus, and some or all of the vagina is feasible in female patients, with preservation of the bladder, as compared to male patients where tumor invasion of the bladder trigone or prostate usually

---

Surgical Management of Advanced Pelvic Cancer, First Edition.
Edited by Michael E. Kelly and Desmond C. Winter.
© 2022 John Wiley & Sons Ltd. Published 2022 by John Wiley & Sons Ltd.

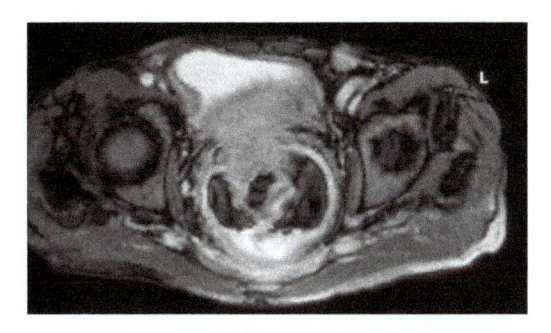

Figure 10.1 Coronal MRI of the pelvis demonstrating extensive primary rectal cancer extending from the rectum to involve a significant part of the posterior bladder wall and trigone. This patient required a TPE to ensure an R0 resection margin. *Source:* Satish K. Warrier, Andrew C. Lynch, and Alexander G. Heriot.

necessitates a TPE (Figure 10.1). Recurrent rectal cancer is a more frequent indication for TPE, with the nature of recurrence requiring "Beyond TME" surgery in order to maximize the likelihood of obtaining clear resection margins [3]. This has been consistently demonstrated to be the most important predictive factor to minimize local recurrence and for long-term survival [11, 12]. The contraindications to TPE have softened since 2010, with consistent outcomes and reducing morbidity despite extending the indications, resulting in prior contraindications such as resectable metastatic disease becoming relative (Table 10.1).

Whilst locally advanced and recurrent rectal cancer are the commonest indications for TPE, it can be applied to any advanced pelvic malignancy. There is experience in pelvic squamous cell cancers including recurrent rectal cancer and a range of gynecological cancers including cervical, vagina, and vulval, though more commonly for recurrent tumors rather than primary. It may also be undertaken for palliation, including uncontrollable malignant masses with small and large bowel to vesical or vaginal fistula, or for unmanageable malignant cutaneous/vaginal wounds.

Who Should Be Performing these Procedures? Selecting the Right Team and Plan

It is important that surgeons who perform regular exenterations build a dedicated team. Cases can be technically challenging and having a team that regularly works together can reduce operator stress, with the hope for better patient outcomes.

The team will usually involve an exenterative surgeon (usually a colorectal surgeon with an exenterative interest), a specialist urologist, vascular surgeon, plastic surgeon, and orthopedic and or neurosurgeon for select cases. In addition, good communication and planning with anesthetic colleagues is important in ensuring that the operation progresses well and without unexpected incidents.

Specialist Centers

the topic of specialist centers is slightly controversial. In general, we believe complex extended resections are best performed in

Table 10.1 Contraindications for TPE.

Relative contraindication	Absolute contraindication
Distant metastases	Encasement of external iliac vessels
Extensive pelvic sidewall involvement	Tumor extension through greater sciatic notch
Predicted R1 or R2 resection	Lower limb edema
Sacral invasion above S2	Poor performance status

specialized centers so that theater staff are familiar with the nuances of the surgery and have the correct equipment to hand. Centralization has been a theme in Europe, with some healthcare systems centralizing rectal cancers to maintain experience. The PelvEx Collaborative recently reviewed 1170 patients who had undergone a pelvic exenteration for LRRC. Centers were split into low volume and high volume centers (> 20 exenterations per year). The results showed there was no significant difference between high volume and low volume centers in overall outcomes and that the R0 resection margin rates in both low and high volume centers (51–60% and 49–65% respectively) improved over the 10 years of the study period [4].

Getting Patients Right – Fitness for Surgery (Prehabilitation)

Patients who undergo advanced pelvic surgery are at risk of major thromboembolic, cardiac, and respiratory as well as wound complications. To mitigate this risk, appropriate selection and pre-optimization is imperative. There is good evidence that a dedicated prehabilitation program can reduce the risks of surgery. The program involves thorough early assessment of the patient's cardiopulmonary status, with exercise programs tailored to their physiological status. This is discussed in more detail in the preoperative planning chapter (see Chapter 5). Ultimately the aim is to build up the patient's exercise tolerance, hence reducing the impact of stressors intraoperatively.

Preoperative Planning

Pelvic magnetic resonance imaging (MRI) is considered the gold standard assessment tool for locally advanced disease, and for providing a "roadmap" for surgical planning in order to determine exenterative margins. It is also the best imaging tool for soft tissue, lymph nodes, and tumor boundaries. The tumor extent and involvement of adjacent viscera (urogenital structures, reproductive structures), vessels,

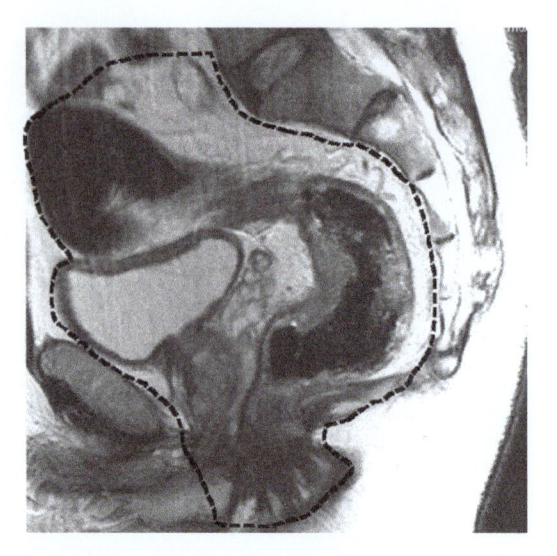

Figure 10.2 .Resection margins for TPE as demonstrated on a sagittal MRI scan. *Source:* Satish K. Warrier, Andrew C. Lynch, and Alexander G. Heriot.

and bony structures can be determined by this technique. The specific pelvic compartments (central, anterior, posterior, lateral, perineal, superior) involved by the tumor can be determined, facilitating the surgical plan. Tumor margin involvement as well as delineation of possible fibrosis can be determined with this technique (Figure 10.2).

All patients at our institution also have diagnostic computed tomography–positron emission tomography (CT-PET) scans as part of their workup. The functional imaging can be useful in determining the appropriateness of resection. In particular, right-sided para-aortic lymph node or higher lymph node disease or multisite metastatic disease may mean that any attempts at local control are deemed palliative.

Examination under Anesthesia/Flexible Sigmoidoscopy/Colonoscopy

Every patient due to have a TPE should have an examination under anesthesia and flexible sigmoidoscopy (if appropriate). The assessment includes the height of the tumor (if rectal) and relationship to the sphincter muscle and/or levator muscle/endo pelvic fascia.

In females a formal vaginoscopy is performed to assess the relationship to the posterior vagina/anterior vagina and cervix.

At the time, an assessment of fixity posteriorly to the sacrum/coccyx and/or a bladder evaluation via cystoscopy can be performed.

Neoadjuvant Therapy

Though outlined in Chapter 4, it is worth stating that the majority of patients with locally advanced pelvic cancer receive neoadjuvant therapy prior to TPE. In some cases this will be their first exposure to radiotherapy; however, a number of centers will also re-irradiate patients if it has been a reasonable duration of time since their previous radiotherapy. This will also depend on the pathology involved.

Surgical Technique

The patient is placed in a modified Lloyd-Davies position with both arms tucked by the side. Where a sacrectomy is being considered, the patient is placed on two saline bags placed beneath the distal lumbar region to elevate the distal sacrum. At the commencement of the procedure ureteric catheters are inserted. A midline laparotomy and appropriate adehesiolysis is performed. A thorough explorative laparotomy is carried out to assess for peritoneal disease. We preferentially use a Balfour Doyen retractor to help exposure. In a scenario where the small bowel is stuck to the mass, this is taken en-bloc with the tumor resection. In some cases where multiple loops are stuck to the tumor, these are stapled off earlier to facilitate small bowel packing. Once the small bowel package has been freed, the dissection initially is commenced, with mobilization of the sigmoid and left colon including splenic flexure if reconstruction is considered feasible.

The ureters are identified and are slung with a vascular sling (vessel loop) to identify and retract them. Both ureters are mobilized down to the pelvi-ureteric junction. Careful consideration is made of the plane of surgery required to facilitate a TPE, with the aim of dissection in a plane beyond the tumor to maximize the potential of an R0 resection margin. The total mesorectal excision (TME) plane is well recognized around the fascia propria of the rectum. Outside of this, the ureteric plane will lead to inclusion of the bladder, and either the prostate or uterus/vagina, and is the usual plane required for TPE. Branches of the internal iliac artery and vein will cross this plane to supply the pelvic organs and must be divided to provide delivery of the pelvic organs. Beyond the ureteric plane is the vascular plane, containing the iliac vessels. The sacral nerve roots lie outside of the vascular plane, with nerves exiting the sacral foramina and joining to form the sciatic nerve which passes into the greater sciatic notch. Beyond the nerves are the pelvic muscles including piriformis, and this is surrounded by the bony pelvis. Whilst a standard TPE requires dissection is the ureteric plane, extension of tumor beyond this plane at any site would require extending the resection into the other planes, such as a vascular resection if there is lateral pelvic sidewall involvement.

The pelvis is usually entered posteriorly behind the rectum in the TME plane, then moving anteriorly, and then laterally. If there is extension beyond the central organs at any point such as into the sacrum or pelvic sidewall, the rest of the dissection is undertaken and then the specific area of extension is focused on.

The anterior dissection involves dissection along the retropubic space down to the levator plate and deep pelvic fascia anteriorly. While urological input can be helpful at this point, the point of division of the urethra must be directed by the exenterative surgeon, as the risk of R1 in a complex anterior tumor is often at the site of division of the urethra.

Perineal dissection will be necessary if a non-restorative procedure is to be undertaken. The ability of the abdominal surgeon and the perineal surgeon to work together in order to identify the correct planes of dissection facilitates the procedure (Figure 10.3).

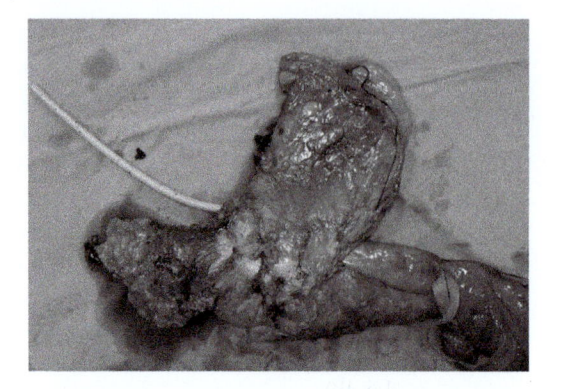

Figure 10.3 Male TPE specimen, including rectum, bladder, and prostate. Note catheter extending from prostate. *Source:* Satish K. Warrier, Andrew C. Lynch, and Alexander G. Heriot.

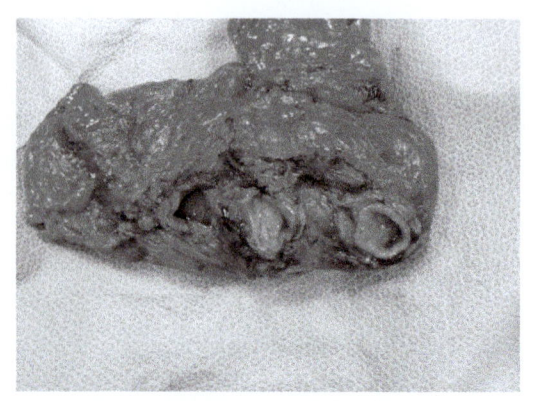

Figure 10.4 Female TPE specimen, shown from below, demonstrating opening into bladder, vagina, and rectum, from left to right. *Source:* Satish K. Warrier, Andrew C. Lynch, and Alexander G. Heriot.

Uterus and Vagina Involvement

If the uterus and vagina are involved, an R0 resection is achieved with en-bloc hysterectomy and partial vaginectomy +/− posterior vaginectomy. The round ligament, broad ligament, and feeding vessels are sequentially ligated. A swab or metallic retractor in the vagina can be used to help isolate the anterior vaginal wall below the cervix. Where the tumor is low with involvement of the posterior vagina, a complete posterior vaginectomy may be required with abdomino-perineal resection (APR) en bloc. The anterior vagina is opened as described with electrocautery and a dual-surgeon approach from above and below is adopted for the subsequent dissection. Extensive tumors may require removal of the whole vagina, with or without the bladder (Figure 10.4).

Anterior Recurrences: Beyond the Normal Planes

There are unique challenges with anterior located tumors, particularly when it is a recurrence. The central axis of the anterior compartment at the pelvic floor is the urethra. It is bounded by the pubic symphysis and the superior and inferior rami. Locally advanced rectal cancers can often abut this margin, however. The authors believe there is a significant risk of having a positive anterior margin if transection of the urethra is pursued through an anterior approach. Ligation of the dorsal venous plexus anteriorly in an irradiated field also provides a separate challenge. In such cases where the margin is believed to be at risk we recommend a perineal approach to access the urethra.

Posterior Compartment and Extended Bony Resections

Our favored approach for composite bone resections below or at the level of S3 is to use an abdomino-lithotomy approach. The technique's full description is beyond the scope of this chapter but is described in Chapter 11. For composite resections of bone involving S3 and above, a prone approach is preferential. For this approach the iliac vessels need to be mobilized off the sacrum. Again, this is described in further detail in Chapter 12.

Lateral Pelvic Recurrences

The technique of lateral pelvic sidewall dissection is beyond the scope of this chapter. It is worth noting that in some instances the obturator internus and nerve can be taken en bloc if required. Vascular structures including proximal ligation of the internal iliac artery or vein or in conjunction with common iliac resections (and therefore external iliac and internal iliac vessels) can be taken with appropriate reconstructions. In advanced cases the obturator nerve or sciatic nerve can be removed en bloc to ensure a clear margin.

Intraoperative Radiation Therapy

Intraoperative radiation allows for boost radiation to the tumor bed following surgical resection. Customized flexible applicators are applied with precise delivery of a single fraction of radiotherapy to the surgical bed. Usually this is an additional 10 Gy. The penetration is for a short distance (5 mm) and is considered an adjunct treatment where an R0 resection is not possible due to bony limitations, or where a close margin is considered likely due to nerve and vascular preservation attempts. It is not considered an alternative to an aggressive surgical resection.

Utilizing intraoperative radiotherapy (IORT) is considered low toxicity, with relative sparing of adjacent tissues. The ureters and neurovascular structures can be protected with appropriate packing and shields. The existing literature demonstrates considerable heterogeneity; however, data suggest improved five-year local control [13].

Reconstruction

Large defects are common following pelvic exenteration surgery. Many options exist to close these defects, including the use of myocutaneous abdominal, gluteal-based, or thigh-based pedicelled flaps. Our initial series of reconstructions involved the use of vertical rectus myocutaneous (VRAM) flaps. These flaps are robust, are desirable for partial vaginal reconstruction, and can fill a sizable defect. However, they come at a significant cost and morbidity for the patient. More recently, our unit has transitioned to an inferior gluteal artery myocutaneous (IGAM) island transposition flap, with anterolateral thigh flaps used as a second option where the internal iliac vessels have been ligated bilaterally.

For the perineal defect there are select cases where a biosynthetic mesh is used to help aid the perineal closure.

Adjuncts to Care: Urinary and Sexual Function and Ostomy Placement

Sexual function, urinary function, and ostomy placement and care are all impacted by exenterative surgery. Specialist nurses and clinics help to deal with the patient's needs and set appropriate expectations and aid in problem solving.

Stomal siting is important. The ostomy should be at least 3 cm from the costal margin in the mid rectus and away from the iliac crest. Examination in both a standing and sitting position is empirical. Where dual ostomies are required, the urostomy should be placed higher. Where a VRAM flap is used, fixed anatomical landmarks provide a guide due to the variability in the final skin position.

Summary Box

- TPE involves the en-bloc removal of all the pelvic organs, rectum, prostate, and bladder in male patients, and the rectum, uterus, ovaries, vagina, and bladder in female patients.
- Modifications of TPE to achieve negative margins including bony resection and/or vascular resection and reconstruction are important skills for the exenterative team.
- TPE is more common in male patients as compared to female in the case of rectal cancer, as the vagina acts as a barrier to bladder trigone invasion.
- TPE may rarely be considered for the palliative management of advanced pelvic malignancy or for unmanageable malignant cutaneous/vaginal wounds.
- There are several reconstructive options to consider and tailor for each individual patient.

A dedicated sexual function clinic is available in our center. Appropriate aids such as phosphodiesterase type 5 (PDE5) inhibitors and injectable agents can help with the sexual health of patients. Psychological counseling is also necessary.

References

1 Brunschwig, A. (1949). Complete excision of pelvic viscera in the male for advanced carcinoma of the sigmoid invading the urinary bladder. *Ann. Surg.* 129 (4): 499–504.
2 Brown, K.G.M., Solomon, M.J., and Koh, C.E. (2017). Pelvic exenteration surgery: the evolution of radical surgical techniques for advanced and recurrent pelvic malignancy. *Dis. Colon Rectum* 60 (7): 745–754.
3 Beyond TME Collaborative (2013). Consensus statement on the multidisciplinary management of patients with recurrent and primary rectal cancer beyond total mesorectal excision planes. *Br. J. Surg* 100 (8): 1009–1014.
4 PelvEx Collaborative (2019). Surgical and survival outcomes following pelvic exenteration for locally advanced primary rectal cancer: results from an international collaboration. *Ann. Surg.* 269 (2): 315–321.
5 Hafner, G.H., Herrera, L., and Petrelli, N.J. (1992). Morbidity and mortality after pelvic exenteration for colorectal adenocarcinoma. *Ann. Surg.* 215 (1): 63–67.
6 Ferenschild, F.T.J., Vermaas, M., Verhoef, C. et al. (2009). Total pelvic exenteration for primary and recurrent malignancies. *World J. Surg.* 33 (7): 1502–1508.
7 Moore, H.G., Shoup, M., Reidel, E. et al. (2004). Colorectal cancer pelvic recurrences: determination of resectability. *Dis. Colon Rectum* 47: 1599–1606.
8 Hahnloser, D., Nelson, H., Gunderson, L.L. et al. (2003). Curative potential of multimodality therapy for locally recurrent rectal cancer. *Ann. Surg.* 237 (4): 502–508.
9 Yamada, K., Ishizawa, T., Niwa, K. et al. (2001 July). Patterns of pelvic invasion are prognostic in the treatment of locally recurrent rectal cancer. *Br. J. Surg.* 88 (7): 988–993.
10 Davies, M.L., Harris, D., Davies, M. et al. (2011;2011:678506). Selection criteria for the radical treatment of locally advanced rectal cancer. *Int. J. Surg. Oncol.*
11 PelvEx Collaborative (2018 May). Factors affecting outcomes following pelvic exenteration for locally recurrent rectal cancer. *Br. J. Surg.* 105 (6): 650–657.
12 Heriot, A.G., Byrne, C.M., Lee, P. et al. (2008). Extended radical resection – the choice for locally recurrent rectal cancer. *Dis. Colon Rectum* 51 (3): 284–291.
13 Skandarajah, A.R., Lynch, A.C., Mackay, J.R. et al. (2009 Mar). The role of intraoperative radiotherapy in solid tumors. *Ann. Surg. Oncol.* 16 (3): 735–744.

11

Extended Exenterative Resections Involving Bone

Timothy Chittleborough[1], Gordon Beadel[2], and Frank Frizelle[3]

[1] *Colorectal Surgery Unit, The Royal Melbourne Hospital, Melbourne, Victoria, Australia*
[2] *Department of Orthopedic Surgery, Christchurch Hospital, Christchurch, New Zealand*
[3] *Department of Surgery, University of Otago and Christchurch Hospital, Christchurch, New Zealand*

Background

The pelvis has long posed challenges for pelvic surgeons by providing a bony cage that limits surgical access. The close proximity of bony structures to pelvic viscera, such as the close proximity of the sacrum to the extraperitoneal rectum, places the sacrum and other bony pelvic structures at risk of involvement in primary or recurrent malignancy. Composite resection, when malignancy extends into the sacrum, means that any pelvic exenteration to be undertaken will require the addition of bone resection in order to obtain clear margins.

While pelvic exenteration was first described in 1948 by Brunschwig [1], bony resection with extenuation was not described until over 20 years later in 1969 by Brunschwig and Barber [4]. Following this, bony resection was not described in the literature until reports by Wanebo and Marcove in 1981 [5] and Takagi et al. in 1983 [6], both describing series of exenteration with en-bloc sacrectomy for recurrent rectal cancer. These series demonstrated acceptable mortality for the times and some cases of long-term survival, leading to more widespread adoption of the technique. Improved outcome over decades can be attributed to improvements in patient selection, radiological assessment of extent of disease, surgical technique, and anesthetic and perioperative care.

The aim of an extended resection involving bone is to achieve an oncological (R0) resection, while maintaining acceptable function and minimizing operative morbidity. Bony resection is indicated in cases where soft tissue resection alone would pose a risk to positive surgical margins. When disease is localized in the pelvis it is almost always technically possible to resect it; however, the extent of resection should also be based on patient considerations and impact on quality of life.

Patients with advanced primary or recurrent rectal cancer comprise the majority of patients undergoing bony resection. Less common indications include advanced primary or recurrent anal squamous cell cancer (SCC), presacral/retrorectal tumors including chordomas, and advanced malignancy arising from other pelvic viscera (Table 11.1).

The close proximity of the sacrum to locally advanced or recurrent rectal cancer can place margin status at risk, even if there is no evidence of direct bone involvement. Retrospective data from 27 centers contributing over one-thousand cases to the PelvEx Collaborative suggest that bony resection is associated with a significantly lower margin positivity rate [2]. These data

Surgical Management of Advanced Pelvic Cancer, First Edition.
Edited by Michael E. Kelly and Desmond C. Winter.
© 2022 John Wiley & Sons Ltd. Published 2022 by John Wiley & Sons Ltd.

Table 11.1 Bony exenteration: indications and contraindications.

Indications	Contraindications
Common	Metastatic disease
• Locally advanced primary rectal cancer	Poor premorbid state
• Recurrent rectal cancer	Poor psychological state
Uncommon	Unacceptable functional outcome
• Advanced/recurrent anal SCC	
• Rare presacral tumors	
– Bone sarcomas (Ewing's, osteogenic sarcoma, chondrosarcoma, myeloma)	
– Soft tissue sarcomas (liposarcoma, fibrosarcoma, leiomyosarcoma)	
– Spinal/neurogenic tumors (chordoma, neuroblastoma, ganglioneuriblastoma, MPNSTs)	
– Germ cell tumors (teratocarcinoma)	
– Benign tumors and cystic lesions	
• Bony metastasis[1] (i.e. melanoma, renal cell carcinoma)	
• Lymphoma[1]	
• Sacral osteomyelitis	

MPNST, Malignant peripheral nerve sheath tumor.
[1] Considered controversial.

demonstrate that appropriate bony resection can contribute to improved oncological outcome.

Presacral/retrorectal tumors represent a heterogenous group of rare tumors extending along a spectrum from benign to malignant conditions [7]. Whilst previous en-bloc surgical excision was undertaken for such tumors given diagnostic uncertainty and malignant potential, improved imaging with magnetic resonance imaging (MRI) has improved preoperative diagnosis. Cystic lesions with no concerning features on MRI can be monitored radiologically without resection [8]. Such rare tumors need discussion within the multidisciplinary team (MDT) in a center with experience and interest in this area [7].

Anatomical Considerations

The morbidity and long-term function of bony exenteration are directly related to the extent of bony resection and resulting functional and neurological impairment. The majority of bony exenterations involve resection of the sacrum; however, anterior and lateral bony pelvic resections are technically possible in order to obtain clear margins.

Sacral Resection

The majority of the sacrum can be resected during bony exenteration. Pelvic stability requires the presence of the upper half of S1 vertebrae, and thus this level is considered the limit for sacrectomy without internal fixation. Whilst the authors would caution against resection above this level, there are reports of spinopelvic fixation facilitating total sacrectomy; however, this is usually reserved for chordomas and bony sarcomas [9]. Following high sacrectomy there is a risk of subsequent stress fractures that may require delayed internal fixation.

High Sacrectomy (S1/S2) Versus Low Sacrectomy (S3 and Below)

The level of sacral transection has implications for operative planning as well as morbidity and complications. Sacrectomy can be divided into "low sacrectomy" to denote resections at or below the level of S3 or "high sacrectomy" for resections above this level (S1/S2).

High sacrectomy can result in bladder dysfunction due to division of the S2 and S3 nerve roots [10, 11]. The division of sacral nerve roots results in motor function disturbance, with increased morbidity resulting from high sacrectomy [11]. Bowel disfunction may also be an issue due to the nerve supply (S2–S3) being damaged, leaving the patient with a flaccid anus; however, in reality most patients have their rectum resected and as such end up with a permanent colostomy.

In addition, the close proximity of the iliac vessels to the upper sacrum increases the risk of major hemorrhage at the time of sacrectomy. Surgical planning can mitigate this risk and is discussed in detail in the section 'Lateral Pelvic Resection'.

Despite the aforementioned anatomical considerations posing a risk with increased morbidity of high sacrectomy, some high-volume centers can achieve good results with high sacrectomy, with no increased complication rate when compared to low sacrectomy [12, 13].

Anterior Pubic Resection

Solomon et al. demonstrated that partial and even complete pubic bone resection is possible in cases of advanced malignancy involving the pubis [14]. The pelvis remains structurally stable despite complete excision of the pubic bone, although these authors do report utilizing polypropylene mesh to reconstruct the pelvic contour. Anterior pubic resection is not an overly difficult procedure and is most likely underutilized. Solomon et al. [14] report similar experience to the authors with no perioperative mortality with this procedure and an acceptable R0 rate (76%) and five-year survival (53%) in a cohort comprising mostly recurrent rectal adenocarcinoma and recurrent anal SCC [15].

Lateral Pelvic Resection

The close proximity of iliac vessels, ureter, and nerves in the pelvic sidewall has resulted in historical high margin rates and poor prognosis following exenteration for disease in the lateral pelvic compartment [16]. Progression of surgical technique has led to en-bloc resection of lateral pelvic sidewall structures, resulting in improved outcomes for recurrent rectal cancer in this region [17]. The en-bloc technique described by Solomon et al. includes bony resection where appropriate, with excision of the ischium and/or pubis to obtain clear margins.

Hemipelvectomy is a most radical form of pelvic resection. External hemipelvectomy (hindquarter amputation) results in significant morbidity, whilst internal hemipelvectomy with internal reconstruction with titanium hemipelvis can allow limb salvage. Whilst hemipelvectomy is rarely performed for sarcoma, the reported results for pelvic visceral carcinoma extending laterally are dismal [18]. For this reason, extensive disease requiring such a major bony resection should generally be considered unresectable.

Patient Workup Specific to Bony Resection

Patients being considered for bony exenteration require thorough preoperative workup/assessment to assess:

- Extent of disease (resectability)
- Presence of metastatic disease (futility)
- Premorbid function and suitability for major exenteration (fitness)

History and Examination

Reviewing the symptoms and investigations with particular attention to the presence of bowel, bladder, and neurological dysfunction with the patient is important. It is valuable to discuss preoperative continence and sexual function prior to planning any exenterative procedure as this may influence decision-making. This is especially so when dealing with a recurrent tumor, as it is important to understand and document what has been done previously and what level of pre-existing treatment/disease-related collateral injury exists.

A pelvic and lower limb neurological examination will help identify pre-existing neurological deficits from tumor invasion or nerve compression and will provide clues as to the degree of nerve root involvement. This may also guide discussion with patients about the potential for neurological deficit following bony exenteration.

Rectal examination will allow some assessment of tumor size, location, and extent of fixation to bony structures. Assessment of the prostate should be undertaken in men and assessment of the vagina in women to determine tumor involvement. At times this may be best done with a formal examination under anesthetic (EUA).

Radiology

Local staging of pelvic tumor should be undertaken with both a computed tomography (CT) of the abdomen and pelvis and MRI of the pelvis. Of these modalities, MRI provides more accurate assessment of pelvic disease burden and bone involvement (Figures 11.1–11.3). If there is concern for vascular involvement, CT angiography/venography assists in operative planning. CT-PET is most helpful in avoiding futile operations by ensuring localized disease [19] (Figure 11.3).

Our pratice is to re-image and restage 48 hours prior to surgery. Given the morbidity of sacrectomy, repeating the staging just prior to surgery will in some instances identify new metastatic disease, precluding bony exenteration. Furthermore, restaging can identify local progression that would prevent an R0 resection, where more extensive surgery may be required or to the extent that patients are best managed non-operatively.

Imaging-guided biopsy is sometimes of use where there is uncertainty about what bony lesion is. With recurrent or primary rectal cancers the use of clinical information, such as carcinoembryonic antigen (CEA), CT, and PET, and if necessary sequential imaging with MRI usually clarifies the clinical issue. As an alternative diagnosis, however, will often alter treatment choices, where there is uncertainty that there is a metastases to the sacrum (Figure 11.1), as opposed to local invasion, image-guided biopsy might be considered. Primary presacral lesions not

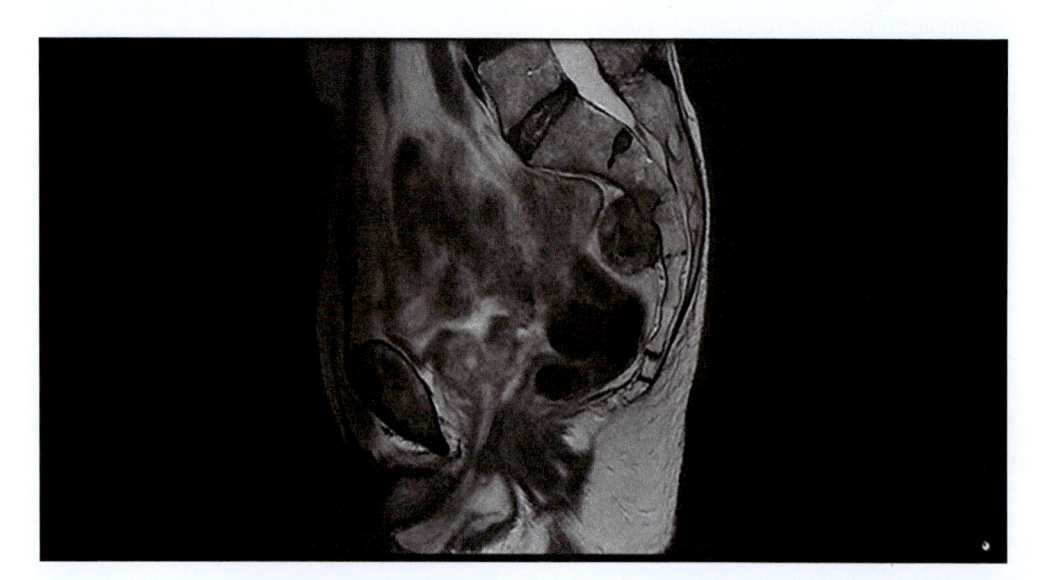

Figure 11.1 Colorectal metastasis to S2/3. *Source:* Timothy Chittleborough, Gordon Beadel, and Frank Frizelle.

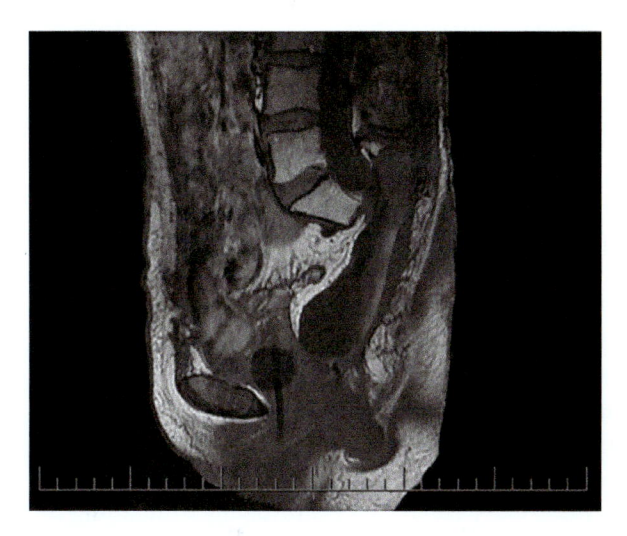

Figure 11.2 Postoperative MRI following S1/2 sacrectomy. *Source:* Professor Timothy Chittleborough, Gordon Beadel, and Frank Frizelle.

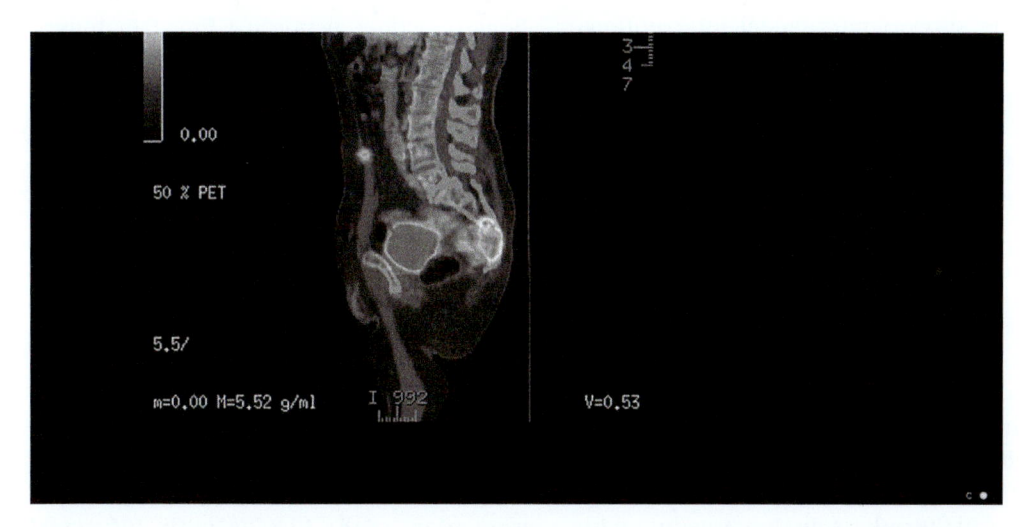

Figure 11.3 CT-PET showing involvement of the distal sacrum with recurrent rectal cancer. *Source:* Timothy Chittleborough, Gordon Beadel, and Frank Frizelle.

involving the rectum may also be considered for biopsy. The concerns, however, about biopsy are the issues of contamination of the biopsy tract and management around interpretation of a negative biopsy. When electing to perform imaging-guided percutaneous biopsy it should be performed in consultation with the treating surgical team so that the biopsy tract can be tattooed at the time of biopsy for subsequent excision with the surgical specimen at time of pelvic exenteration. A transrectal, parasacral, or perineal approach usually facilitates en-bloc excision of the tract at time of surgery.

Anesthetic Assessment

Patients being considered for pelvic exenteration should undergo a high-risk anesthetic pre-assessment clinic. It is essential that the assessing anesthetist has experience of high-risk surgery that involves sacral resections, internal iliac vessel mobilization and/or ligation, substantial blood loss, and multiple patient repositioning.

Concerns about cardiovascular fitness are not uncommon given the age of the patients. Cardiopulmonary exercise testing (CPET) can be useful when there is concern as it provides an objective assessment of fitness for surgery [20–22]. CPET should be considered as part of preoperative assessment for patients being considered for bony resection/pelvic exenteration to provide patients and clinicians with an accurate assessment of operative risk.

Prehabilitation is a vital process to optimize nutritional status, physical fitness, and psychological preparedness prior to major surgery. Though there is a paucity of evidence to support multimodal interventions in major colorectal surgery [23], there is evidence from a retrospective cohort study that a structured exercise program prior to major cancer surgery results in improvement in cardiopulmonary function as assessed by CPET [23].

Multidisciplinary Meeting

Cases being put forward for bony resection should be reviewed in a multidisciplinary meeting (MDM) setting which has expertise in advanced pelvic malignancy. Bony resections typically require the assistance of an orthopedic/spinal surgeon, who should be involved in the MDM discussion regarding suitability for surgery and extent of bony resection. Bony resection usually results in a large tissue defect and preoperative planning for flap reconstruction should be undertaken with a plastic/reconstructive surgeon.

In referral-type practices, many patients travel a distance for this surgery; as a result it is the authors' practice to admit patients at 24–48 hours prior to planned bony exenteration to allow for discussion with team members, inpatient bowel preparation (when needed), stoma site marking, and restaging CT chest/abdomen and pelvis and MR pelvis imaging to be conducted.

Neoadjuvant treatment

Our practice is to utilize neoadjuvant chemoradiotherapy where appropriate. This is more so with bone resect patients having extenuative procedures than those having soft tissue alone resections, because close margins can be an issue with bony resection. Advanced primary rectal cancers involving or abutting the sacrum should undergo long-course chemoradiotherapy, as should recurrent carcinomas that have not been previously irradiated [24]. Bony resections performed for other indications (i.e. sarcoma) can also benefit from irradiation, but this will depend on the particular tumor type.

If the patient requires a defunctioning stoma formed prior to radiation due to local symptoms, careful consideration needs to be given to the type of stoma(s) required at the final resection, what type of flaps may be required for reconstruction, and what surgical damage has already occurred to the abdominal wall/musculature.

Patients who have undergone previous pelvic irradiation are usually not candidates for re-irradiation. A multicenter trial of re-irradiation with 40.8 Gy with infusional fluorouracil (5-FU) in recurrent cancer demonstrated acceptable side effects and a response rate of 41% [25]). Our [25] own experience is that neoadjuvant chemoradiotherapy provides an increase in R0 resection [26]. Despite this, the larger PelvEx Collaborative series demonstrated that neoadjuvant chemoradiotherapy conferred no survival advantage in recurrent rectal cancer, and was indeed associated with increased complication and readmission rates [2]. Our usual practice is not to re-irradiate the pelvis in cases of recurrent rectal cancer, although we routinely involve a radiation oncologist in each case discussion in our advanced pelvic malignancy MDM. In select circumstances where re-irradiation is considered, this is dependent on previous radiation dosage/fractionation and radiation field.

There is no survival benefit from neoadjuvant chemotherapy alone in recurrent rectal cancer patients intended for curative surgery [26], and this does not form part of our treatment algorithm.

Operative Technique

Thorough consideration needs to be given to the extent of resection and surgical approach in order to maximize the chances of successful resection with clear margins. Our surgical exenterative team consists of a colorectal surgeon, orthopedic surgeon, urologist, vascular surgeon, gynecological oncological surgeon, and plastic surgeon. For such major procedures we schedule an all-day theater session, and book an intensive care bed for postoperative care. A prolonged, major resection of this nature can result in surgeon fatigue, and our team is cognizant of human factors that can reduce performance. The multidisciplinary nature of exenterative surgery allows surgeons to scrub out to minimize the risk of fatigue.

Surgical Approach

Surgery is usually initially undertaken in Lloyd-Davies position, and when undertaking rectal resection with en-bloc sacrectomy it is not the intent to reconstruct enteric continuity. For low sacrectomy/coccycectomy the patient can be repositioned following abdominal dissection to the prone jack knife position or resection can occur without turning in some circumstances [27]. Tumor involvement above the S3 level necessitates high sacrectomy and this can only be performed in the prone jack-knife position.

Thromboembolic-deterrent stockings and sequential compression devices are routine to mitigate the risk of venous thromboembolism during the procedure. Bilateral ureteric catheters are inserted in appropriate cases requiring sacrectomy and secured to an indwelling urinary catheter. Prior to incision the abdomen is marked for a vertical rectus abdominis myocutaneous (VRAM) flap to ensure that midline incision does not impair subsequent flap formation. The institutional preference is to use a rectus muscle flap without skin where possible, reserving flaps involving skin for larger tumors in which there is a significant perineal skin defect present. This approach helps prevent perineal herniation whilst minimizing flap-related complications and preserving perineal skin sensation.

A full-length midline laparotomy is performed, as this incision facilitates access to the pelvis and splenic flexure and is required for VRAM flap formation. Initial assessment is undertaken for evidence of radio occult metastatic disease, which if present would suggest exenteration and sacrectomy to be futile. Adhesiolysis is undertaken to access the pelvis in reoperative cases. Prior to embarking on pelvic dissection, the ureters are identified as they cross the bifurcation of the iliac arteries.

The common practice is to perform the anterior dissection including division of the upper rectum, construction of the urinary conduit (if required), and harvesting the myocutaneous flap before temporary abdominal closure to allow repositioning to the prone jack-knife position for sacrectomy and en-bloc removal of the specimen. The patient is then repositioned in the supine position to allow formation of an end colostomy and definitive closure of the abdominal cavity.

Negative surgical margins are the key to successful exenteration with sacrectomy. Pelvic dissection is undertaken following considered operative planning and review of the preoperative imaging. Whilst there is the temptation for colorectal surgeons to dissect in the mesorectal plane, doing so may result in compromised margins in cases of advanced and recurrent pelvic malignancy. The correct plane of dissection for recurrent disease is different than for primary disease and is deeper, leading to skeletonization of vessels and other structures. The exact extent of resection and approach will depend on the location and burden of pelvic disease.

When undertaking a high sacrectomy (S2 and above) the iliac vessels are fully mobilized as part of the anterior dissection. The internal iliac arteries and veins are ligated at their origins. An alternative to this is to undertake preoperative angioembolization of the internal iliac arteries, although this may not be as helpful as surgical ligation. The common and external iliac artery and vein are fully mobilized and a pack is placed posterior to these vessels (between the iliac vessels and sacrum) to provide protection during subsequent sacrectomy.

By comparison, when undertaking a low sacrectomy (S3 and below) the iliac branches can be segmentally ligated at the level of sacral division. Both low and high sacrectomy may be performed in the prone position following the anterior dissection. Low sacrectomy can, however, be performed in the modified Lloyd-Davies position without the need to reposition into the prone position. This approach has several advantages, including avoiding the need to reposition an anesthetized patient, improved vascular control, and improved access to the lateral compartments [27].

The extent of the lateral dissection from the anterior position is critical. Seldom are cancers exactly in the midline, they are commonly off to one side of other. The need for an extended dissection laterally on one side is common, and we find that this is best done from behind. It is therefore important to take advantage on the contralateral side by dissection further, while restricting dissection on the tumor side.

If possible it is worth making a perineal incision anterior to the rectum joining the abdominal cavity to the perineum and therefore allowing for a finger to be inserted during the initial stages of the sacrectomy to palpate the lateral aspects of dissection. As the dissection moves proximally this incision can be extended, allowing tactile input to deciding the extent of the lateral margins.

If the bladder has been resected, the ileal conduit may be constructed at this stage, leaving it free in the abdominal cavity, as the small bowel will swell with time and subsequent anastomosis is more challenging.

Once all anterior and lateral dissection is completed, the rectum is divided, the VRAM flap is harvested, and temporary closure of the abdominal wall is undertaken with skin clips to allow repositioning to the prone position. Following sacrectomy the patient is returned to the supine position to allow definitive closure of the abdominal wall, formation of an end colostomy in the left iliac fossa, and formation of a urostomy (where required).

Technique for Sacrectomy

Following repositioning to the prone position and further skin preparation and draping, a "tennis racquet" incision is made to encircle the anus and extend superiorly in the midline to above the desired level of sacral division. Dissection continues through the ischiorectal fossa inferiorly, and superiorly the deep fascia and gluteus maximus are released laterally from the posterior sacrum. The dissection is then continued through the superiorly ischiorectal fossa on each side and to where the greater sciatic notch is exposed and the sacrospinous and sacrotuberous ligaments are divided at a safe distance laterally from the tumor mass. Where possible the sciatic nerve should be mobilized at this time and preserved, although it should be sacrificed in cases of direct tumor invasion.

Anterior dissection is then undertaken to meet the abdominal dissection – either in the retropubic space (in the case of total exenteration) or with a standard mesorectal excision with or without posterior vaginectomy (in cases where bladder preservation is possible).

Once all other aspects of the dissection are complete, the sacrum is exposed at the desired level of division (this can be confirmed with image intensified if desired). The posterior laminar is removed with rongeurs. The sacral nerve roots are exposed using Kerrison Rongeur to preserve the nerve roots just superior to the level of resection. The spinal cord is ligated distal to the preserved nerve roots with a heavy ligature before sharp division is undertaken. The sacrum is then divided with an osteotome to reach the presacral tissue. The presacral tissue is divided with diathermy to reach the abdominal dissection and allow extraction of the specimen.

Following sacrectomy and extraction of the specimen, meticulous pelvic hemostasis is undertaken. Careful hemostasis throughout this operation is important using suture, energy devices, and/or hemostatic agents. Major exenteration frequently results in significant blood loss and transfusion requirements, which may need hematology input and thromboelastography (TEG) monitoring.

Reconstruction

Exenteration in particular that involves bony resection/sacrectomy results in a large tissue defect that is not possible to be closed primarily. Flap reconstruction functions to cover the defect with healthy tissue and prevent perineal herniation by reducing pelvic "dead space." The VRAM is advantageous as it is robust and not from the radiation fields, and confers relatively little morbidity. A series of VRAMs following major pelvic exenteration demonstrated a relatively low rate of 16% of major flap complications requiring return to theater [28]. When compared to other pedicled myocutaneous flaps such as gluteal flaps, we prefer the VRAM as it is derived from tissue distant from the site of radiotherapy, ensuring healthy flap tissue with adequate perfusion.

In addition to VRAM, we find other techniques to prevent herniation of the small bowel into the pelvic cavity are useful, including a pedicled omental flap. In cases where anterior structures remain (bladder/uterus) following exenteration, these are positioned to further reduce the risk of pelvic/perineal herniation.

Intraoperative Radiotherapy

Intraoperative radiotherapy (IORT) may be a useful on-table adjunct for patients with borderline resectable disease. In cases in which there is suspicion of a macroscopically close or involved margin or minimal residual disease in an unresectable location (e.g. abutting S1), IORT can be applied to the remaining sacrum following excision of the surgical specimen [10].

There is a paucity of quality evidence regarding the effectiveness of IORT due to small sample sizes and heterogeneity in series reporting its use in conjunction with sacrectomy. When considering IORT as an adjunct to surgical management it is important to consider the morbidity associated with IORT in this population, including impaired wound healing, wound breakdown, fistula, infection, and late effects such as ureteric stenosis, neuropathy, and osteonecrosis [10]. A series of IORT in locally advanced or recurrent rectal cancer in which 10 Gy was delivered to the tumor bed reported significant toxicity in 37% of patients, comprising wound breakdown, abscesses, soft tissue toxicity, bowel obstructions, ureteric obstructions, and sensory neuropathies [29].

Novel Approaches in Sacrectomy

Partial Anterior Sacrectomy

A partial sacrectomy has been reported, in which only the anterior cortex is excised en bloc with the specimen [30, 31]. This is described as a technique for tumor that involves/abuts the upper sacrum that would otherwise require a high sacrectomy. Proposed advantages of such a technique include maintaining pelvic stability and minimizing neurological deficit. One group reporting anterior sacrectomy concede that the procedure will compromise oncological resection when compared to a traditional sacrectomy [31].

Laparoscopic Sacrectomy

Reports of laparoscopic pelvic exenteration involving sacrectomy have been reported [32]. The authors consider complex reoperative pelvic surgery, prolonged operative time, and need for a sacrectomy as contraindications to a laparoscopic approach; however, this may change with the use of robotics in the future.

Outcomes

Bony resection and achieving clear margins have been shown to confer positive prognostic significance in pelvic exenteration [2, 3, 26]. Mean survival following exenteration in the PelvEx Collaborative series of exenteration for recurrent rectal cancer has been shown to be 36 months for patients that underwent bony resection, compared to 29 months for patients without bony resection [2].

Of note, there is no significant survival difference between patients undergoing high versus low sacrectomy. A large international sacrectomy series for rectal cancer demonstrated no significant difference in overall survival at five years following high and low sacrectomy (52.6 and 44.1% respectively). Only margin positivity and advanced age were significant predictors of mortality [33]. Whilst a series from a high-volume exenteration center demonstrated no difference in complications between high and low sacrectomy [12], a subsequent systematic review of 220 sacrectomies for recurrent rectal cancer demonstrated incremental increase in complications and length of stay with a higher level of sacral division [3]. This review did, however, demonstrate increased margin positivity with distal sacrectomy, encouraging the adoption of high sacrectomy where required in order to achieve clear surgical margins (Table 11.2).

Morbidity following bony resection is high, with the majority of patients suffering a complication. An Australian series of sacrectomy for recurrent rectal cancer reported major complications in 39% of patients, with 24% requiring return to theater and 14% requiring placement of a radiologically guided drain. Eighty-two percent of patients suffered some form of complication [12].

Functional impairment following sacrectomy can be predicted by premorbid impairment, tumor extent, and level of sacrectomy/nerve division [11]. Persisting morbidity includes sensory and motor deficits and neurogenic bladder. High sacrectomy with division of the S1/S2 nerve roots will result in neurogenic bladder requiring either long-term catheterization or intermittent self-catheterization. Motor deficits from high nerve root division and/or sciatic nerve division can be managed with orthotics. Almost all patients undergoing sacrectomy will suffer from sexual dysfunction. Given the morbidity of high sacral nerve root division, consideration should be given to the unilateral preservation of the S1/S2 nerve roots where possible to minimize functional impairment.

A prospective cohort study of quality of life following pelvic exenteration for rectal cancer from two Australian centers demonstrated an expected drop in quality of life immediately following surgery, with improvement occurring from 3 months and continuing until 12 months following surgery. This group found that premorbid quality of life was the best predictor of postoperative quality of life, and that bony resection was associated with lower quality of life scores at 12 months [34].

Table 11.2 Series of en-bloc sacrectomy for recurrent rectal adenocarcinoma. Summary of data extracted from studies included in the review by Sasikumar [3].

	Khaled et al., 2014 [35]	Melton et al., 2006 [36]	Moriya et al., 2004 [13]	Milne et al., 2013 [12]	Bhangu et al., 2012 [37]	Dozois et al., 2011 [38]	Uehara et al., 2015 [39]	Summary[1]
Total, n	19	29	57	49	22	9	35	220
Median age, years	62	60	55	59	61.3	63	66	60 (55–66)
High sacrectomy	13	0	9	20	5	9	6	62 (28)
Low sacrectomy	6	29	48	29	17	0	26	155 (70)
Operation time, minutes	624	–	709	725	570	822	992	717 (570–992)
Blood loss, ml	5000	5000	3046	6200	1725	3700	2653	3700 (1725–6200)
R0	19	18	48	36	15	9	27	172 (78)
R1	0	10	9	11	7	0	8	45 (20)
R2	0	1	0	2	0	0	0	3 (1)
Mortality	1	1	2	0	0	0	0	4 (2)
Morbidity	15	13	31	19	15	3	18	114 (52)
LOS median	20	18	35.1	37	15	22	46	22 (15–46)
DFS R0	13	9	26	25	9	3	20	95 (55)
DFS R1	0	0	0	0	0	0	0	0
OS R0	14	14	27	34	11	3	20	123 (72)
OS R1	0	0	0	0	1	0	7	8 (18)
F/U, months	38	23	42	17	26	60	33	33 (17–60)

DFS, Disease-free survival; F/U, follow-up; LOS, length of stay; OS, overall survival.
[1] Values stated are n (percentage) and/or median (range).
Source: Sasikumar A, Bhan C, Jenkins JT, Antoniou A, Murphy J Systematic Review of Pelvic Exenteration With En Bloc Sacrectomy for Recurrent Rectal Adenocarcinoma: R0 Resection Predicts Disease-free Survival. Dis Colon Rectum. 2017;60:346-352. © 2017, The American Society of Colon and Rectal Surgeons.

Summary Box

- Centers embarking on extended exenterative surgery involving bone require a committed MDM to achieve good results.
- Patient selection is critical. Workup should include a thorough anesthetic/medical workup and consideration should be given to preoperative optimization (prehabilitation).
- Extensive counseling of the patient is necessary regarding the morbidity of bony resection, especially important when considering high sacrectomy.
- Accurate staging and multidisciplinary operative planning are the key to achieving clear margins. Stage appropriately and plan radical resection to achieve an R0 resection
- Neoadjuvant radiotherapy can improve the rate of R0 resection.

References

1. Brunschwig, A. (1948). Complete excision of pelvic viscera for advanced carcinoma; a one-stage abdominoperineal operation with end colostomy and bilateral ureteral implantation into the colon above the colostomy. *Cancer* 1 (2): 177–183.
2. PelvEx Collaborative (2018). Factors affecting outcomes following pelvic exenteration for locally recurrent rectal cancer. *Br. J. Surg.* 105 (6): 650–657.
3. Sasikumar, A., Bhan, C., Jenkins, J.T. et al. (2017). Systematic review of pelvic exenteration with en bloc sacrectomy for recurrent rectal adenocarcinoma: R0 resection predicts disease-free survival. *Dis. Colon Rectum* 60 (3): 346–352.
4. Brunschwig, A. and Barber, H.R. (1969). Pelvic exenteration combined with resection of segments of bony pelvis. *Surgery* 65 (3): 417–420.
5. Wanebo, H.J. and Marcove, R.C. (1981). Abdominal sacral resection of locally recurrent rectal cancer. *Ann. Surg.* 194 (4): 458–471.
6. Takagi, H., Morimoto, T., Kato, T. et al. (1983). Pelvic exenteration combined with sacral resection for recurrent rectal cancer. *J. Surg. Oncol.* 24 (3): 161–166.
7. Ghosh, J., Eglinton, T., Frizelle, F., and Watson, A. (2007). Presacral tumours in adults. *Surgeon* 5 (1): 31–38.
8. Hopper, L., Eglinton, T.W., Wakeman, C. et al. (2016). Progress in the management of retrorectal tumours. *Colorectal Dis.* 18 (4): 410–417.
9. Zhang, H.Y., Thongtrangan, I., Balabhadra, R.S. et al. (2003). Surgical techniques for total sacrectomy and spinopelvic reconstruction. *Neurosurg. Focus* 15 (2): E5.
10. Heriot, A.G., Tekkis, P.P., Darzi, A., and Mackay, J. (2006). Surgery for local recurrence of rectal cancer. *Colorectal Dis.* 8 (9): 733–747.
11. Moran, D., Zadnik, P.L., Taylor, T. et al. (2015). Maintenance of bowel, bladder, and motor functions after sacrectomy. *Spine J.* 15 (2): 222–229.
12. Milne, T., Solomon, M.J., Lee, P. et al. (2013). Assessing the impact of a sacral resection on morbidity and survival after extended radical surgery for locally recurrent rectal cancer. *Ann. Surg.* 258 (6): 1007–1013.
13. Moriya, Y., Akasu, T., Fujita, S., and Yamamoto, S. (2004). Total pelvic exenteration with distal sacrectomy for fixed recurrent rectal cancer in the pelvis. *Dis. Colon Rectum* 47 (12): 2047–2054.
14. Solomon, M.J., Austin, K.K.S., Masya, L., and Lee, P. (2015). Pubic bone excision and perineal urethrectomy for radical anterior compartment excision during pelvic exenteration. *Dis. Colon Rectum* 58 (11): 1114–1119.
15. Austin, K.K.S., Herd, A.J., Solomon, M.J. et al. (2016). Outcomes of pelvic exenteration with en bloc partial or complete pubic bone excision for locally advanced primary or recurrent pelvic cancer. *Dis. Colon Rectum* 59 (9): 831–835.
16. Heriot, A.G., Byrne, C.M., Lee, P. et al. (2008). Extended radical resection: the choice for locally recurrent rectal cancer. *Dis. Colon Rectum* 51 (3): 284–291.
17. Solomon, M.J., Brown, K.G., Koh, C.E. et al. (2015). Lateral pelvic compartment excision during pelvic exenteration. *Br. J. Surg.* 102 (13): 1710–1717.
18. Baliski, C.R., Schachar, N.S., McKinnon, J.G. et al. (2004). Hemipelvectomy: a changing perspective for a rare procedure. *Can. J. Surg.* 47 (2): 99–103.
19. Watson, A.J., Lolohea, S., Robertson, G.M., and Frizelle, F.A. (2007). The role of positron emission tomography in the management of recurrent colorectal cancer: a review. *Dis. Colon Rectum* 50 (1): 102–114.
20. Older, P., Hall, A., and Hader, R. (1999). Cardiopulmonary exercise testing as a screening test for perioperative management of major surgery in the elderly. *Chest* 116 (2): 355–362.
21. Colson, M., Baglin, J., Bolsin, S., and Grocott, M.P.W. (2012). Cardiopulmonary exercise

testing predicts 5 yr survival after major surgery†. *Br. J. Anaesth.* 109 (5): 735–741.

22 Lee, A., Kong, J., Ismail, H. et al. (2018). Systematic review and meta-analysis of objective assessment of physical fitness in patients undergoing colorectal cancer surgery. *Dis. Colon Rectum* 61 (3): 400–409.

23 Bolshinsky, V., Li, M.H.G., Ismail, H. et al. (2018). Multimodal prehabilitation programs as a bundle of care in gastrointestinal cancer surgery: a systematic review. *Dis. Colon Rectum* 61 (1): 124–138.

24 Harji, D.P., Griffiths, B., McArthur, D.R., and Sagar, P.M. (2013). Surgery for recurrent rectal cancer: higher and wider? *Colorectal. Dis.* 15 (2): 139–145.

25 Valentini, V., Morganti, A.G., Gambacorta, M.A. et al. (2006). Preoperative hyperfractionated chemoradiation for locally recurrent rectal cancer in patients previously irradiated to the pelvis: a multicentric phase II study. *Int. J. Radiat. Oncol. Biol. Phys.* 64 (4): 1129–1139.

26 Harris, C.A., Solomon, M.J., Heriot, A.G. et al. (2016). The outcomes and patterns of treatment failure after surgery for locally recurrent rectal cancer. *Ann. Surg.* 264 (2): 323–329.

27 Solomon, M.J., Tan, K.K., Bromilow, R.G. et al. (2014). Sacrectomy via the abdominal approach during pelvic exenteration. *Dis. Colon Rectum* 57 (2): 272–277.

28 Creagh, T.A., Dixon, L., and Frizelle, F.A. (2012). Reconstruction with vertical rectus abdominus myocutaneous flap in advanced pelvic malignancy. *J. Plast. Reconstr. Aesthet. Surg.* 65 (6): 791–797.

29 Tan, J., Heriot, A.G., Mackay, J. et al. (2013). Prospective single-arm study of intraoperative radiotherapy for locally advanced or recurrent rectal cancer. *J. Med. Imag. Radiat. Oncol.* 57 (5): 617–625.

30 Shaikh, I., Holloway, I., Aston, W. et al. (2016). High subcortical sacrectomy: a novel approach to facilitate complete resection of locally advanced and recurrent rectal cancer with high (S1–S2) sacral extension. *Colorectal Dis.* 18 (4): 386–392.

31 Evans, M.D., Harji, D.P., Sagar, P.M. et al. (2013). Partial anterior sacrectomy with nerve preservation to treat locally advanced rectal cancer. *Colorectal Dis.* 15 (6): e336–e339.

32 Uemura, M., Ikeda, M., Kawai, K. et al. (2018). Laparoscopic surgery using a Gigli wire saw for locally recurrent rectal cancer with concomitant intraperitoneal sacrectomy. *Asian J. Endosc. Surg.* 11 (1): 83–86.

33 Lau, Y.C., Jongerius, K., Wakeman, C. et al. (2019). Influence of the level of sacrectomy on survival in patients with locally advanced and recurrent rectal cancer. *Br. J. Surg.* 106 (4): 484–490.

34 Choy, I., Young, J.M., Badgery-Parker, T. et al. (2017). Baseline quality of life predicts pelvic exenteration outcome. *ANZ J. Surg.* 87 (11): 935–939.

35 Khaled, F., Smith, M.J., Moises, C. et al. (2014). Single-stage anterior high sacrectomy for locally recurrent rectal cancer. *Spine* 39: 443.

36 Melton, G.B., Paty, P.B., Boland, P.J. et al. (2006). Sacral resection for recurrent rectal cancer: analysis of morbidity and treatment results. *Dis. Colon Rectum* 49: 1099–1107.

37 Bhangu, A., Brown, G., Akmal, M., and Tekkis, P. (2012). Outcome of abdominosacral resection for locally advanced primary and recurrent rectal cancer. *Br. J. Surg.* 99: 1453–1461.

38 Dozois, E.J., Privitera, A., Holubar, S.D. et al. (2011). High sacrectomy for locally recurrent rectal cancer: can long-term survival be achieved? *J. Surg. Oncol.* 103: 105–109.

39 Uehara, K., Ito, Z., Yoshino, Y. et al. (2015). Aggressive surgical treatment with bony pelvic resection for locally recurrent rectal cancer. *Eur. J. Surg. Oncol.* 41: 413–420.

12

Exenterative Resections Involving Vascular and Pelvic Sidewall Structures

Brian K. Bednarski and George J. Chang

Department of Surgical Oncology, University of Texas MD Anderson Cancer Center, Houston, Texas, USA

Background

Pelvic exenteration is a critical operative strategy in the multidisciplinary management of locally advanced primary and recurrent rectal cancer. Pelvic exenteration surgery can take many forms. Traditionally, it involves the removal of part or all of the pelvic viscera including the rectum, bladder, prostate, uterus, and/or vagina. These complex radical surgical procedures have a high associated morbidity but have been shown to yield meaningful oncologic benefits. In specialized centers, overall survival and disease-free survival of 60–80% and 50–70% respectively have been reported for patients undergoing pelvic exenteration for rectal cancer [1–4]. Margin-negative resection remains the cornerstone of advanced pelvic surgery for rectal cancer, as this consistently is recognized as the factor that influences the oncologic outcomes following exenterative surgery [1–4].

Historically, complex pelvic tumors were considered unresectable based on an assessment of the balance between associated morbidity and oncologic outcomes. For example, tumors involving the sacrum above the S3 level or tumors involving the pelvic sidewall were placed in this category secondary to a higher risk of positive margins and worse oncologic outcomes [5–7]. However, understanding the benefit of extended surgery for patients with locally advanced primary and recurrent rectal cancer, interest has grown in applying radical surgery to tumors that were previously considered unresectable. This includes management of tumors that involve the lateral pelvis. The lateral pelvis presents a number of operative challenges secondary to the presence of the internal and external iliac vessels, the femoral, sciatic, and obturator nerves, as well as muscular and bony structures. As a result, there were concerns over the ability to balance the oncologic benefit with the morbidity of the necessary surgical procedure while still being able to obtain a negative margin [8].

However, since 2009 a few specialized centers have begun to perform increasingly complex resections of tumors involving the lateral pelvis. One of the earliest reports described en-bloc resection of the internal iliac vessels as a means to provide access to the lateral pelvic structures to enable resection of additional neuromuscular or bony structures as needed. In a report of 36 patients who underwent lateral pelvic resection, R0 resection was achieved in 53% of patients with these advanced tumors with a 28% re-recurrence rate in the site of resection [9]. More recently, Solomon et al. [6]

Surgical Management of Advanced Pelvic Cancer, First Edition.
Edited by Michael E. Kelly and Desmond C. Winter.
© 2022 John Wiley & Sons Ltd. Published 2022 by John Wiley & Sons Ltd.

have updated their series including 197 patients requiring this type of radical surgery for cancer. R0 resection was completed in 66.5% of the patients, while median disease-free survival was 27 months and three- and five-year survival rates were 46 and 35% respectively. This included a variety of malignancies, including primary and recurrent colorectal cancer. An additional smaller series described the outcomes of six patients undergoing a combination of prone and supine positioning to remove tumors involving the lateral pelvis including with sciatic nerve resection (extended lateral pelvic sidewall excision (ELSiE)) [10].

Others have also reported on outcomes of extended lateral pelvic resections. Mariathasan et al. [11] noted that patients undergoing beyond total mesorectal excision (TME) surgery for locally advanced rectal cancer with pelvic sidewall involvement had a lower R0 resection rate (75%) compared to other organ involvement (84%) and resections in the TME group (93.5%). Additionally, they noted shorter disease-free survival and shorter overall survival in this group, although it was not significant on multivariate analysis. Similarly, Kusters et al. [12] examined the role of induction chemotherapy in patients with a lateral pelvic recurrence. They reported an R0 resection rate of 55%. This was increased in patients who underwent induction chemotherapy (85% in that subgroup). This was attributed to the increased pathologic complete response rate in patients treated with induction chemotherapy. While successful resection of these tumors can be achieved, these various groups highlight many of the challenges in tumors involving the lateral pelvic sidewall, including risks for margin-positive resections secondary to the lack of space and the difficulty identifying the extent of tumor infiltration.

To efficiently and safely resect tumors involving the lateral pelvis, the surgical team must possess a detailed understanding of the anatomy. Specifically, the operating surgeon must have comfort with the technical approaches to accessing and resecting the relevant structures such as the pelvic vasculature, nerves, and bones. Additionally, the team must understand the associated morbidity and dysfunction that comes with surgical procedures in the lateral pelvis. Finally, beyond the surgical team, the management of patients requiring exenterative surgery necessitates a multidisciplinary approach – from the preoperative treatment and preparation to the intraoperative execution to the postoperative recovery.

This chapter details our approach to the resection of locally advanced primary tumors and recurrent rectal cancers that involve structures in the lateral pelvis through either direct extension or metastatic disease to the lymph nodes in the lateral pelvis. Topics covered include preoperative preparation, intraoperative technical approaches, and postoperative management.

Anatomy

Surgeons undertaking exenterative surgery that includes the removal of lateral pelvic structures must have an in-depth understanding of vascular, neurologic, urologic, and muscular anatomy. Command of pelvic anatomy is an essential prerequisite for interpreting imaging to determine resectability and generate an operative plan. The ability to translate the two-dimensional images to an understanding of their three-dimensional relationships in the pelvis greatly aids the surgeon by facilitating a margin-negative resection and avoidance of preventable hemorrhage. Beyond the technical requirements during the operation, knowledge of anatomy and its related function serves an important role in setting expectations for the patient regarding potential postoperative disability. The surgical anatomy of the lateral pelvis is reviewed in the following sections including vascular, neurologic, urologic and gynecologic, and muscular structures.

Vascular

The external or internal iliac vessels and their branches may be associated with tumors involving the lateral compartment. The common iliac artery gives rise to the external iliac artery and the internal iliac artery which courses medially, before giving rise to its numerous branches, including the superior gluteal and the umbilical artery and culminating in the pudendal vessels. The branches and tributaries to the internal iliac vessels are organized as those arising anteriorly, medially, and posteriorly. The internal iliac artery and vein provide the blood supply to and from the pelvic viscera and the gluteus muscles. The entire internal iliac vessels and their branches can be resected unilaterally without compromising the pelvic viscera provided the branches of the opposite side remain intact. Therefore resection of these vessels unilaterally may not mandate the removal of the pelvic viscera.

Anatomy of the iliac vessels and their branches is highly variable and recognizing the major named branches is essential. For instance, the initial posterior branch off of the internal iliac vessels is the superior gluteal artery and vein. These vessels typically traverse posteriorly through the piriformis muscle between the L5 and S1 nerve roots to supply the gluteus muscles. Anteriorly, the vessels vary slightly in men and women. In a male, the first anterior branch along the artery is the obliterated umbilical artery. This subsequently gives rise to the superior vesical branch. As you continue distally, additional inferior vesical branches and the prostatic pedicle are encountered as well as the middle rectal vessels medially. In a female, an obliterated umbilical with superior vesicle branches can also be seen. The distal branches include the uterine and vaginal vessels along with the middle rectal vessels. Posteriorly, the inferior gluteal and internal pudendal vessels can be seen exiting the pelvis between the distal sacral nerve roots and near the ischial spine respectively. Lastly, the obturator artery and vein, while typically associated with the internal iliac vessels, can arise from the external iliac vessels. However, they are reliably identified coursing laterally along the obturator internus muscle and the obturator nerve prior to exiting the pelvis through the obturator foramen [13]. Recognizing these vascular structures on preoperative imaging and their relationship to the tumor can help the surgeon plan for surgical resection to optimize R0 resection and minimize bleeding risk.

Neurologic

The nerves traversing the lateral pelvis include the components of the sciatic nerve, distal sacral nerves, and obturator nerve. The components of the sciatic nerve include L5, S1, S2, and branches of S3. The L5 nerve root travels high along the lateral pelvis. The S1 and S2 nerve roots traverse the piriformis muscle until they merge with the L5 nerve root to form the sciatic nerve (Figure 12.1). Similarly, the S3 nerve root, which is significantly smaller, will traverse the posterolateral pelvis, giving branches toward the sciatic nerve as well as branches to the pelvic viscera. The sciatic nerve roots will supply motor and sensory innervation to the posterior leg. The S4 and S5 nerve roots are much smaller and traverse some of the levator muscles and will primarily supply the levator ani muscles, anal sphincters, and perineal skin. The obturator nerve arises from lumbar nerve roots and travels higher in the pelvis along the obturator internus muscle before exiting the obturator foramen to innervate muscles of the medial thigh [13].

Urologic and Gynecologic

The primary urologic structure in the lateral pelvis is the ureter. Identifying the location of the ureter is essential. It can be difficult to identify due to postoperative fibrosis or have a varied course following prior mobilization in patients who have had previous pelvic surgery. Given that radiation is commonly utilized in

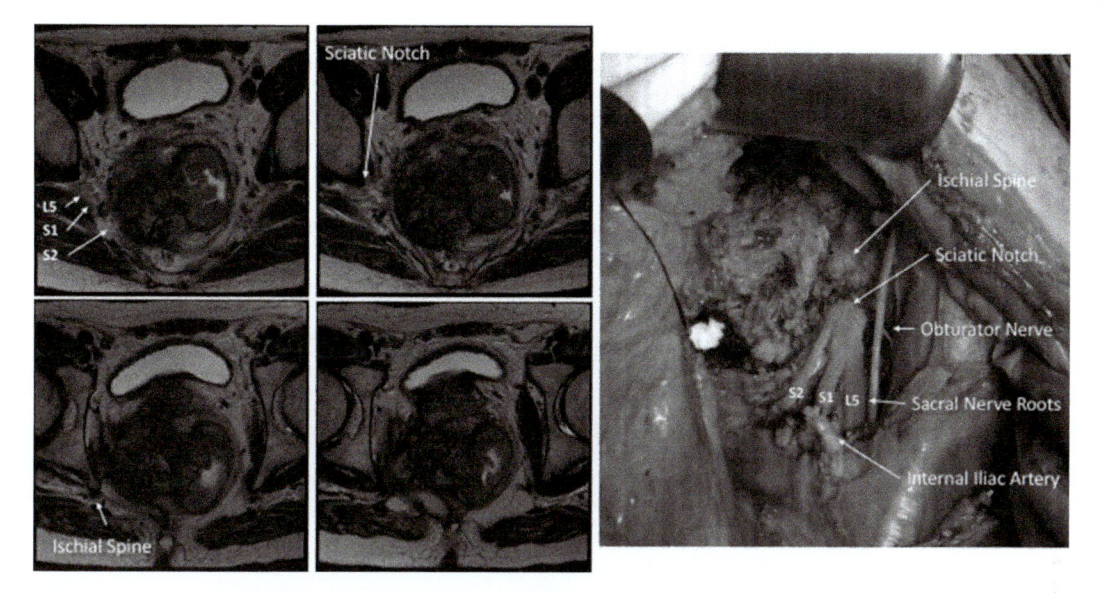

Figure 12.1 MRI demonstrates the extent of a locally advanced primary rectal cancer. The tumor involves the prostate and extends to involve the lateral pelvic sidewall on the right including the obturator internus muscle. The operative photo demonstrates exposure of sacral nerve roots approaching the sciatic notch. It also shows the exposed ischial spine following resection of the obturator internus muscle with preservation of the obturator nerve. This was accomplished with en-bloc resection of the internal iliac vessels and entire right pelvic sidewall. *Source:* Brian K. Bednarski and George J. Chang.

the setting of locally advanced and recurrent rectal cancer and extensive mobilization for lateral pelvic resection is associated with the potential for devascularization of the ureter, it is necessary to be prepared to resect and re-implant the ureter. The ureter may also be involved by tumor and need to be resected with ureteral reconstruction. Additionally, in males, the vas deferens will traverse the lateral pelvis as one of the most superficial/medial structures. In females, the fallopian tube and ovary reside in the lateral pelvis and the gonadal vessels will also traverse the proximal lateral pelvis. Lastly, the round ligament will be identified as a superficial structure in the lateral pelvis.

Muscular

The muscles that are encountered in the lateral pelvis include the piriformis, obturator internus, and levator ani muscles. The piriformis extends from the anterior surface of the sacrum to the trochanter of the femur. The sacral nerve roots course along the anterior aspect of the piriformis to the sciatic notch and this is a common place for nerve root and muscle involvement. The obturator internus extends from the ischium and rim of the pubis to the trochanter of the femur. Lastly, the levator ani muscles, specifically the iliococcygeus component, arise in the lateral pelvis from fascia of the obturator internus and from the ischial spine and traverse medially [13]. Lateral pelvic compartment tumor resection may require detachment of the levator ani at the ischial spine which serves as a landmark for the lateral extent of soft-tissue resection (Figure 12.2).

Preoperative Evaluation

Imaging

In determining the suitability of patients with locally advanced primary or recurrent rectal cancer for exenterative surgery, patients should undergo complete staging evaluation. The preoperative staging evaluation can be divided into two components: (i) evaluation for

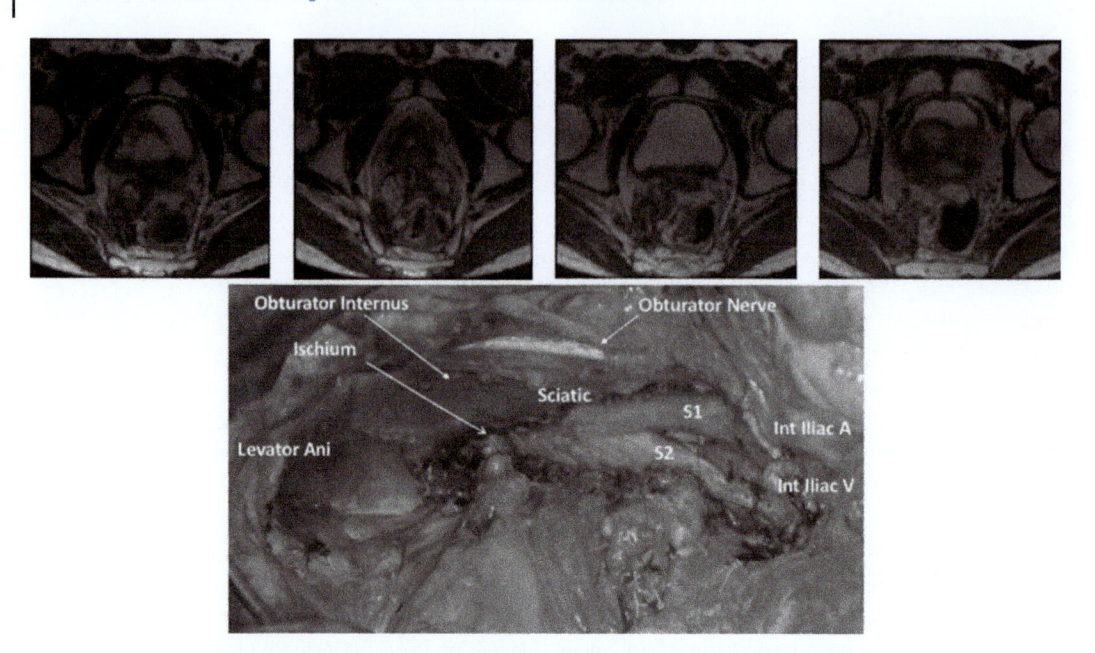

Figure 12.2 This case illustrates a recurrent rectal cancer involving the right lateral pelvis. The tumor involves the right seminal vesicle, abuts the internal iliac vessels, and involves the lateral portion of the presacral fascia. Resection of internal iliac vessels en bloc with the specimen resulted in exposure of sacral nerve roots and access to the ischial spine. In this case the tip of the spine was exposed together with lateral-most insertions of levator ani muscles. The obturator internus and obturator nerve did not require resection but were exposed, and the tissues medial to those structures were removed. *Source:* Brian K. Bednarski and George J. Chang.

distant disease and (ii) evaluation of local tumor extent and resectability [5]. This is discussed at length in Chapter 3.

Relating to this specific topic, high-definition magnetic resonance imaging (MRI) of the pelvis is the gold standard for assessing local tumor extent (Figures 12.1 and 12.2) [5, 14]. These images can provide insight into the ability to achieve a margin-negative resection. This includes the preoperative identification of the need to resect urologic, vascular, neurologic, and/or muscular anatomy and the need for other multidisciplinary service involvement such as vascular surgery, plastic surgery, or urology to assist in the extirpation of the tumor and reconstruction [14].

Functional Status

Beyond the considerations of locoregional and distant disease, evaluation of the functional status of the patient and their associated comorbidities is also necessary. The impact of the patient's functional status on outcomes of complex oncologic surgery has been demonstrated in other malignancies where the risk of recurrent and metastatic disease is high, including pancreas cancer and adrenal cancer [15, 16]. Patients with locally advanced pelvic malignancies warrant a similar approach. This is especially true when the resection of the tumor may require neurologic or muscular resections that can have direct impacts on mobility.

Informed Consent

Patient understanding of the magnitude of pelvic exenteration and its associated morbidity is an important consideration for surgical teams. While informed consent is part of any surgical procedure, the discussion with the patient prior to exenterative surgery warrants additional attention. Resection of anatomic structures involving the lateral pelvis is associated with the typical complications of extended pelvic surgeries, including infectious complications, bleeding and the need for blood transfusion, urologic dysfunction, sexual dysfunction, damage to normal structures, need for reoperation, cardiac and pulmonary complications, venous thromboembolism, and death [4, 11, 17]. In addition, dissection along the sacral nerve roots or resection of the nerve roots may have implications for mobility of the associated lower extremity, pain in the sciatic nerve distribution, and numbness [18]. The high incidence of postoperative complications and associated morbidity should be discussed with the patient and their family to ensure that all involved parties are prepared for the associated risks, the potential for prolonged recovery, and/or the need for physical rehabilitation. Lastly, given the complexity of the surgery and its associated recovery, we also discuss the need for a prolonged stay in the immediate area following discharge for patients that travel from out of town. This enables ongoing care to occur, with frequent postoperative clinic visits to identify and manage early any complications that arise in the first two to four weeks following hospital discharge.

Intraoperative Management

Preparation and Positioning

When amenable, the use of epidural anesthesia can help with early postoperative pain management. This is placed prior to induction. Once anesthetized, patients are positioned in low lithotomy, ensuring proper positioning of the lower extremities with appropriate padding to avoid pressure-related nerve injuries. Preoperative antibiotics covering skin and bowel flora are administered. Venous thrombosis prophylaxis is addressed with sequential compression devices as well as pharmacologic prophylaxis with either subcutaneous heparin or low molecular weight heparin. For patients requiring pelvic sidewall resection, the patients will undergo cystoscopy and bilateral ureteral stent placement. The patient's abdomen and perineum are prepped and the Foley catheter included in the operative field to provide access during urologic assessment or reconstruction.

Equipment

In addition to routine operative equipment including self-retaining retractors and electrocautery, we typically have bipolar cautery available secondary to the proximity of the neurologic structures. A vessel-sealing device can assist with management of the small lateral branches of the internal iliac vessels and division of fibromuscular soft tissue. Additionally, we would consider utilizing saline-linked electrocautery in cases necessitating dissection along the sacrum posteriorly.

Operative Approach

A midline incision provides adequate access to the pelvis and bifurcation of the aorta and vena cava. For any lateral pelvic resection, having access to the common iliac vessels and the origin of the internal and external iliac vessels is essential to be able to maintain core vascular surgery principles of proximal and distal control. Once access to the abdomen is established, the pelvis is exposed and the small bowel is retracted cranially.

Initial dissection begins posteriorly when possible. In primary or recurrent disease that does not involve posterior pelvic anatomy, posterior dissection can create some mobility and will enable the surgeon to establish a distal target for lateral pelvic dissection. After the posterior plane is started, dissection proceeds on the uninvolved lateral plane. The operation continues anteriorly. This enables dissection in the non-tumor-involved tissue planes to occur as distally as possible. This can help identify the target for the distal side of the tumor involved in lateral pelvic resection. Additionally, it reserves the most challenging and highest risk portion of the operation for last. Working in the lateral pelvis can result in bleeding and in some cases removal of the tumor is necessary to gain adequate control. By approaching the lateral pelvic sidewall resection involved by tumor last, this can help decrease the extent of bleeding as the majority of the pelvic dissection has already been completed.

Our approach to the lateral pelvis is guided by the anatomic landmarks as outlined above. In terms of exposure, for all tumors involving the lateral pelvis the common iliac is identified and the origins of the internal and external iliac vessels are dissected. At the same time, the ureter is mobilized and is encircled with a vessel loop. The bladder is mobilized in the space of Retzius. The peritoneum overlying the external iliac vessels is incised. The vas deferens or the round ligament will also be transected to help expose the lateral pelvis. These maneuvers provide initial access to the anterolateral pelvis.

For cases requiring dissection in the extravascular plane, the extent of the vascular resection is determined by preoperative MRI. When possible, the superior gluteal branches are preserved and the internal iliac vessels are isolated and divided just distal to the first posterior branch. The vessels can be controlled with prolene suture ligatures or an Endo GIA™ stapler at the discretion of the operating surgeon. Occasionally, with more superior involvement of the posterior lateral pelvis or in the presence of anatomical variations resulting in additional arterial or venous branches at the level of the superior gluteal, it is necessary to control the posterior superior gluteal in order to avoid accidental injury. Once the vessels are divided, the dissection proceeds along posterior and lateral to the internal iliac vessels. The individual branches exiting between the sacral nerve roots and at the level of the sciatic notch are controlled with clamps and ties or with a vessel-sealing device. Additionally, attention should be paid to the distal branches of the posterior branch of the internal iliac vessels, pudendal, and inferior gluteal. Failure to obtain appropriate control of these vessels prior to division can result in significant blood loss.

Review of preoperative MRI can significantly aid in understanding the number and extent of lateral branches and provide insight into aberrant vascular anatomy. Being prepared for lateral vascular branches enables careful dissection while minimizing bleeding risk. This can be very challenging in re-operative pelvic surgery, but remains a focal point of preparation and execution of extended lateral pelvic resections.

Tumors extending to the sacral nerve roots or the sciatic nerve require division of the internal iliac vessels to provide access to those structures. The dissection can then proceed along the nerves, including the nerve sheath as necessary. Sharp dissection and the use of bipolar cautery can minimize surgical trauma to the nerves. Additionally, the nerve roots and sciatic nerve proper can be resected en bloc as necessary (Figure 12.1). Resection of the individual L5 or S1 nerve roots, or the sciatic nerve itself, will have impacts on postoperative ambulatory function. While there is a paucity of literature regarding the functional outcomes of this type of radical resection, there is evidence that it is feasible and that while patients may have some impairment, they remain ambulatory with support [18]. In addition to impacts on mobility, operative dissection along the sacral nerve roots and sciatic nerve can result in chronic pain and/or numbness. Posterior and lateral to the internal iliac vessels, the piriformis muscle is identified together with the more distal sacral nerve roots, including S2 and S3 (Figure 12.2).

For more anterolateral tumors, the surgeon needs to be prepared to resect the obturator nerve and vessels as well as the obturator internus. Approach to this anterolateral area is done by dissecting just posterior to the external iliac vein. This enables the dissection to stay anterior to the obturator nerve and vessels. It provides access to the obturator internus muscle and the medial wall of the acetabulum laterally. Resection of the vessels and nerve can be accomplished with this approach. Ligating the vasculature will have little consequence for the patient. Transecting the nerve can result in some weakness in the adductor muscles of the medial thigh. It will also result in numbness of the skin of the medial thigh secondary to its cutaneous branch.

Lastly, a wide resection of the levator ani muscles can be aided by a lateral approach. By dividing the internal iliac vessels and incising the obturator internus fascia posterior to the external iliac vein, access is provided to the sciatic notch, ischial spine, and sacral spinous ligament (Figure 12.2). This enables division of the levators at their posterior and lateral insertions. It can also allow the ischial spine to be resected en bloc with bone shears to exit the pelvis a bit higher along the lateral wall. Additionally, this technique provides access to the inferior pubic ramus as it traverses anterolaterally. This will allow further transection of the levator ani muscles widely. This is often aided by an approach from both the abdomen and perineum. This two-team approach enables for better exposure and direct division of the pelvic floor laterally. It is important to be aware of the pudendal vessels as they typically exit the pelvis near the ischial spine.

Once the specimen is removed, any additional hemostasis can be confirmed with close inspection of the divided vasculature. Margins are evaluated. Reconstruction can then commence. Gastrointestinal continuity is re-established if the pelvic floor is spared and only a unilateral resection of the lateral pelvic structures is required. Alternatively, an ostomy is sited. The urology team will then prepare the ileal conduit as necessary for bladder reconstruction. Finally, our group routinely performs these operations in collaboration with plastic and reconstructive surgery specialists. The defect created in patients requiring resection of the lateral pelvis as well as the bladder and rectum is significant. Being able to adequately fill the defect is an important consideration, especially in the setting of neoadjuvant radiation. The use of qualified plastic and reconstructive surgeons enables the space to be filled with viable, well-perfused, and non-irradiated tissue. The most common flap utilized is the vertical rectus abdominus muscle (VRAM) flap. Alternatives include bilateral gricilis flaps, gluteal advancement flaps, and omental flaps. The decision of which flap is best is guided by the size of the defect, extent of skin resection required, and availability of healthy flaps. An additional option includes the utilization of mesh for closure.

Postoperative Management

Postoperative management is consistent with other operative procedures in the pelvis and is discussed in Chapter 18. Essential to postoperative management after these complex cases is the involvement of supportive services, including physical therapy, occupational therapy, and wound ostomy continence nurses (WOCN). As noted, the magnitude of this type of surgery and subsequent reconstruction may include resection of neuromuscular structures. Therefore postoperative mobilization can be challenging but is essential.

Complications

Operative resections of this magnitude are associated with a high incidence of postoperative morbidity. The incidence of postoperative complications has been reported in 55–65% of cases. Postoperative deaths can occur but are uncommon, representing 2–4% of patients undergoing exenterations [2–4, 6, 8, 11].

There are some unique issues that can arise following operative resections of the lateral pelvis. Specifically, resection of the internal iliac vessels can result in rare but life-threatening hemorrhage in the postoperative period. This can result from the breakdown of the staple or suture line. It can also result from pseudoaneurysm formation. This scenario can present with sentinel bleeding that is large volume but initially ceases on its own. However, significant ongoing hemorrhage and shock can be the sole presenting event. Early recognition and rapid control is essential to avoid fatal bleeding. This is best managed with endovascular approaches to embolize or stent across the internal iliac artery depending on the length of the stump. The risk is raised in patients with postoperative pelvic infectious complications. It is essential to treat any pelvic infectious complication aggressively to try to mitigate the risk for pseudoaneurysm formation and rupture. Additionally, the ability to spare the internal iliac vessels proximal to the superior gluteal provides a stump that can be embolized in the event that any significant bleeding occurs.

> **Summary Box**
> - Exenterative surgery involving the lateral pelvis presents significant challenges with added morbidity.
> - Incorporating knowledge of the anatomy together with high-quality preoperative imaging can allow the operating surgeon to organize the necessary team to safely extirpate tumors involving these vascular and/or neuromuscular structures.
> - While this area remains particularly challenging in exenterative surgery, surgical management of this disease can be accomplished with experience in specialized centers.

References

1 Gannon, C.J., Zager, J.S., Chang, G.J. et al. (2007). Pelvic exenteration affords safe and durable treatment for locally advanced rectal carcinoma. *Ann. Surg. Oncol.* 14 (6): 1870–1877.

2 Kusters, M., Austin, K.K., Solomon, M.J. et al. (2015). Survival after pelvic exenteration for T4 rectal cancer. *Br. J. Surg.* 102 (1): 125–131.

3 PelvEx Collaborative (2018). Factors affecting outcomes following pelvic exenteration for locally recurrent rectal cancer. *Br. J. Surg.* 105 (6): 650–657.

4 PelvEx Collaborative (2019). Surgical and survival outcomes following pelvic exenteration for locally advanced primary rectal cancer: results from an international collaboration. *Ann. Surg.* 269 (2): 315–321.

5 Beyond TME Collaborative (2013). Consensus statement on the multidisciplinary management of patients with recurrent and primary rectal cancer beyond total mesorectal excision planes. *Br. J. Surg.* 100 (8): E1–E33.

6 Solomon, M.J., Brown, K.G., Koh, C.E. et al. (2015). Lateral pelvic compartment excision during pelvic exenteration. *Br. J. Surg.* 102 (13): 1710–1717.

7 Yamada, K., Ishizawa, T., Niwa, K. et al. (2001). Patterns of pelvic invasion are prognostic in the treatment of locally recurrent rectal cancer. *Br. J. Surg.* 88 (7): 988–993.

8 Lee, D.J., Sagar, P.M., Sadadcharam, G., and Tan, K.Y. (2017). Advances in surgical management for locally recurrent rectal cancer: how far have we come? *World J. Gastroenterol.* 23 (23): 4170–4180.

9 Austin, K.K. and Solomon, M.J. (2009). Pelvic exenteration with en bloc iliac vessel resection for lateral pelvic wall involvement. *Dis. Colon Rectum* 52 (7): 1223–1233.

10 Shaikh, I., Aston, W., Hellawell, G. et al. (2014). Extended lateral pelvic sidewall excision (ELSiE): an approach to optimize complete resection rates in locally advanced or recurrent anorectal cancer involving the

pelvic sidewall. *Tech. Coloproctol.* 18 (12): 1161–1168.
11 Mariathasan, A.B., Boye, K., Giercksky, K.E. et al. (2018). Beyond total mesorectal excision in locally advanced rectal cancer with organ or pelvic side-wall involvement. *Eur. J. Surg. Oncol.* 44 (8): 1226–1232.
12 Kusters, M., Bosman, S.J., Van Zoggel, D.M. et al. (2016). Local recurrence in the lateral lymph node compartment: improved outcomes with induction chemotherapy combined with multimodality treatment. *Ann. Surg. Oncol.* 23 (6): 1883–1889.
13 Mahadevan, V. (2018). Anatomy of the pelvis. *Surgery (Oxford)* 36 (7): 333–338.
14 Brown, W.E., Koh, C.E., Badgery-Parker, T., and Solomon, M.J. (2017). Validation of MRI and surgical decision making to predict a complete resection in pelvic exenteration for recurrent rectal cancer. *Dis. Colon Rectum* 60 (2): 144–151.
15 Bednarski, B.K., Habra, M.A., Phan, A. et al. (2014). Borderline resectable adrenal cortical carcinoma: a potential role for preoperative chemotherapy. *World J. Surg.* 38 (6): 1318–1327.
16 Katz, M.H., Pisters, P.W., Evans, D.B. et al. (2008). Borderline resectable pancreatic cancer: the importance of this emerging stage of disease. *J. Am. Coll. Surg.* 206 (5): 833–846; discussion 46–8.
17 Bird, T.G., Ngan, S.Y., Chu, J. et al. (2018). Outcomes and prognostic factors of multimodality treatment for locally recurrent rectal cancer with curative intent. *Int. J. Color. Dis.* 33 (4): 393–401.
18 Brown, K.G.M., Solomon, M.J., Lau, Y.C. et al. (2019). Sciatic and femoral nerve resection during extended radical surgery for advanced pelvic tumours: long-term survival, functional, and quality-of-life outcomes. *Ann. Surg.* **Jun 7; doi:**https://doi.org/10.1097//SLA.000000000003390.

13

Extended Exenterative Resections for Recurrent Neoplasm
Peter Sagar

The John Goligher Department of Colorectal Surgery, St. James's University Hospital, Leeds, UK; University of Leeds, Leeds, UK

Background

The principal aim of the surgical treatment of local recurrence of rectal cancer is to achieve a clear resection margin, as it is the most significant prognostic factor in predicting long-term survival. However, this is not always technically feasible, especially in the setting of recurrent disease. The desire to resect higher and wider can come at considerable morbidity and functional loss to the patient. This is particularly relevant with regard to pelvic sidewall masses and tumors involving the upper part of the sacrum. Nonetheless, the development and technical innovations related to resection of locally recurrent pelvic cancer have led to a paradigm shift in what surgeons would consider absolute versus relative contraindications since the mid-1990s. Situations once considered an absolute contraindication to resection such as high sacral involvement, encasement of the iliac vessels, and extension of tumor through the sciatic foramen would now be considered relative contraindications.

It should be appreciated, however, that the morbidity and associated functional deficits should not be considered trivial or dismissed lightly. This chapter explores the surgical principles and nuances that underpin the operative management of locally recurrent pelvic cancer.

Strategies for Tackling Involvement of Posterior Compartment Including Sacrum

The level of sacral involvement is critical, with considerable differences in management strategies of upper and lower levels of sacral invasion.

Low Sacrectomy

In low sacrectomy, a lower abdominal midline incision is made to provide good access, and the use of a retractor system like Omni-Tract® or a Goligher-style retractor is utilized. The majority of local recurrences involving the distal sacrum (i.e. below S3) can be tackled by means of an abdominal approach [1]. Mobilization of the rectum/neorectum abdomen is required and continues into the lower pelvis, either dislocating the urogenital organs from the neorectum if there is a plane of dissection that is not involved with the malignant process, or progressing anteriorly such that the plane of dissection encompasses the urogenital organs as a total pelvic exenteration with sacrectomy.

There is no absolute requirement to devascularize the sacrum by means of ligating the internal iliac arteries and veins in cases where

---

Surgical Management of Advanced Pelvic Cancer, First Edition.
Edited by Michael E. Kelly and Desmond C. Winter.
© 2022 John Wiley & Sons Ltd. Published 2022 by John Wiley & Sons Ltd.

the distal sacral is to be resected unless there is concomitant involvement of these vessels by the tumor. The pelvic dissection should stop about 2–3 cm above the cephalad extent of the tumor and attention should then be turned to the perineum. The surgical team may choose between completing the procedure with the patient remaining in the Lloyd-Davies position or closing the abdominal wound with the maturation of the colostomy (and urostomy where indicated) and turning the patient prone jackknife. The preference for the latter facilitates the surgeon making a longitudinal incision over the sacrum, reflecting the gluteal muscles off the posterior aspect of the sacrum and detaching the sacrospinous and sacrotuberous ligaments before detaching the distal sacrum from the proximal sacrum with an osteotome. Placement of a small swab behind the neorectum at completion of the abdominal component allows the surgeon using the perineal approach to cut down onto the swab and prevent inadvertent slippage with the potential to damage iliac vessels. The dissection is completed by the division of any residual anterior attachments, with the perineal approach providing excellent visualization and protection of the prostate/bladder/urethra and finishing with careful hemostasis.

High Sacrectomy

High sacrectomy provides a greater surgical challenge than low sacrectomy, in particular with the risk of significant intraoperative bleeding and the potential reconstruction difficulties to ensure a stable pelvic ring [2] (Figures 13.1 and 13.2). The previously described abdominal and perineal parts of the surgical procedure are completed before attention is turned to the upper sacrum; however, attention is turned to the upper sacrum and it is obligatory to control and be able to ligate the internal iliac arteries and veins bilaterally. With the abdominal part of the operation complete, the patient is turned prone. Again, abdominal swabs may be left in the pelvis to

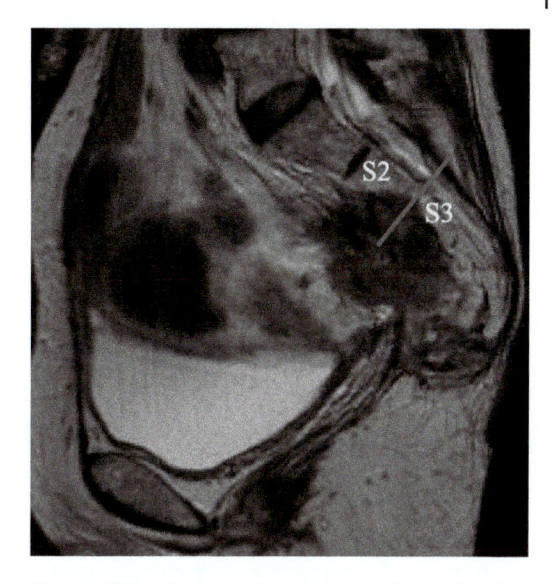

Figure 13.1 Recurrent rectal cancer involving S2 and S3. A high sacrectomy was required with S1 maintaining the integrity of the pelvic bony ring. Red line indicates junction between S2 and S3.

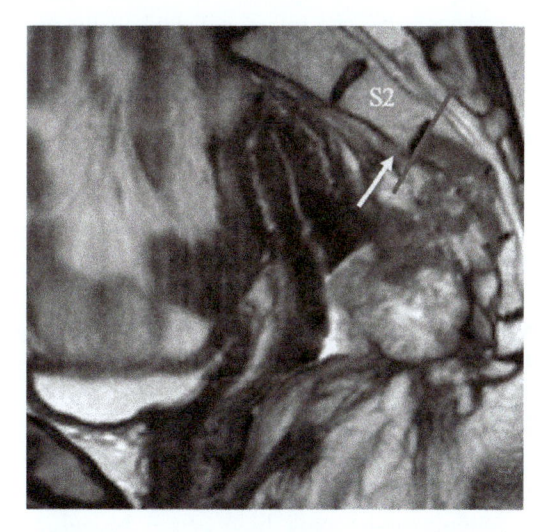

Figure 13.2 Recurrence mainly involving S2, but a small deposit in the anterior–inferior corner of S2 also required excision, albeit with most of S2 left in situ. Line lies between between S2 and S3; The arrow indicates involvement of S2. *Source:* Peter Sagar.

keep the loops of the small bowel out of the way to minimize the risk of accidental damage when the sacrum is divided from the posterior approach. It is helpful to tackle the upper sacral resections with the help of either a neurosurgeon or an orthopedic surgeon with an interest in spinal surgery. A vertical incision is made and deepened onto the sacrum with reflection of the gluteal muscles giving full exposure of the sacrum. The sacrospinous, sacrotuberous, and sacrococcygeal ligaments are divided and the piriformis muscles exposed. The dissection is deepened with protection of the sacral nerve roots and the sciatic nerve before the level of transection of the sacrum is identified. Much care must be taken at this point to prevent error in the choice of level of transection, and this can be facilitated by placement of a staple or pin into the sacrum 2–3 cm above the cephalad extent of the recurrent tumor, or during the abdominal part of the operation with a screening X-ray used to confirm the level. The dural sac is ligated with a non-absorbable suture to prevent subsequent leakage of cerebrospinal fluid (CSF) and division of the sacrum is achieved using an oscillating saw, avoiding undue pressure that may allow the saw to inadvertently damage pelvic structures. The tumor and adjacent involved organs may then be removed through the perineal wound. Hemostasis is achieved with a combination of cautery set at a relatively high level, suture ligation of vessels, and judicious use of hemostatic agents. Bone wax is helpful to control bleeding from the proximal end of the sacrum. Closure of the perineal wound is usually feasible by a primary suture, but if this would lead to tension on the wound, gluteal flaps based on the inferior gluteal artery pedicle (IGAP flaps) are a useful option.

Patients undergoing high sacral resection that removes more than half of the first sacral body or higher will require spinopelvic stabilization, and a number of techniques have been advocated to maintain the pelvic ring including fibular grafts, metallic supports, and the use of cages. Spinopelvic reconstruction and stabilization can be achieved with the Synthes MATRIX Spine System (DuPuySynthes Spine Company, Oberdorf, Switzerland) with the placement of bilateral pedicle screws between L3 and L5 into the iliac wings. X-ray guidance should be used to confirm correct placement of instrumentation and a titanium rod can be contoured and fixed to the pedicle screws and the iliac bolts. A cross-link placed between both of the titanium rods facilitates some rotational stability.

High transection of the sacrum is associated with specific risks of injury to the posteriorly sited nerves and the potential breach to the dural sac with leakage of CSF. One option is to use an ultrasonic bone aspirator (Sonopet® (Stryker, USA)) for bony dissection [3]. The Sonopet uses ultrasonic vibrations at the tip to permit precise surgical incisions, while stopping as it reaches vascular or neural structures, thereby minimizing risk. This is of particular help with resection of a diseased S1 and/or S2 vertebra. Excision of either S1 or S2 alone can be facilitated by the use of an expandable cage to restore the vertebral column and maintain the integrity of the pelvic ring to support the torso while preserving the lumbar lordosis, height, and alignment. One such expandable cage is the FORTIFY® Spacer implant (Globus Medical, USA). This device is made up of a central core and two end plates with integrated titanium screws to facilitate fixation into the recipient vertebra. Crucially, the implant is able to expand within the sacral defect to provide appropriate height. Bone grafts positioned around the implant provide additional stability.

There are cases where the involvement of the upper sacrum only involves the anterior portion of the bone and the remaining part is clear of disease. The anterior table of the first or second part of the sacrum can be resected without compromising the stability of the pelvis by leaving the majority of each sacral vertebrae [4] (Figure 13.3). Excision of the anterior table involves stripping the presacral fascia from the sacral promontory to the inferior end of the involved sacrum, and the cortex of the bone is incised with a chisel, noting a change in tension as the softer medullary bone is reached. A rongeur is then used to develop the

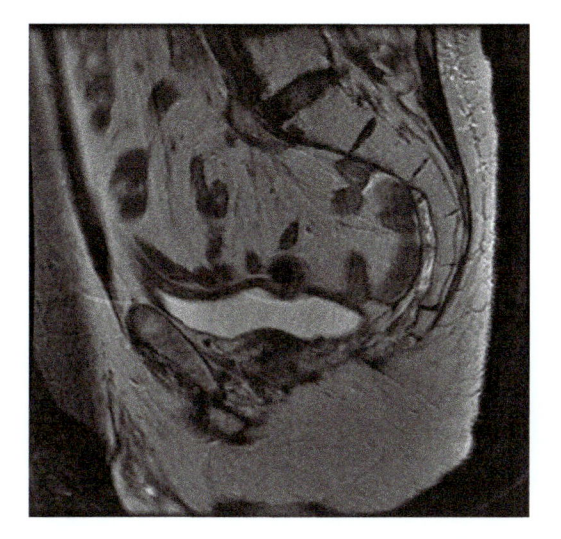

Figure 13.3 Invasion of S1 suitable for resection of the anterior table of the bone. *Source:* Peter Sagar.

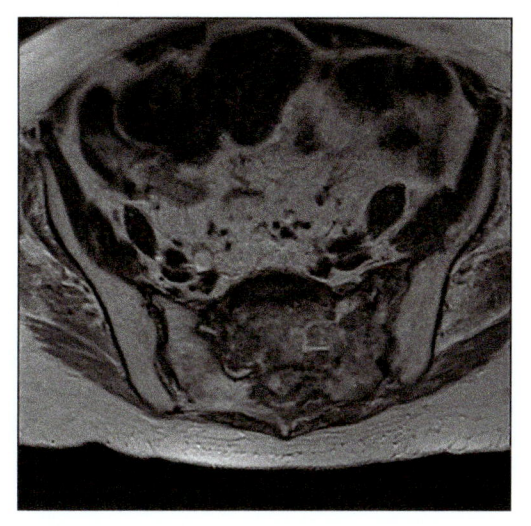

Figure 13.4 Bulky but low recurrence that required resection of right piriformis and gluteal muscles together with obturators to achieve a clear margin. An IGAP flap was used to close the defect. *Source:* Peter Sagar.

plane with its sharp-edged, scoop-shaped tip, taking care to stay posterior to the recurrent tumor on the anterior cortex of the bone. This technique preserves both the dura and the posterior nerve roots, avoiding the need for any subsequent pelvic stabilization. Bleeding with such cases is not usually troublesome, but bone wax or hemostatic agents are useful to control any ooze.

Perineal Closure

In patients that have a large perineal defect after an extended resection of locally recurrent tumor, often reconstruction using a flap is needed (Figure 13.4). The choice of flap reconstruction is ideally made prior to the operation and the availability of a plastic reconstruction surgeon confirmed. The flap will provide not only skin to cover the defect but also well-nourished muscle to help fill the dead space within the pelvic cavity. Vertical rectus abdominus myocutaneous (VRAM) flap satisfies these requirements as it provides sufficient bulk to fill the pelvic defect, but care must be taken to ensure the inferior epigastric vessels remain viable and not compromised by abdominal wall incision or stoma formation. Alternatively, myocutaneous flaps based on the gracilis muscles are easy to harvest but provide little in the way of bulk in filling the potential dead space.

Strategies for Tackling Involvement of Pelvic Sidewall

The principal concept in tackling recurrent tumors involving the pelvic sidewall is understanding that the sidewall is structured in a series of layers [5]. Preoperative imaging using magnetic resonance imaging (MRI) is vital to plan the surgical approach (Figure 13.5) Parts of this include the following, working outwards: pelvic peritoneum, ureter, iliac arteries and veins, sidewall nerves that include the lumbosacral trunk, branches that constitute the sciatic nerve, obturator muscles, and finally the bony pelvis. Anatomy of the vessels provides a rich plethora of arterial branches and a highly variable venous anatomy that can when injured cause brisk hemorrhage. It is for this reason that proximal and distal control of the arteries and veins must be secured before

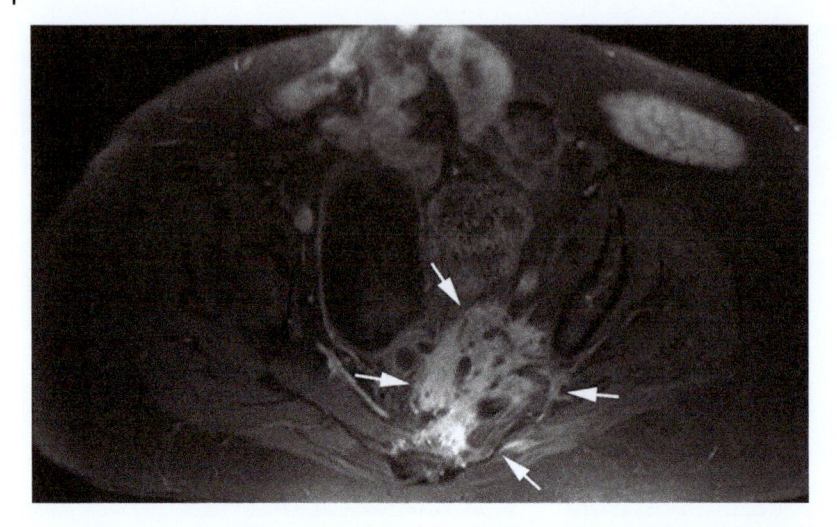

Figure 13.5 Left pelvic sidewall recurrence that had responded to preoperative chemotherapy with fibrosis on the left side of the mass and an R0 resection was obtained. *Source:* Peter Sagar.

directing attention to the tumor mass to minimize intraoperative blood loss.

A sequential approach to the recurrent tumor sited on the pelvic sidewall includes identifying the ureter which is mobilized, dissecting the iliac artery, and securing it with vessel loops [6]. The internal iliac vein is then similarly dissected and looped, with mobilization of the common and external veins according to the location of the recurrence. Once the arteries and veins had been mobilized, the nerves can be visualized and, in particular, the sciatic nerve identified and protected. The lumbosacral trunk provides a major contribution to the innervation of the muscles of the lower limb and preservation of this trunk is therefore important in maintaining quality of life.

Recurrent tumors spreading up or through the greater sciatic notch present a particular challenge (Figure 13.6). Division of the sacrospinous ligament provides wider access to the pelvis when required, with the ischial spine acting as the boundary into the anterior/caudal portion of the pelvis. By carefully working through each of the layers of the pelvis and by tackling the tumor by working above, from the sides, and below, one can gradually mobilize the tumor whilst maintaining a clear margin and maintaining hemostasis.

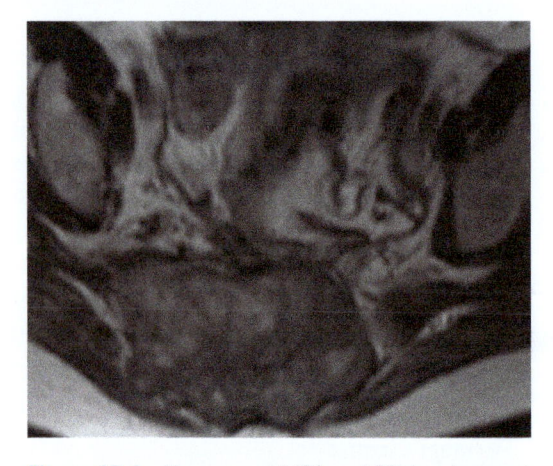

Figure 13.6 Upper sacral (S1 and S2) involvement with spread across the left sacroiliac joint deemed too advanced to justify attempted resection. *Source:* Peter Sagar.

Bleeding can be substantial, and having preliminary control of the vessels prior to tumor dissection minimizes significant hemorrhage. Accurate hemorrhage control is enabled with the use of suture ligation or application of metallic clips. Bleeding from presacral vessels may be controlled by turning up the cautery and/or by use of commercial products. Encasement of the external iliac vessels is particularly challenging, but adherence to basic surgical principles with careful mobilization of arteries and veins and reconstruction with a vein graft allows en-bloc removal of the tumor mass. In the absence of a clearly visualized bleeding vessel, careful packing of the region with firm pressure allows time to consider options and for anesthetic colleagues to optimize physiological issues. With major hemorrhage, packing should be maintained for at least 15–20 minutes or longer as needed. There are occasions when abandoning the procedure with pelvic packing and a plan to return to the operating room over 24–48 hours is necessary.

Strategies for Tackling Involvement of Anterior Compartment

Involvement of the urogenital organs by a recurrence typically requires resection of the anterior pelvic structures, especially if there is direct invasion into the bladder, prostate, or urethra in the male or if the tumor extends beyond the posterior vaginal wall/uterus in the female to involve the bladder [7]. En-bloc resection of the tumor mass and adjacent involved organs usually proceeds with an initial dissection posteriorly, assuming the tumor is clear of the sacrum, with lateral mobilization of the tumor with any involved or encased pelvic vessels. Attention is then turned to the anterior plane of dissection and the retropubic space of Retzius is opened and the plane of dissection developed inferiorly and then swung posteriorly to meet the previous plane of lateral dissection. The dorsal veins of the penis may bleed briskly and, whilst the original urinary catheter will have been divided to remove the proximal urethra, an aid to control bleeding from this area is the reinsertion of a wide-bore urinary catheter with inflation of the balloon and connection to a urine bag with a liter of fluid to provide tension/pressure on these veins. Ultimately, suture ligation of the dorsal vein complex will suffice. In the relatively unusual case of the tumor involving the pubic rami, the dissection may be continued anteriorly, dividing the pubic rami to facilitate en-bloc resection. Reconstruction with the involvement of an orthopedic surgeon is necessary.

> **Summary Box**
> - Extended exenterative resection for locally recurrent pelvic neoplasms offers control of symptoms and potential for long-term survival.
> - Recurrent cancers needing multiviseral resection should be referred to specialist tertiary units that have expertise in surgical oncology, spinal orthopedics, and advanced reconstructive services.
> - Multidisciplinary review and specific planning is needed to tailor each resection to the individual patient and their recurrence.
> - High-quality imaging with magnetic resonance of the pelvis and computed tomography–positron emission tomography (CT-PET) is critical to establishing surgical strategy.
> - Thorough counseling with patient appreciation of the implications of the operation is vital.

References

1 Solomon, M.J., Tan, K.K., Bromilow, R.G. et al. (2014). Sacrectomy via abdominal approach during pelvic exenteration. *Dis. Colon Rectum* 57: 272–277.

2 Dozois, E.J., Privitera, A., Holubar, S.D. et al. (2011). High sacrectomy for locally recurrent rectal cancer: can long-term survival be achieved? *J. Surg. Oncol.* 103: 105–109.

3 Lee, D.J.K., Wang, K.Y., Sagar, P.M., and Timothy, J. (2018). S1 sacrectomy for re-recurrent rectal cancer: our experience with reconstruction using an expandable vertebral body replacement device. *Dis. Colon Rectum* 61: 261–265.

Describes a useful reconstructive technique.

4 Evans, M.D., Harji, D.P., Sagar, P.M. et al. (2013). Partial anterior sacrectomy with nerve preservation to treat locally advanced rectal cancer. *Colorectal Dis.* 15: e336–e339.

5 Maslekar, S., Sagar, P.M., Mavor, A.I.D. et al. (2013). Resection of recurrent rectal cancer with encasement of external iliac vessels. *Tech. Coloproctol.* 17: 131–132.

6 Austin, K.K.S. and Solomon, M.J. (2009). Pelvic exenteration with en bloc iliac vessel resection for lateral pelvic wall involvement. *Dis. Colon Rectum* 52: 1223–1233.

7 Austin, K.S.S., Herd, A., Solomon, M.J. et al. (2016). Outcomes of pelvic exenteration with en bloc partial or complete pubic excision for locally advanced or recurrent pelvic cancer. *Dis. Colon Rectum* 59: 831–835.

14

Pelvic Exenteration in the Setting of Peritoneal Disease

Niels Kok, Arend Aalbers, and Geerard Beets

Netherlands Cancer Institute, Amsterdam, The Netherlands

Background

Peritoneal metastases occur in up to 10% of patients with colorectal cancer. Cytoreductive surgery and hyperthermic intraperitoneal chemotherapy (CRS-HIPEC) with or without perioperative systemic chemotherapy is the most aggressive strategy to treat peritoneal metastases. CRS-HIPEC and adjuvant chemotherapy is associated with a significant better survival than systemic chemotherapy alone [1]. In select patients, long-term survival and cure can be achieved. However, the potential survival benefit must be balanced with the risk of surgical complications. Extensive peritoneal metastases, reflected as a high peritoneal cancer index (PCI), are associated with increased perioperative morbidity and mortality, with poor overall survival. The combination of limited peritoneal metastases and locally advanced or recurrent colorectal cancer requiring pelvic exenteration is rare and the literature is extremely scarce. In selected patients there may be a role for combining pelvic exenteration with HIPEC

Traditionally, the main mechanism for developing peritoneal metastases of colorectal cancer is full-thickness penetration of the bowel wall by the primary tumor and transcoelomic spread. As peritoneal fluid flows, seeding of tumor cells to the pelvis, the paracolic gutters, the hemidiaphragms, and/or the omentum occurs. The mechanism of spread is not fully understood, but tumor spill and seeding occur in the setting of obstruction and perforation and have a predilection for old scars, stomas, or prior anastomosis sites [2].

Peritoneal metastases may present synchronously with the primary tumor or present as a recurrence. Segelman et al. performed a population-based study in Sweden in the Stockholm county [3]. They observed synchronous and metachronous peritoneal metastases in 4.3 and 4.2% respectively of all patients with colorectal cancer. Lemmens et al. observed similar findings in a Dutch population study, with 4.8% of new colorectal cancer diagnosis having synchronous peritoneal metastases [4].

There is now a belief that all T4 tumors may harbor occult peritoneal disease, which is difficult to detect. The Dutch COLOPEC trial randomized patients with T4 tumors without peritoneal metastases to standard treatment with or without adjuvant HIPEC [5]. In a minority of patients, some underwent HIPEC simultaneously with primary resection, but the majority had HIPEC at five to eight weeks after primary surgery. Interestingly, peritoneal metastases were detected in 10% of the

---

Surgical Management of Advanced Pelvic Cancer, First Edition.
Edited by Michael E. Kelly and Desmond C. Winter.
© 2022 John Wiley & Sons Ltd. Published 2022 by John Wiley & Sons Ltd.

patients, supporting the idea that the risk of synchronous peritoneal disease is higher than previously thought in T4 disease. However, peritoneal metastases seem to occur less frequently in rectal cancer than in colon cancer. This seems logical as only a third of the rectum is proximal of the peritoneal fold. Therefore the need for pelvic exenteration and CRS-HIPEC is limited.

Treatment Options of Colorectal Peritoneal Metastases

Current treatment options for patients with colorectal peritoneal metastases include supportive care, palliative systemic chemotherapy, pressurized intraperitoneal aerosol chemotherapy (PIPAC), CRS, and CRS-HIPEC. Survival of patients with colorectal peritoneal metastases is poor. These patients have a median survival of 13 months when treated with modern systemic chemotherapy [6]. This was significantly shorter compared to patients with metastatic colorectal cancer without peritoneal metastases who had a median survival of 18 months. Poor survival is due to the poor response patients have to systemic chemotherapy. Chemotherapy has limited penetration of peritoneal metastases.

Patients with low-volume peritoneal disease may be candidates for surgery (CRS-HIPEC) with curative intent. Alternatively, those with higher-volume disease are given treatment in an attempt to either downstage their disease or palliate it.

In the French PRODIGE-7 trial [7] patients with peritoneal metastases were randomized to either CRS or CRS-HIPEC. All patients were treated with oxaliplatin-based systemic chemotherapy for at least six months and received HIPEC with oxaliplatin during 30 minutes. Median overall survival was 41.7 and 41.2 months with and without HIPEC respectively. From this trial it can be deducted that surgery has an important role in treating peritoneal metastases and that in a highly selected group of patients who underwent substantial systemic treatment short oxaliplatin-based HIPEC does not further improve survival.

PIPAC has been proposed in patients with more extensive disease, mainly for improving quality of life. An aerosol containing pressurized chemotherapy is insufflated during a laparoscopy. This procedure can be repeated several times [8]. Alyami et al. [9] showed that PIPAC may downstage peritoneal metastases; 14% of 146 patients with a variety of peritoneal surface malignancies where downsized to a point whereby CRS-HIPEC was possible.

Pelvic Exenteration, Cytoreductive Surgery, and HIPEC

Locally advanced or recurrent rectal cancer is the most frequent indication for pelvic exenteration. As two-thirds of the rectum is located below the peritoneal fold, peritoneal metastases are rare in those cancers. Simkens et al. published a study of 317 patients with colorectal cancer who underwent CRS-HIPEC at their institute [10]. Only 29 patients (9%) had rectal cancer. The median distance of the lower border of the tumor to the anus was 10 cm (range 4–15 cm). An abdomino-perineal resection was performed in two patients. Some patients were treated for recurrent rectal cancer with peritoneal metastases. The authors did not observe a poorer survival for patients who underwent CRS-HIPEC for peritoneal metastases of rectal cancer versus patients who underwent CRS-HIPEC for metastases of colonic cancer as opposed to other reported studies [11]. Shinde et al. [12] performed a systematic review and did not find studies including patients who underwent pelvic exenteration and CRS-HIPEC. However, though there is little evidence on this topic it does not mean that performing pelvic exenteration with CRS-HIPEC is not considered. A posterior exenteration with removal of the rectosigmoid and uterus and ovaries en bloc is common in CRS-HIPEC procedures, so as to clear the pelvis of peritoneal metastases. In some instances, to take part or all of the bladder is also necessary to clear disease in the vesico-uterine/rectal pouch.

There is evidence of cases that have observed a high recurrence rate when only a limited resection of peritoneal metastases is performed [13, 14]. Therefore, in the setting of locally or recurrent pelvic disease with peritoneal involvement only, a pelvic exenteration with complete CRS-HIPEC is needed, if feasible. Patient selection is vital, including consideration of associated morbidity and mortality of both procedures. The PelvEx Collaborative has observed a perioperative mortality of 1.5% and a severe complication rate of > 35% [15], while the PROPHYLOCHIP study had a severe complication rate of > 40% following CRS-HIPEC [14]. Logic suggests that combining these procedures will be associated with an increased morbidity and mortality.

To balance potential morbidity and potential oncological benefit and select patients, it seems reasonable to stick to rules learnt from patients with the combination of peritoneal metastases and liver metastases. Elias et al. retrospectively reviewed the outcomes of patients who were treated for both liver and peritoneal metastases [16]. Patients received systemic chemotherapy first, and subsequently CRS-HIPEC plus local treatment of the liver. Their survival was compared with patients who underwent local treatment of liver metastases only or CRS-HIPEC only. Although median survival of patients who underwent both local treatment of the liver and CRS-HIPEC was lower, 26% of patients were alive at five years postoperatively. Thus, for carefully selected patients the combined treatment offered an advantage over systemic chemotherapy alone [6]. Elias et al. proposed a nomogram in which PCI and number of liver metastases are important [16]. The combined operation is most likely to benefit patients with a low PCI and few liver metastases.

The same principles are probably sensible for the selection of patients for pelvic exenteration and CRS-HIPEC. Patients should be fit, resections should be technically feasible, the morbidity of either operation should be limited, and the PCI should be low. PCI has a linear correlation with survival [17]; however, it is difficult to ascertain an exact PCI cut-off point.

Ultimately, the treatment of colorectal peritoneal metastases has significantly evolved over the last decades from palliative management to curative intent. There is a considerable lack of evidence of the role of pelvic exenteration and synchronous CRS-HIPEC. Tailoring this treatment approach to individual patients is needed, including good perioperative counseling and expectation management.

Summary Box

- Peritoneal penetration is the main mechanism by which colorectal tumors can cause peritoneal metastases.
- CRS-HIPEC plus systemic therapy improved survival as compared to systemic chemotherapy in selected patients with colorectal cancer and peritoneal metastases.
- Locally advanced or recurrent rectal cancers with accompanying peritoneal metastases are underrepresented in the current literature on CRS with or without HIPEC.
- Pelvic exenteration and CRS-HIPEC is feasible in carefully selected patients. Potential survival benefit must be weighed against additional morbidity.

References

1. Verwaal, V.J., van, Ruth, S., de, Bree, E. et al. (2003). Randomized trial of cytoreduction and hyperthermic intraperitoneal chemotherapy versus systemic chemotherapy and palliative surgery in patients with peritoneal carcinomatosis of colorectal cancer. *J. Clin. Oncol.* 21 (20): 3737–3743.
2. Yoshida, M., Sugino, T., Kusafuka, K. et al. (2016). Peritoneal dissemination in early gastric cancer: importance of the lymphatic route. *Virchows Arch.* 469 (2): 155–161.
3. Segelman, J., Granath, F., Holm, T. et al. (2012). Incidence, prevalence and risk factors for peritoneal carcinomatosis from colorectal cancer. *Br. J. Surg.* 99 (5): 699–705.
4. Lemmens, V.E., Klaver, Y.L., Verwaal, V.J. et al. (2011). Predictors and survival of synchronous peritoneal carcinomatosis of colorectal origin: a population-based study. *Int. J. Cancer* 128 (11): 2717–2725.
5. Klaver, C.E.L., Wisselink, D.D., Punt, C.J.A. et al. (2019). Adjuvant hyperthermic intraperitoneal chemotherapy in patients with locally advanced colon cancer (COLOPEC): a multicentre, open-label, randomised trial. *Lancet Gastroenterol. Hepatol.* 4 (10): 761–770.
6. Franko, J., Shi, Q., Goldman, C.D. et al. (2012). Treatment of colorectal peritoneal carcinomatosis with systemic chemotherapy: a pooled analysis of north central cancer treatment group phase III trials N9741 and N9841. *J. Clin. Oncol.* 30 (3): 263–267.
7. Quenet, F., Elias, D., Roca, L. et al. (2018). A UNICANCER phase III trial of hyperthermic intra-peritoneal chemotherapy (HIPEC) for colorectal peritoneal carcinomatosis (PC): PRODIGE 7. *J. Clin. Oncol.* 36 (18 Suppl).
8. Willaert, W., Van de Sande, L., Van Daele, E. et al. (2019). Safety and preliminary efficacy of electrostatic precipitation during pressurized intraperitoneal aerosol chemotherapy (PIPAC) for unresectable carcinomatosis. *Eur. J. Surg. Oncol.* 45 (12): 2302–2309.
9. Alyami, M., Mercier, F., Siebert, M. et al. (2019). Unresectable peritoneal metastasis treated by pressurized intraperitoneal aerosol chemotherapy (PIPAC) leading to cytoreductive surgery and hyperthermic intraperitoneal chemotherapy. *Eur. J. Surg. Oncol.* Jun 21:S0748-7983(19)30522-0.
10. Simkens, G.A., van Oudheusden, T.R., Braam, H.J. et al. (2016). Cytoreductive surgery and HIPEC offers similar outcomes in patients with rectal peritoneal metastases compared to colon cancer patients: a matched case control study. *J. Surg. Oncol.* 113 (5): 548–553.
11. Tonello, M., Sommariva, A., Pirozzolo, G. et al. (2019). Colic and rectal tumors with peritoneal metastases treated with cytoreductive surgery and HIPEC: one homogeneous condition or two different diseases? A systematic review and meta-analysis. *Eur. J. Surg. Oncol.* 45 (11): 2003–2008.
12. Shinde, R.S., Acharya, R., Kumar, N.A. et al. (2019). Pelvic exenteration with cytoreductive surgery and hyperthermic intraperitoneal chemotherapy (CRS + HIPEC) for rectal cancer-case series with review of literature. *Indian J. Surg. Oncol.* 10 (Suppl 1): 80–83.
13. Honore, C., Gelli, M., Francoual, J. et al. (2017). Ninety percent of the adverse outcomes occur in 10% of patients: can we identify the populations at high risk of developing peritoneal metastases after curative surgery for colorectal cancer? *Int. J. Hyperth.* 33 (5): 505–510.
14. Goere, D., Glehen, O., Quenet, F. et al. (2018). Results of a randomized phase 3 study evaluating the potential benefit of a second-look surgery plus HIPEC in patients at high risk of developing colorectal peritoneal metastases (PROPHYLOCHIP- NTC01226394). *J. Clin. Oncol.* 36 (15 Suppl).

15 PelvEx Collaborative (2019). Surgical and survival outcomes following pelvic exenteration for locally advanced primary rectal cancer: results from an international collaboration. *Ann. Surg.* 269 (2): 315–321.

16 Elias, D., Faron, M., Goere, D. et al. (2014). A simple tumor load-based nomogram for surgery in patients with colorectal liver and peritoneal metastases. *Ann. Surg. Oncol.* 21 (6): 2052–2058.

17 Faron, M., Macovei, R., Goere, D. et al. (2016). Linear relationship of peritoneal cancer index and survival in patients with peritoneal metastases from colorectal cancer. *Ann. Surg. Oncol.* 23 (1): 114–119.

15

Minimally Invasive Pelvic Exenteration

Danielle Collins[1], Christos Kontovounisios[2,3,4], Shahnawaz Rasheed[4], and Paris Tekkis[2,3,4]

[1] *Edinburgh Colorectal Unit, Western General Hospital, Edinburgh, UK*
[2] *Department of Colorectal Surgery, Chelsea and Westminster NHS Foundation Trust, London, UK*
[3] *Department of Surgery and Cancer, Imperial College, London, UK*
[4] *Department of Colorectal Surgery, Royal Marsden Hospital, London, UK*

Background

The surgical approach to advanced pelvic malignancy or recurrent pelvic disease has largely depended on open surgical techniques. Recurrent disease is generally associated with re-operative surgery in an irradiated field with distortion of surgical planes making a minimally invasive approach extremely challenging. In addition, there is debate regarding the role of minimally invasive surgery (MIS) in the management of advanced disease or recurrence. However, in the last decade (since 2010) advances in technology (ergonomic instruments, improved vessel sealers, better optics, 3D imaging) have evolved to facilitate more minimally invasive approaches to complex pelvic surgery.

In cases of locally advanced pelvic malignancy or disease recurrence, achieving a negative resection margin (R0) is the most important factor for disease survival [1–4]. Multivisceral resection, extended lymphadenectomy, or total pelvic exenteration (TPE) involving en-bloc resection of the rectum, bladder, and internal genital organs provides the best chance for cure [5, 6]. However, extended pelvic resections beyond normal anatomical planes are technically demanding procedures, often requiring a multidisciplinary surgical input which may include urology, gynecology, neurosurgery, vascular, orthopedic, and plastic surgeons [7]. Given these technical considerations and varying levels of expertise in minimally invasive techniques between disciplines, a minimally invasive approach to complex pelvic malignancy represents a unique challenge. Incomplete resection rates for a laparoscopic approach for locally advanced rectal cancer have been reported in the range of 20–30% [8, 9]. However, with the advent of robotic surgery, a minimally invasive approach is more feasible [10, 11], with good results in expert hands.

History of Minimally Invasive Pelvic Exenterative Surgery

A significant amount of the available literature relating to minimally invasive exenterative surgery is derived from the laparoscopic management of advanced gynecological disease. One of the first cases of a laparoscopic exenteration was reported in 2004 describing an anterior exenteration with continent bladder

Surgical Management of Advanced Pelvic Cancer, First Edition.
Edited by Michael E. Kelly and Desmond C. Winter.
© 2022 John Wiley & Sons Ltd. Published 2022 by John Wiley & Sons Ltd.

reconstruction for a locally advanced cervical cancer with a vesico-vaginal fistula [12]. A large case series of laparoscopic anterior exenteration for locally advanced or recurrent cervical cancer has been reported from an Indian group with good oncological outcomes [13]. In their approach, a laparoscopic uretero-sigmoidostomy was performed for urinary diversion.

The majority of reports of laparoscopic exenteration in colorectal cancer come from Japan, where laparoscopic pelvic sidewall lymphadenectomy is routine [14, 15]. In addition, laparoscopic radical cystectomy and ileal conduit formation may be necessary. It has been shown that patients undergoing laparoscopic exenteration have a shorter length of stay, although mean operating times can be longer. The ability to perform laparoscopic urinary diversion has been an important step in progressing to a totally minimally invasive pelvic exenteration [16].

The first robotic exenteration was described in 2009 for a recurrent cervical cancer with a malignant recto-vaginal fistula [17]. The patient underwent a robotic-assisted TPE with omentoplasty, end colostomy, and formation of a robotic-assisted ileal conduit. The authors recorded an operating time of just over six hours. The earliest report in the colorectal literature was in 2003 when Shin et al. described three cases of robotic-assisted multivisceral resection for locally advanced rectal cancers involving the prostate and bladder [18]. Subsequently there have been several case series detailing single-institution experiences with robotic pelvic exenteration. Data from the University of Texas MD Anderson Cancer Center describe 36 patients undergoing robotic multivisceral resection or extramesorectal lymph node dissection for locally advanced rectal cancers [19]. Results from this cohort demonstrated a 100% R0 resection rate, with a median hospital stay of four days despite operative times of nearly seven hours. There was only one conversion to open surgery and this was due to inability of the patient to tolerate the Trendelenburg position. Winters et al. describe a case series of three patients undergoing a robotic-assisted TPE with minimally invasive rectus flap reconstruction of the perineum [20]. Operative time in this series ranged from 9.5 to 11 hours with an estimated blood loss of 500 cc which compares favorably to open TPE.

Rectal Cancer Beyond TME

There is likely to be an increasing role for robotic rectal cancer resection beyond total mesorectal excision (TME). A subset of patients requiring extra-levator abdomino-perineal resection (ELAPE) may benefit from a robotic abdominal approach [21]. ELAPE involves total mesorectal excision up to the coccyx and pelvic peritoneal dissection anterior to Denonvillier's fascia with either mesh or soft tissue reconstruction of the perineal defect [22]. ELAPE is a more radical approach for locally advanced or recurrent low rectal cancers. Feasibility of robotic resection for recurrent rectal cancer has also been demonstrated; however, careful patient selection is paramount [23].

Advantages of a Robotic Approach to Exenteration

Robotic surgery has several benefits over traditional laparoscopic surgery particularly for pelvic work. A 3D magnified view that can be controlled by the surgeon and not the assistant is a major advantage. In addition, the robotic platform offers fixed traction, multiple ports, and better ergonomics for the surgeon which is important in a long procedure. Precise dissection of pelvic sidewall nodes and para-aortic nodes as well as nerve sparing procedures are all facilitated by a robotic approach. Furthermore, EndoWrist technology allows for articulated instruments that have greater degrees of freedom than traditional laparoscopic instruments as well as providing excellent vessel-sealing capabilities [24]. The surgeon may, however, be disadvantaged from a lack of haptic feedback and, in the early learning phases, the time taken to dock and undock the robot. This could potentially be an issue if a rapid conversion to open surgery is required in case of an intraoperative catastrophe.

Surgical Planning and Reconstruction

There are several factors that should be considered to ensure patient suitability for minimally invasive exenteration. These can be subdivided into patient factors, disease factors, and technical factors.

Patient Factors

Patients who have undergone previous open surgery may not be candidates for a minimally invasive approach due to formation of adhesions or loss of planes in a re-operative/irradiated field. In addition, patient comorbidities may preclude a laparoscopic/robotic approach due to inability to tolerate a pneumo-peritoneum or steep Trendelenburg for several hours. As with all patients undergoing pelvic exenteration, preoperative assessment is essential to minimize postoperative morbidity.

Disease Factors

It is crucial that staging is accurate and up to date prior to embarking on a multivisceral resection. In addition to good cross-sectional imaging, endoscopic (colonoscopy/cystoscopy) may be necessary. Evidence of distant metastatic disease is generally a contraindication to exenteration. All cases should be discussed at a multidisciplinary meeting involving pathologists, radiologists, radiation and medical oncologist, and surgeons.

For the purposes of exenterative surgery, the pelvis is divided into four anatomical compartments: axial, anterior, posterior, and lateral [25]. The axial compartment consists of the vagina, uterus, ovaries, fallopian tubes, broad ligament, round ligament of the uterus, rectum, and pelvic floor muscle (iliococcygeus part of levator ani). The anterior compartment comprises the bladder, prostate, seminal vesicles, vas deferens, urethra, urogenital diaphragm, dorsal vein complex, obturator internus and externus muscles, anterior pelvic floor muscles, pelvic bone (pubic symphysis, superior and inferior pubic rami), and obturator nerves and vessels. The posterior compartment consists of the rectum, pelvic floor (coccygeus muscle), internal iliac vessels, piriformis muscle, sacral nerves S1–S4, pelvic bone (sacrum and coccyx), anterior sacrococcygeal ligament, and medial sacrotuberous and sacrospinous ligaments. The lateral compartment equates to the pelvic sidewall structures: ureters, internal, and external iliac vessels, piriformis, obturator internus and coccygeus muscles, lateral sacrotuberous and sacrospinous ligaments attached to the ischium, ischium (including tuberosity and spine), lumbosacral trunk, and sciatic nerve distal to ischial spine [22].

In terms of surgical approach, an anterior exenteration involves removal of the reproductive organs, bladder, and urethra. A posterior exenteration often involves excision of the rectum as well as the reproductive organs. A TPE removes all pelvic organs as well as ligamentous and muscular supports. This may be extended to bony structures and nerves [26, 27].

Technical Factors

Technical factors involve determining whether the tumor is resectable as well as the operative approach. If a large perineal defect necessitating extensive soft tissue reconstruction is required (e.g. VRAM flap), a minimally invasive approach would not be advisable. Also, if an incision is required for specimen extraction or ileal conduit formation, a minimally invasive approach may be redundant. It is therefore important to have a preoperative discussion with relevant specialties (plastic surgeons, urologist, gynecologists, vascular surgeons, neurosurgeons) prior to defining the operative approach.

Robotic Surgical Approach

Patients are placed in the Lloyd-Davies position in varying degrees of Trendelenburg according to surgeon preference. Consideration should be given to preoperative ureteric stenting in certain cases. Attention should be paid to patient positioning and any pressure areas should be padded. Surgeons should be conscious of the length of the operation and the risk for compartment syndrome or deep vein thrombosis (DVT) with prolonged surgery. Port placement is very much up to surgeon preference; however, fortunately the same ports can generally be used to perform the rectal dissection as dissection of the anterior and lateral compartments. Often the posterior rectal dissection is performed first as mobilization of the anterior structures (bladder, uterus) may lead to an obstructed view. A perineal incision is often made and this can therefore be used as a site for specimen extraction. Shin et al. describe a minimally invasive rectus abdominus flap which requires a small fascial incision and can keep the abdominal scars to a minimum [19].

Outcomes

To date, the majority of published evidence on minimally invasive exenterative surgery has been retrospective, single-institution series of carefully selected patients. Nonetheless, MIS has been shown to confer benefits in terms of less postoperative pain, shorter hospital stay, and earlier recovery [28, 29]. In addition, there appears to be a lower rate of blood loss [14]. Operative times, however, are longer, although this does not appear to translate to an increase in morbidity. Most importantly, there does not appear to be a compromise in terms of oncological resection with a minimally invasive approach. The PelvEx Collaborative recently conducted a meta-analysis of the current literature [30] which comprised four studies totaling 170 patients. A comparison of minimally invasive (20%) to open surgery (80%) was performed. The current evidence consists of mainly low-volume case series and differs in terms of disease subtypes. Nevertheless, this meta-analysis observed that a minimally invasive approach seemed to confer a lower rate of morbidity and blood loss at a cost of longer operating times. Surgeons, however, should be cognizant of the fact that MIS exenteration may be unsuitable or unsafe in cases where sacrectomy, nerve involvement, or extensive soft tissue reconstruction is required.

Future Directions

Robotic pelvic exenteration provides a unique platform for the minimally invasive multidisciplinary management of advanced and recurrent pelvic cancers. It is interesting that surgical techniques have been borrowed and refined from various specialties to be able to tackle these complex cases. Although the operative times may be longer than the current gold standard open approach, we are only at the upstroke of the learning curve. Clearly, patient selection is key in MIS exenteration, but as technology and surgical skill advance, a robotic multivisceral approach to complex pelvic malignancy may become more mainstream.

Summary Box

- Minimally invasive exenteration is feasible in highly selected cases.
- Preoperative planning with up-to-date imaging and MDT discussion is important in identifying suitable candidates.
- An experienced MDT should be involved including colorectal surgeons, gyne-oncologists, urologists, plastic surgeons, and anesthetists.
- Similar outcomes compared to the gold standard of open surgery have been achieved at high-volume centers.
- Advantages may include less blood loss, shorter length of stay, and decreased morbidity compared to open surgery. This is at the expense of longer operative times.

References

1 Kusters, M., Austin, K.K.S., Solomon, M.J. et al. (2015). Survival after pelvic exenteration for T4 rectal cancer. *Br. J. Surg.* 102: 125–131.
2 Harris, D.A., Davies, M., Lucas, M.G. et al. (2011). Multivisceral resection for primary locally advanced rectal carcinoma. *Br. J. Surg.* 98: 582–588.
3 Radwan, R.W., Jones, H.G., Rawat, N. et al. (2015). Determinants of survival following pelvic exenteration for primary rectal cancer. *Br. J. Surg.* 102: 1278–1284.
4 Bhangu, A., Ali, S.M., Darzi, A. et al. (2012). Meta-analysis of survival based on resection margin status following surgery for recurrent rectal cancer. *Colorectal Dis.* 14 (12): 1457–1466.
5 PelvEx Collaborative (2019). Surgical and survival outcomes following pelvic exenteration for locally advanced primary rectal cancer: results from an international collaboration. *Ann. Surg.* 269 (2): 315–321.
6 PelvEx Collaborative (2018). Factors affecting outcomes following pelvic exenteration for locally recurrent rectal cancer. *Br. J. Surg.* 105 (6): 650–657.
7 Beyond TME Collaborative (2013). Consensus statement on the multidisciplinary management of patients with recurrent and primary rectal cancer beyond total mesorectal excision planes. *Br. J. Surg.* 100 (8): E1–E33.
8 Bretagnol, F., Dedieu, A., Zappa, M. et al. (2011). T4 colorectal cancer: is laparoscopic resection contraindicated? *Colorectal Dis.* 13: 138–143.
9 Kim, K.Y., Hwang, D.W., Park, Y.K., and Lee, H.S. (2012). A single surgeon's experience with 54 consecutive cases of multivisceral resection for locally advanced primary colorectal cancer: can the laparoscopic approach be performed safely? *Surg. Endosc.* 26: 493–500.
10 Shin, U.S., Nancy You, Y., Nguyen, A.T. et al. (2016). Oncologic outcomes of extended robotic resection for rectal cancer. *Ann. Surg. Oncol.* 23 (7): 2249–2257.
11 Reddy, S.S., Smith, R.K., Viterbo, R. et al. (2014). 465 robotic assisted laparoscopic total pelvic Exenteration. *Gastroenterology* 146 (5): S1015.
12 Pomel, C. and Castaigne, D. (2004). Laparoscopic hand-assisted Miami pouch following laparoscopic anterior pelvic exenteration. *Gynecol. Oncol.* 93 (2): 543–545.
13 Puntambekar, S., Sharma, V., Jamkar, A.V. et al. (2016). Our experience of laparoscopic anterior exenteration in locally advanced cervical carcinoma. *J. Minim. Invasive Gynecol.* 23 (3): 396–403.
14 Nagasue, Y., Akiyoshi, T., Ueno, M. et al. (2013). Laparoscopic versus open multivisceral resection for primary colorectal cancer: comparison of perioperative outcomes. *J. Gastrointest. Surg.* 17 ((7): 1299–1305.
15 Uehara, K., Nakamura, H., Yoshino, Y. et al. (2016). Initial experience of laparoscopic pelvic exenteration and comparison with conventional open surgery. *Surg. Endosc.* 30 (1): 132–138.
16 Ogura, A., Akiyoshi, T., Konishi, T. et al. (2016). Safety of laparoscopic pelvic exenteration with urinary diversion for colorectal malignancies. *World J. Surg.* 40 (5): 1236–1243.
17 Lim, P.C. (2009). Robotic assisted total pelvic exenteration: a case report. *Gynecol. Oncol.* 115 (2): 310–311.
18 Shin, J.W., Kim, J., Kwak, J.M. et al. (2014). First report: robotic pelvic exenteration for locally advanced rectal cancer. *Colorectal Dis.* 16 (1): O9–O14.
19 Shin, U.S., Nancy You, Y., Nguyen, A.T. et al. (2016). Oncologic outcomes of extended robotic resection for rectal cancer. *Ann. Surg. Oncol.* 23 (7): 2249–2257.
20 Winters, B.R., Mann, G.N., Louie, O., and Wright, J.L. (2015). Robotic total pelvic exenteration with laparoscopic rectus flap: initial experience. *Case Rep. Surg.* 2015: 835425.

21 Baird, D.L.H., Simillis, C., Kontovounisios, C. et al. (2017). A systematic review of transabdominal levator division during abdominoperineal excision of the rectum (APER). *Tech. Coloproctol.* 21 (9): 701–707.

22 Singh, P., Teng, E., Cannon, L.M. et al. (2015). Dynamic article: tandem robotic technique of extralevator abdominoperineal excision and rectus abdominis muscle harvest for immediate closure of the pelvic floor defect. *Dis. Colon Rectum* 58 (9): 885–891.

23 Nanayakkara, P.R., Ahmed, S.A., Oudit, D. et al. (2014). Robotic assisted minimally invasive pelvic exenteration in advanced rectal cancer: review and case report. *J. Robot. Surg.* 8 (2): 173–175.

24 Lin, S., Jiang, H.G., Zhi-Heng, C. et al. (2011). Meta-analysis of robotic and laparoscopic surgery for treatment of rectal cancer. *World J. Gastroenterol.* 17 (47): 5214–5220.

25 Kontovounisios, C. and Tekkis, P. (2017). Locally advanced disease and pelvic exenterations. 30 (05): 404–414.

26 Dresen, R.C., Gosens, M.J., Martijn, H. et al. (2008). Radical resection after IORT-containing multimodality treatment is the most important determinant for outcome in patients treated for locally recurrent rectal cancer. *Ann. Surg. Oncol.* 15 (07): 1937–1947.

27 Suzuki, K., Dozois, R.R., Devine, R.M. et al. (1996). Curative reoperations for locally recurrent rectal cancer. *Dis. Colon Rectum* 39 (07): 730–736.

28 Jayne, D.G., Guillou, P.J., Thorpe, H. et al. (2007). Randomized trial of laparoscopic-assisted resection of colorectal carcinoma: 3-year results of the UK MRC CLASICC trial group. *J. Clin. Oncol.* 25: 3061–3068.

29 Clinical Outcomes of Surgical Therapy Study Group (2004). A comparison of laparoscopically assisted and open colectomy for colon cancer. *N. Engl. J. Med.* 350: 2050–2059.

30 PelvEx Collaborative (2018). Minimally invasive surgery techniques in pelvic exenteration: a systematic and meta-analysis review. *Surg. Endosc.* 32: 4707–4715.

16

Stoma Considerations Following Exenteration
Gabrielle H. van Ramshorst[1] and Jurriaan B. Tuynman[2]

[1] *Department of Gastrointestinal Surgery, Ghent University Hospital, Ghent, Belgium*
[2] *Department of Surgery, Amsterdam UMC, Amsterdam, The Netherlands*

Background

The majority of patients who undergo exenterative surgery for urological, gynecological, or colorectal cancer will require urinary and/or fecal diversion. The decision-making and formation of a stoma can be complex, with major impact on the quality of life (QoL) of patients. As large pelvic defects are created, the harvest of myocutaneous abdominal wall flaps adds extra complexity to the reconstruction of the abdominal wall and the placement of one or more stomas. Previous (chemo)radiation therapy is widely used as neoadjuvant treatment and is a major risk factor for early and late complications [1]. Patients needing pelvic exenteration have a QoL heavily influenced by morbidity relating to stoma complications. In a prospective study among gynecologic cancer patients who underwent pelvic exenteration, stoma-related QoL was inversely correlated with body image distress scores and sexual discomfort scores [2]. The complexity of exenterative procedure often needs tailoring to consider the restorative part of the surgery (including abdominal wall repair and stoma formation). This chapter describes various possible urinary and/or combined fecal diversion methods.

Urinary Diversion

The standard urinary diversion made by urologists is the ileal conduit placed in the right part of the lower abdomen, often being part of a Bricker procedure for bladder resection. Since the complexity of exenterative surgery often requires other possibilities, a range of procedures have been described and used. Diversion of urine can be performed and the creation of urinary pouches using the ileum, sigmoid, or transverse colon. A tailor-made approach and informing patients preoperatively of the various treatment options and the outcomes with regard to body image, complications, and revisional surgery is essential.

Incontinent Urinary Diversions

Ileal Conduit

Ileal conduit, first described by Bricker in 1950, has remained the popular option for urinary diversion [3]. A 10- to 12-cm ileal segment is isolated approximately 20 cm proximal to the ileocecal valve. After enteroenterostomy of the proximal and distal ileum, the segment is

---

Surgical Management of Advanced Pelvic Cancer, First Edition.
Edited by Michael E. Kelly and Desmond C. Winter.
© 2022 John Wiley & Sons Ltd. Published 2022 by John Wiley & Sons Ltd.

placed posterior to the anastomosis. The mesenteric window is closed and the left ureter is brought beneath the sigmoid mesocolon inferior to the level of the inferior mesenteric artery. Both ureters are anastomosed with the ileal conduit over stents. The distal end of the ileal segment is fashioned as an ileostomy in the right lower abdominal quadrant [3, 4].

Few reports have been published on variations of this technique, including presence of ileostomy, flap reconstruction, and limited ureter length. Previously created loop ileostomies can be converted in urinary conduits by stapling of the efferent ileum and creation of a new enteroenterostomy proximal to the conduit. In case of myocutaneous rectus abdominis flap reconstruction, the ileal conduit can be brought out through the internal oblique muscle, lateral to the (right) rectus muscle sheath above the level of the arcuate line [5]. If one or both ureters are short, the conduit can be placed anterior to the enteroenterostomy ("water over the bridge") through the mesentery of the right colon. The ureters are then anastomosed to the retroperitoneal tail of the conduit and stented [6].

Russo et al. reported on a series of 47 patients who underwent urinary diversion after total pelvic exenteration for rectal cancer (44 of whom had ileal conduits) [7]. Median follow-up was 17 months. Complications occurred in 17%. Long-term complications such as skin excoriation (parastomal dermatitis), parastomal hernia, and uretral stenosis are relatively common after Bricker deviation with rates > 60% of cases [8].

Transverse Colon Urinary Diversion

The rational of using transverse colon for urinary diversion is the use of non-irradiated bowel. Ten to twenty centimeters of the transverse colon is isolated and used as a conduit, with intact blood supply from the mesentery including the middle colic artery [9]. The proximal and distal transverse colon are reanastomosed after creation of a mesenteric defect for the left ureter. The conduit is then secured to the peritoneum. This technique can also be used in case of short ureters. In a series of 86 patients (and 165 ureterocolic anastomoses) published by Segreti et al., early stent dislodgment (< 24 hours) occurred in five patients, of whom three developed ureteral stricture and one patient eventually had loss of kidney function [9].

Distal Colon Urinary Diversion

Teixeira et al. reported the results of 27 patients who had a colonic conduit following pelvic exenteration compared with 47 patients having an ileal conduit [10]. Initially, the colonic conduit was preferred if the ileum had significant radiotherapy effects. Colonic conduit was also the preferred method if a colostomy was already in place. The ureters were spatulated and anastomosed end-to-end and end-to-side to the distal part of the remaining colon. Stents were placed and the colon conduit and end colostomy were sutured to the skin at separate sites. If there was already a colostomy in place, a conduit was created after transsection of the proximal bowel. A new colostomy was created at the contralateral side. The combined incidence of conduit-related complications (fistula, leakage, drained collections, sepsis) was significantly higher in the ileal conduit group compared to the colonic conduit group (40% vs. 19%, $p < 0.001$) [10].

A series of 21 patients by Meijer et al. also described the use of the distal colon (sigmoid) as a conduit [11]. Short-term complications were found in 11/21 patients, with five patients requiring stents or nephrostomy for management of post-renal obstruction. One patient with persistent urinary leakage required revision [11]. There are also concerns of colorectal cancer developing in the pouch, which is reportedly higher if the sigmoid colon is used instead of the ileum. This mechanism has been related to nitrosamine bacterial production in the reservoir, warranting long-term surveillance/follow-up [12, 13].

Comparative studies on urinary diversion are scarce. Tabbaa et al. compared short-term outcomes for incontinent ileal (n = 129), sigmoid (n = 26), and transverse (n = 11) colonic conduits in a retrospective series of 166 patients with gynecological malignancies [14]. Significant conduit-related complications included ureteral stricture or anastomotic leak, conduit leak or obstruction, ischemia or stent obstruction requiring reinterventions, and/or renal failure. Complication rates for the ileal, sigmoid, and transverse colon groups were 22, 29, and 0% respectively. Eight of the 34 patients had complications within 90 days requiring reoperation (7/27 ileal group; 1/7 sigmoid group) and 16 required an interventional radiology procedure (11/27 ileal group; 5/7 sigmoid group). In the long term, 9/129 patients in the ileal group developed complications; four ureteral strictures, two renal failures, two ureteral obstructions, and one conduit leak/obstruction. Two patients were affected in the transverse group (one ureteral obstruction and one renal failure) and none in the sigmoid colon group. The transverse colon group had a statistically significant lower rate of general complications than the ileal group (19% vs. 40%, p < 0.001) [14].

Soper et al. reported a series of 69 women following pelvic exenteration for gynecologic malignancy [15]. They found significantly more surgical morbidity in patients who had an ileal conduit without gracilis flap reconstruction compared to patients who had a transverse colon conduit (42% vs. 23%). Also, 61% of patients with sigmoid colon conduits developed serious complications (mainly stomal strictures, fistula formation, small bowel obstruction, and ureteral obstruction) [15].

Direct Cutaneous Ureterostomy

This technique has been associated with high long-term morbidity (> 50%), including stenosis of the cutaneous ureteral meatus. Stenosis will often require dilatation and/or revisional surgery. These diversions have been associated with leaking external stomal appliances. In addition due to the high incidence of complications, including obstruction-related renal failure, this technique has been abandoned [1].

Continent Urinary Diversions

Continent diversion options for urinary diversions include the use of the appendix as the continence mechanism (Mitrofanoff valve, Penn pouch), the intussuscepted nipple valve (Kock, Mainz, UCLA pouch), tapered terminal ileum, ileocecal valve and right colon (Indiana pouch, Florida pouch, and Miami pouch), or the orthotopic neobladder.

Accumulation of urine in continent urinary reservoirs can result in metabolic acidosis by reabsorption of ammonia, chloride, and hydrogen and secretion of bicarbonate and sodium. These disturbances are more common if the jejunum is used instead of the ileum. A long conduit can also result in stasis of urine, resulting in hyperchloremic and hypocalcemic metabolic acidosis. The most commonly reported complications relating to continent reservoirs are urinary tract infections, ureteral strictures, and difficulty in self-catheterization [16]. In the long term, use of irradiated ureter and/or bowel can cause excessive fibrosis. Ureteral stenosis can occur at the uretero-ileal anastomosis. Stenosis or fistulization can be symptoms of cancer recurrence. Patients are advised to irrigate the pouch regularly (daily–weekly) to prevent accumulation of mucus. Ureteral obstructions can be managed with percutaneous nephrostomy and ureteral stenting [1]. Other long-term problems include ureteral stones, related to presence of foreign body such as staples, ureteral stenosis, and renal insufficiency [17]. An overview of techniques for continent catheterizable pouches was published by Rink et al. [18].

Miami Pouch

The Miami pouch technique was introduced in 1988 by Bajany and Politano, and involves the creation of a pouch using the terminal ileum and ascending colon [19]. A 10-cm segment of terminal ileum is isolated along with the ascending colon. The appendix is removed and the colon segment is irrigated and detubularized. A catheter is inserted into the cecum through the ileocecal valve. The distal ileum is tapered by stapling, and the valve mechanism is reinforced with three purse-string sutures. Stents are placed in both ureters, which are anastomosed to the colon. A lateral opening is created in the pouch, allowing insertion of a 24-Fr catheter, and the pouch is secured to the abdominal wall.

Ramirez et al. published a series of 40 patients with gynecologic malignancies [20]. Sixty percent of patients developed postoperative conduit reservoir complications, including urinary tract infections or pyelonephritis (n = 12), urinary stomal stricture, acute renal failure, ureteral stricture, or anastomotic leak (all n = 1). Fifteen patients had to undergo surgical procedures for reservoir stones, stomal strictures, ureteral anastomotic stricture, or fistula formation. Late complications included recurrent urinary tract infections or pyelonephritis (n = 14), urinary stomal strictures (n = 9), stones (n = 7), ureteral strictures (n = 2), acute renal failure (n = 1), and pouch-cutaneous fistula (n = 1). However, at a median follow-up of 28 months, 90% of patients were continent for urine [20].

In a series of 41 patients with gynecologic malignancies, late urinary complications were found in 66% of Miami pouch patients [21]. Eight patients needed uretero-renal dilatation and five patients were reoperated for, respectively, urine leakage, stomal stenosis, and pouch perforation, and two patients with pouch stones. Sanchez-Valdivieso et al. reported continency in 22/23 patients (96%) who had a Miami pouch after anterior or total pelvic externation for gynecological malignancy after a median follow-up of 25 months [22].

Indiana Pouch

Rowland's first description of the Indiana pouch technique dates from 1985 [23, 24]. This pouch consists of a detubularized right colon segment with a plicated ileocecal valve and tapered distal ileum. The hydraulic valve design relies on a fixed resistance to outflow. Stomal incontinence occurs once the internal reservoir pressure rises [25].

Mannel et al. described a series of 37 patients [26]. After a median follow-up of 11 months, urinary tract infections or pyelonephritis were observed in four patients, strictures in two patients, and reflux in four patients. Mild to moderate hydronephrosis was also reported in five patients, none of whom developed renal failure. Daytime continence was achieved in all patients and 89% had nocturnal continence. Three patients required revisional surgery for stomal stenosis and catheterization difficulties [26].

Castillo et al. reported on continent urinary reservoirs following exenteration [27]. Postoperative complications occurred in 19% of patients, including urinary sepsis, surgical wound infection, and ileocolonic fistula with peritonitis, requiring reconstruction of an ileostomy and mucous fistula. After a mean follow-up of 56 months, 32% of patients developed reservoir-related complications: ureteral anastomosis stenosis (n = 11), cutaneous stoma stenosis (n = 9), and renal stone formation (n = 6). Interventions for these complications were not reported [27]. Husain et al. reported on 33 patients with gynecologic malignancies who received Indiana pouches, 13 of whom had a low rectal anastomosis [28]. Alarmingly, 7 of these 13 patients developed anastomotic leakage, one of whom died. Two patients developed rectovaginal fistulas and required end colostomies, leaving only four patients with bowel continuity [28].

Uretero-ileocecal Appendicostomy

Uretero-ileocecal appendicostomy could be considered as a modification of the Penn pouch, using a detubularized colonic segment folded into a U-shape. The tip of the appendix is removed and a 14- to 16-Fr catheter is inserted into the lumen. Then the appendix is folded cephalad and buried in a cecal submucosal tunnel. The ureters are anastomosed to a connected 15-cm segment of terminal ileum and stented. The appendiceal stoma is formed at the umbilicus or right lower quadrant. Bochner et al. published a series of 14 patients who underwent total or anterior pelvic exenteration [25]. After a median follow-up of 10 months, four patients developed stoma-related complications, including stenosis requiring dilatation and false passage requiring an indwelling catheter, and two patients disruption of the stomal–umbilical anastomosis. One patient underwent surgical revision of the stoma and the other patient died before revision could be performed. All patients reported continence with catheterization intervals of three to six hours [25].

Orthotopic Neobladder

Orthotopic neobladder is well known for reconstruction after cystectomy. It is an alternative for patients without disease of the urethra requiring uretherectomy. The technique allows voiding via the urethra with urinary continence. The pressure within the reservoir needs to be lower than the resting pressure of the urethra. Transsection of the musculature of the ileal loop, also called detubularization, increases the compliance of the N- or Y-shaped reservoir by avoiding intestinal peristalsis [29]. Omentum can be placed between a colorectal anastomosis and the neobladder to reduce the risk of fistulization. Though this technique is well known for reconstruction after cystectomy, it has only been described in three case series after pelvic exenteration. Yamamoto et al. described five patients with rectal carcinoma, with one patient needing an ileal conduit because of partial neobladder necrosis and minor leakage of the neobladder [29]. Koda et al. reported on five patients with advanced colorectal cancer [30]. One patient developed a fistula between the coloanal and neobladder–urethral anastomoses, and a transverse colostomy was created. Another patient developed minor anastomotic leakage of the coloanal anastomosis, which was managed conservatively [30]. Finally, Chiva et al. published a series of six patients with cervical cancer, all trained in self-catheterization of the bladder [31]. One patient developed a neobladder anastomotic leak which was managed conservatively, two patients suffered from episodes of metabolic acidosis due to bicarbonate loss, and two patients developed late neobladder anastomotic leaks [31]. When compared with ileal conduit, the formation of an orthotopic neobladder extends operative time by approximately one hour [29]. Both Yamamoto and Koda reported that daytime continence was achieved in all of their patients, with nighttime voiding needed to maintain nocturnal continence [29, 30]. Chiva et al. reported satisfactory to good continence after six months of follow-up [31].

Comparison of Continent and Incontinent Urinary Diversions

Comparative studies on continent and incontinent urinary diversion techniques are scarce. Martinez et al. compared QoL after pelvic exenteration for gynecologic malignancy in a French multicenter prospective study [32]. Patients with continent urinary diversion had worse overall QoL scores than patients with incontinent urinary diversion at one month after surgery. This effect is thought to be related to the learning curve of self-catheterization, which has been reported to be a source of psychological stress [33]. However, after one year, similar scores were found for both groups for overall QoL, physical, cognitive, and social function [32].

Forner et al. compared outcomes of 33 gynecologic oncology patients with a variation of a continent ileocecal pouch, using the appendix as stoma at the umbilicus, to 67 patients with an ileal conduit [34]. Operation time and postoperative hospital stay were significantly longer in the pouch group. The pouch group reported significantly more complications than the ileal conduit group (48% vs. 31%, p = 0.03). Surgical treatment was needed for seven patients with an ileal conduit and six patients with an ileocecal pouch. One patient in the ileal conduit group developed renal failure [34].

Goldberg et al. surveyed 103 patients regarding their satisfaction after total pelvic exenteration. Fourteen patients developed anastomotic leaks, without a difference between ileal conduit and continent conduits (Indiana or Miami pouch variation) [35]. Eighty-nine percent of 38 patients with continent conduits were continent. Six patients (16%) with continent conduits reported persistent problems with self-catheterization and 21 patients (54%) with continent conduits would prefer an ileal conduit if they could make the choice again. Self-catheterization is reportedly more difficult in case of a long ileal segment and adherence to the pelvic floor, for which anchoring to the abdominal wall is advised [35].

Urological Leaks

Urological leaks can be demonstrated by contrast extravasation on radiological imaging such as computer tomography (CT) scans or conduitograms. Leakage can occur due to ischemia, stomal stenosis, technical error, or iatrogenic perforation, and tend to be more frequent in patients with a body mass index > 30 kg/m^2 [21, 35]. Urine leaks from the ureteroenteric anastomosis can be considered anastomotic leaks, whereas leakage from other sites can be considered conduit leaks. Brown et al. described a clinical algorithm for the diagnosis and management of urological leaks following pelvic exenteration [36]. They recommend to perform regular drain creatinine studies, and to have a high index of suspicion of urological leaks in patients who remain septic in spite of appropriate treatment. Management may include percutaneous and/or transconduit drainage, insertion of nephrostomy tubes, or, eventually, surgical revision of the conduit. Urinary leakage has been observed to be more common in macroscopic irradical resections (R2) and total pelvic exenteration, involving all four quadrants of the pelvis [10]. Furthermore, Teixeira et al. found increased length of hospital stay and decreased survival (34 vs. 40 months, p = 0.04) [10]. Some have suggested that ongoing sepsis and pro-inflammatory cytokines may enhance tumor growth and proliferation [37, 38].

Fecal Diversion

Almost all patients with exenterative pelvic surgery require a fecal diversion, causing considerable impact on QoL. Having a stoma impacts body image, and sexual and social functioning [39]. Stoma-related problems such as skin erosion, swelling, pain, leakage, and prolapse can result in direct and indirect healthcare implications [40]. There are conflicting data regarding whether one versus two stoma influences overall QoL [41–44].

If patients initially present with symptoms of obstruction, a loop ileostomy, transverse colostomy, or end colostomy may be created to facilitate complete staging and/or neoadjuvant therapy Overall, there are several options for fecal diversion and these must be tailored to each individual patient [45].

Combined Fecal and Urinary Diversion

Wet Colostomy

When first reported in 1948, all pelvic exenterations resulted in a wet colostomy [46]. Both ureters were implanted in the end colostomy proximal to fecal output, causing a mixture of urine and feces. This resulted in electrolyte disturbances, malodour, and recurrent pyleonephritis, causing this technique to fall out of favor [46].

Double-Barreled Wet Colostomy

Double-barreled wet colostomy was first described in 1989 [47, 48]. The ureters are implanted on the antimesenteric side of the distal sigmoid colon. Thereafter, a diverting loop colostomy is created 8-10 cm proximal to the sigmoid stump. Fecal and urine streams are kept separate, reducing the risk of pyelonephritis. Patients can void urine bags when full or when intermittently mixed with feces. Stoma bags with air filter can help to reduce malodour if present.

Gan published a review comparing double-barreled wet colostomy versus ileal conduit with colostomy [49]. A retrospective series of 181 patients observed shorter median operating times for double-barreled wet colostomy compared to ileal conduit (32 vs. 64 minutes, $p < 0.0001$) [50]. Also, overall morbidity was significantly lower in the double-barreled wet colostomy group (11.5 vs. 23.4%, $p = 0.04$). Similarly, Backes et al. noted shorter mean operating times (610 vs. 720 minutes, $p = 0.04$), fewer leakages, less sepsis, and shorter median length of stay (14.5 vs. 26 days, $p = 0.01$) in the wet colostomy cohort when compared with ileal conduit patients [51]. In contrast, Chokshi et al. observed higher 30-day morbidity with double-barreled wet colostomies, and comparable operating times and length of hospital stay [52].

A small prospective series comparing plain wet colostomy and double-barreled wet colostomy in 15 patients observed no significant differences in short-term outcome. The plain wet colostomy was associated with higher rates of pyelonephritis (37% vs. 14%) in the double-barreled colostomy [53].

García-Granero et al. reported on 30 patients who underwent double-barreled wet colostomy, 14 patients with ileal conduit, and 2 patients with uretero-cutaneostomies [54]. Operative time and hospital stay were not reported per type of reconstruction. Urinary leakage was found in three ileal conduit patients (21%) and three double-barreled wet colostomy patients (10%). After a mean follow-up of 8.5 months, late urological complications including pyelonephritis, fistual formation, and stenosis had occurred in five and nine patients respectively [53]. A high incidence of urinary tract infections in double-barreled wet colostomy patients (5/10 patients) was also found by Bloemendaal et al. [55].

In case of a short ureter, creation of the double-barreled wet colostomy may not be possible. Macrí modified the technique by performing a uretero-ureterostomy and uretero-colic anastomosis [56]. In summary, the double-barreled colostomy for both urinary and fecal diversion seems to be associated with less morbidity compared to two stomas and better QoL. Long-term outcome and formation of dysplasia at the ureter–mucosal side needs evaluation.

Parastomal Hernia

The incidence of parastomal hernia is estimated at 50% for end colostomy and 30% for end ileostomy at 10 years [57]. Funahashi et al. reported on a Japanese cohort of 80 patients who underwent abdomino-perineal resection or pelvic exenteration [58]. After a median follow-up of 31 months, parastomal hernias were found in 22 (27.5%) of patients. Independent risk factors for the occurrence of parastomal hernia were body mass index, laparoscopic approach, and transperitoneal route of colostomy formation [58]. Other reported risk factors for parastomal hernia include female gender, age, and enlarged ostomy opening [59, 60]. Fascia defects smaller than 2.5 cm have been reported to lower the risk of developing a parastomal hernia [61].

The 2018 European Hernia Society guidelines on prevention and treatment of parastomal hernias strongly recommend to avoid performing a suture repair for elective parastomal hernia [62]. The use of a prophylactic synthetic non-absorbable mesh during construction of an end colostomy is also strongly recommended. There is not enough evidence to recommend specific surgical techniques (open or laparoscopic) or preferable types of meshes, although a flat mesh is preferred over keyhole meshes in laparoscopic repair [62]. Similar data and recommendations were published in a meta-analysis on this topic with additional trial sequential analysis [63].

Future Developments

The double-barreled wet colostomy technique has gained popularity in recent years. There are no large series comparing outcomes between double-barreled wet colostomy and continent urinary diversion techniques. Randomized studies are lacking and it is presumed that patient participation will be difficult when randomizing between one or two stomas. Data on long-term outcomes, e.g. development of malignancy in the colon reservoir and parastomal hernia, are scarce and will only be attainable for patient registries.

The use of mesh to prevent parastomal and incisional hernia is slowly gaining ground in the surgical community. However, there remains debate on surgical technique and type of mesh utilized.

Summary Box

- Plan the urinary and fecal diversion pre-operatively with multidisciplinary team input.
- Patient education and peri-operative counseling is associated with improved outcomes.
- Single stoma diversion using double-barreled wet colostomy should be considered especially if the rectus muscle is used for reconstruction.
- Factors to consider in decision-making are (i) abdominal wall reconstruction, (ii) extent of radiation, (iii) residual length of ureter, and (iv) patient preference.
- Prospective registry is needed to collect long-term outcome data.

References

1 Bladou, F., Houvenaeghel, G., Delpéro, J.R., and Guérinel, G. (1995). Incidence and management of major urinary complications after pelvic exenteration for gynecological malignancies. *J. Surg. Oncol.* 58: 91–96.

2 Armbruster, S.D., Sun, C.C., Westin, S.N. et al. (2018). Prospective assessment of patient-reported outcomes in gynecologic cancer patients before and after pelvic exenteration. *Gynecol. Oncol.* 149 (3): 484–490.

3 Bricker, E.M. (1950). Bladder substitution after pelvic evisceration. *Surg. Clin. North Am.* 30: 1511–1521.

4 Scherr, D.S. and Barocas, D.A. (2012). Ileal conduit. In: *Hinman's Atlas of Urologic Surgery*, 3rde (eds. J.A. Smith Jr., S.S. Howards, E.J. McGuire and G.M. Preminger), 615–628. Philadelphia: Elsevier Saunders.

5 Moller, F.V., Christensen, P., Rasmussen, P.C., and Laurberg, S. (2006). Ipsilateral ileal conduit placement at vertical rectus abdominis myocutaneous flap donor site in pelvic exenteration. *Dis. Colon Rectum* 49: 1458–1461.

6 Hatano, T., Hayakawa, M., Koyama, Y. et al. (1998). An alternative procedure for the creation of an ileal conduit in patients undergoing pelvic exenteration: dextrotransmesenteric location. *World J. Urol.* 16: 410–412.

7 Russo, P., Ravindran, B., Katz, J. et al. (1999). Urinary diversion after total pelvic exenteration for rectal cancer. *Ann. Surg. Oncol.* 6 (8): 732–738.

8 Sherwani Afak, Y., Wazir, B.S., Hamid, A. et al. (2009). Comparative study of various forms of urinary diversion after radical cystectomy in muscle invasive carcinoma urinary bladder. *Int. J. Health Sci. (Qassim)* 3 (1): 3–11.

9 Segreti, E.M., Morris, M., Levenback, C. et al. (1996). Transverse colon urinary diversion in gynecologic oncology. *Gynecol. Oncol.* 63: 66–70.

10 Teixeira, S.C., Ferenschild, F.T., Solomon, M.J. et al. (2012). Urological leaks after pelvic exenterations comparing formation of colonic and ileal conduits. *Eur. J. Surg. Oncol.* 38: 361–366.

11 Meijer, R.P., Mertens, L.S., Meinhardt, W. et al. (2015). The colon shuffle: a modified urinary diversion. *Eur. J. Surg. Oncol.* 41: 1264–1268.

12 Mundy, A.R. (1999). Metabolic complications of urinary diversion. *Lancet* 353 (9167): 1813–1814.

13 Malone, M.J., Izes, J.K., and Hurley, L.J. (1997). Carcinogenesis: the fate of intestinal segments used in urinary reconstruction. *Urol. Clin. North Am.* 24 (4): 723–728.

14 Tabbaa, Z.M., Janco, J.M.T., Mariani, A. et al. (2014). Short-term outcomes after incontinent conduit for gynecologic cancer: comparison of ileal, sigmoid, and transverse colon. *Gynecol. Oncol.* 133: 563–567.

15 Soper, J.T., Berchuck, A., Creasman, W.T., and Clarke-Pearson, D.L. (1989). Pelvic exenteration: factors associated with major surgical morbidity. *Gynecol. Oncol.* 35: 93–98.

16 Salom, E.M., Mendez, L.E., Schey, D. et al. (2004). Continent ileocolonic urinary reservoir (Miami pouch): the University of Miami experience over 15 years. *Am. J. Obstet. Gynecol.* 190: 994–1003.

17 Vergote, I.B. (1997). Exenterative surgery. *Curr. Opin. Obstet. Gynecol.* 9: 26–28.

18 Rink, M., Kluth, L., Eichelberg, E. et al. (2010). Continent catheterizable pouches for urinary diversion. *Eur. Urol. Suppl.* 9: 754–762.
Excellent overview of benefits and risks of continent pouches for urinary diversion.

19 Bajany, D.E. and Politano, V.A. (1988). Stapled and nonstapled tapered distal ileum for construction of a continent colonic urinary reservoir. *J. Urol.* 140: 491–494.

20 Ramirez, P.T., Modesitt, S.C., Morris, M. et al. (2002). Functional outcomes and complications of continent urinary diversions in patients with gynecologic malignancies. *Gynecol. Oncol.* 85: 285–291.

21 Karsenty, G., Moutardier, V., Lelong, B. et al. (2005). Long-term follow-up of continent urinary diversion after pelvic exenteration for gynecologic malignancies. *Gynecol. Oncol.* 97: 524–528.

22 Sanchez-Valdivieso, E., González Enciso, A., Herrera Gomez, A. et al. (2001). Experiencia preliminar con el reservorio urinario ileocolónico tipo Miami en la práctica de Ginecología Oncológica. *Arch. Esp. Urol.* 54 (4): 327–333.

23 Rowland, R.G., Mitchell, M.E., and Bihrle, R. (1985). The cecoileal continent urinary reservoir. *World J. Urol.* 3: 185–190.

24 Rowland, R.G., Mitchell, M.E., Birhle, R. et al. (1987). Indiana continent urinary reservoir. *J. Urol.* 137: 730–734.

25 Bochner, B.H., McCreath, W.A., Aubey, J.J. et al. (2004). Use of an ureteroileocecal

appendicostomy urinary reservoir in patients with recurrent pelvic malignancies treated with radiation. *Gynecol. Oncol.* 94: 140–146.
26 Mannel, R.S., Manetta, A., Buller, R.E. et al. (1995). Use of ileocecal continent urinary reservoir in patients with previous pelvic irradiation. *Gynecol. Oncol.* 59: 376–378.
27 Castillo, O.A., Aranguren, G., and Campos-Juanatey, F. (2014). Indiana continent catheterizable urinary reservoir. *Actas Urol. Esp.* 38 (6): 413–418.
28 Husain, A., Curtin, J., Brown, C. et al. (2000). Continent urinary diversion and low-rectal anastomosis in patients undergoing exenterative procedures for recurrent gynecologic malignancies. *Gynecol. Oncol.* 78: 208–211.
29 Yamamoto, S., Yamanaka, N., Maeda, T. et al. (2001). Ileal neobladder for urinary bladder replacement following total pelvic exenteration for rectal carcinoma. *Dig. Surg.* 18: 67–72.
30 Koda, K., Tobe, T., Takiguchi, N. et al. (2002). Pelvic exenteration for advanced colorectal cancer with reconstruction of urinary and sphincter functions. *Br. J. Surg.* 89 (10): 1286–1289.
31 Chiva, L.M., Lapuente, F., Nuñez, C., and Ramírez, P.T. (2009). Ileal orthotopic neobladder after pelvic exenteration for cervical cancer. *Gynecol. Oncol.* 113 (1): 47–51.
32 Martinez, A., Filleron, T., Rouanet, P. et al. (2018). Prospective assessment of first-year quality of life after pelvic exenteration for gynecologic malignancy: a French multicentric study. *Ann. Surg. Oncol.* 25: 535–541.
33 Kaur, M., Joniau, S., D'oore, A. et al. (2012). Pelvic exenterations for gynecological malignancies. *Int. J. Gynecol. Cancer* 22 (5): 889–896.
34 Forner, D.M. and Lampe, B. (2011). Ileal conduit and continent ileocecal pouch for patients undergoing pelvic exenteration. *Int. J. Gynecol. Cancer* 21 (2): 403–408.
35 Goldberg, G.L., Sukumvanich, P., Einstein, M.H. et al. (2006). Total pelvic exenteration: the Albert Einstein College of Medicine/Montefiore Medical Center experience (1987 to 2003). *Gynecol. Oncol.* 101: 261–268.
36 Brown, K.G.M., Koh, C.E., Vasilaras, A. et al. (2014). Clinical algorithms for the diagnosis and management of urological leaks following pelvic exenteration. *Eur. J. Surg. Oncol.* 40: 775–781.
37 Balkwill, F. and Mantovani, A. (2001). Inflammation and cancer: back to Virchow? *Lancet* 357 (9255): 539–545.
38 Pidgeon, G.P., Harmey, J.H., Kay, E. et al. (1999). The role of endotoxin/lipopolysaccharide in surgically induced tumour growth in a murine model of metastatic disease. *Br. J. Cancer* 81 (8): 1311–1317.
39 Herrle, F., Sandra-Petrescu, F., Weiss, C. et al. (2016). Quality of life and timing of stoma closure in patients with rectal cancer undergoing low anterior resection with diverting stoma: a multicenter longitudinal observational study. *Dis. Colon Rectum* 59 (4): 281–290.
40 Montgomery, A. (2017). Parastomal hernia. In: *Textbook of Hernia* (eds. W.W. Hope, W.S. Cobb and G.L. Adrales). Cham: Springer.
41 Hawighorst-Knapstein, S., Schonefussrs, G., Hoffmann, S.O. et al. (1997). Pelvic exenteration: effects of surgery on quality of life and body imageea prospective longitudinal study. *Gynecol. Oncol.* 66: 495–500.
42 Roos, E.J., de Graeff, A., van Eijkeren, M.A. et al. (2004). Quality of life after pelvic exenteration. *Gynecol. Oncol.* 93: 610–614.
43 Austin, K.K., Young, J.M., and Solomon, M.J. (2010). Quality of life of survivors after pelvic exenteration for rectal cancer. *Dis. Colon Rectum* 53: 1121–1126.
44 Harji, D.P., Griffiths, B., Velikova, G. et al. (2016). Systematic review of health-related quality of life in patients undergoing pelvic exenteration. *Eur. J. Surg. Oncol.* 42: 1132–1145.

45 De Wever, I., Van de Moortel, M., and Stas, M. (1996). Temporary colostomy in supralevator pelvic exenteration. A comparative study between stapled loop and loop colostomy. *Eur. J. Surg. Oncol.* 22: 84–87.

46 Brunschwig, A. and Pierce, V.K.L. (1950). Partial and complete pelvic exenteraion; a progress report based upon the first 100 operations. *Cancer* 4: 972–975.

47 Carter, M.F., Dalton, D.P., and Garnett, J.E. (1989). Simultaneous diversion of the urinary and fecal strems utilizing a single abdominal stoma: the double-barrelled wet colostomy. *J. Urol.* 141 (5): 1189–1191.

48 Carter, M.F., Kalton, D.P., and Garnett, J.E. (1994). The double-barrelled wet colostomy: long-term experience with the first 11 patients. *J. Urol.* 152 (6 part 2): 2312–2315.

49 Gan, J. and Hamid, R. (2016). Literature review: double-barrelled wet colostomy (one stoma) versus ileal conduit with colostomy (two stomas). *Urol. Int.* 98 (3): 249–254.

50 Pavlov, M.J., Ceranic, M.S., Nale, D.P. et al. (2013). Double-barrelled wet colostomy versus ileal conduit and terminal colostomy for urinary and fecal diversion: a single institution experience. *Scand. J. Surg.* 103: 189–194.

51 Backes, F.J., Tierney, B.J., Eisenhauer, E.L. et al. (2013). Complications after double-barreled wet colostomy compared to separate urinary and fecal diversion during pelvic exenteration: time to change back? *Gynecol. Oncol.* 128 (1): 60–64.

52 Chokshi, R.J., Kuhrt, M.P., Schmidt, C. et al. (2011). Single institution experience comparing double-barrelled wet colostomy to ileal conduit for urinary and fecal diversion. *Urology* 78 (4): 856–862.

53 Yazici, S., Tonyali, S., Bozaci, A.C. et al. (2018). Urinary and fecal diversion following pelvic exenteration: comparison of double-barrelled and plain wet colostomy. *Urol. J.* 15 (5): 290–294.

54 García-Granero, A., Biondo, S., Espin-Basany, E. et al. (2018). Pelvic exenteration with resection for different types of malignancies at two tertiary referral centres. *Cir. Esp.* 96 (3): 138–148.

55 Bloemendaal, A.L.A., Kraus, R., Buchs, N.C. et al. (2016). Double-barreled wet colostomy formation after pelvic exenteration for locally advanced or recurrent rectal cancer. *Colorectal Dis.* 18: O427–O431.

56 Macrí, A. (2017). Modified double-barrelled wet colostomy after total pelvic exenteration. *Updat. Surg.* 69: 545–548.

57 Carne, P.W., Robertson, G.M., and Frizelle, F.A. (2003). Parastoma hernia. *Br. J. Surg.* 90 (7): 784–793.

58 Funahashi, K., Suzuki, T., Nagahima, Y. et al. (2014). Risk factors for parastomal hernia in Japanese patients with permanent colostomy. *Surg. Today* 44: 1465–1469.

59 Hong, S.Y., Oh, S.Y., Lee, J.H. et al. (2013). Risk factors for parastomal hernia: based on radiological definition. *J. Korean Surg. Soc.* 84 (1): 43–47.

60 Pilgrim, C.H., McIntyre, R., and Bailey, M. (2010). Prospective audit of parastomal hernia: prevalence and associated comorbidities. *Dis. Colon Rectum* 53 (1): 71–76.

61 Hotouras, A., Bhan, C., Murphy, J. et al. (2014). Parastomal hernia prevention: is it all about mesh reinforcement? *Dis. Colon Rectum* 57 (112): e443–e444.

62 Antoniou, S.A., Agresta, F., Garcia Alamino, J.M. et al. (2018). European Hernia Society guidelines on prevention and treatment of parastomal hernias. *Hernia* 22 (1): 183–198.

63 López-Cano, M., Brandsma, H.T., Bury, K. et al. (2017). Prophylactic mesh to prevent parastomal hernia after end colostomy: a meta-analysis and trial sequential analysis. *Hernia* 21 (2): 177–189.

17

Reconstructive Techniques Following Pelvic Exenteration

Dimitrios Patsouras, Alexis Schizas, and Mark George

Department of Colorectal Surgery, St. Thomas' Hospital, London, UK

Background

Pelvic exenteration requires multivisceral pelvic dissection, with a considerable destructive phase to remove locally advanced or recurrent pelvic malignancies. Following this phase, reconstruction of the urinary system is always necessary and bowel reconstruction can be considered if the anal canal is spared. One of the major complications following exenterative surgery is the perineal wound which is often large and within an irradiated field. Techniques for bowel, urinary, and perineal reconstruction are discussed within this chapter.

Bowel Reconstruction

If a supralevator exenteration is possible with sparing of the levators and anal canal then a restorative bowel procedure is possible. With the rectum and other organs fully mobilized it is possible to join below the tumor at the anorectal junction. The choice between a hand-sutured or stapled anastomosis depends on surgeon preference. Clinical trials of the various techniques have not shown any to be superior. The double-staple technique has the advantage of simplicity, but there is a risk of increased anastomotic leak from the ends of the transverse suture lying lateral to the anastomosis.

Options

- *Hand-sutured anastomosis*: Given the evidence that no particular technique is superior, a double- or single-layer suture, interrupted or continuous, using absorbable or non-absorbable material may all be used. The choice is usually determined by surgeon preference.
- *Single-staple anastomosis*: Following removal of the specimen, a purse-string suture is placed in the distal rectum and the proximal colon. Points of technical importance include the use of suture, the distance and depth of placement of the purse-strings bites, and avoiding damage to the internal sphincter on inserting the stapler. Good approximation of staple head and anvil without incorporating other tissues, and gentle extraction ensure a well-formed anastomosis.
- *Double-staple anastomosis*: The double-staple technique simplifies stapling, by avoiding the distal purse-string which can be difficult to place. Points of particular importance include the correct application of the transverse staples, their incorporation into the final anastomosis, and the avoidance of

Surgical Management of Advanced Pelvic Cancer, First Edition.
Edited by Michael E. Kelly and Desmond C. Winter.
© 2022 John Wiley & Sons Ltd. Published 2022 by John Wiley & Sons Ltd.

tearing the very short anorectal stump when advancing the staple gun.

- *Endoanal coloanal anastomosis*: This enables restoration of intestinal continuity as far distally as possible. Not all cases are suitable for stapling and occasional technical difficulties can occur. To be able to salvage a failed or impossible stapled anastomosis, coloanal hand suturing is an indispensable option. The colon must be mobilized adequately to descend to the anus. This almost always requires ligation of all vessels to the left colon, leaving perfusion by the marginal artery via the middle colic artery. The anastomosis can be facilitated by a mucosectomy of the anal stump to the dentate line. In some cases previous colectomy or rectal resection may result in inadequate mobility of the colon to permit a tension free, well-vascularized coloanal anastomosis. In these cases Deloyer's reversion can be used. This involves rotating the cecum and ascending colon to allow the ascending colon to reach the anus.
- *Colonic pouch*: After ultra-low anterior resection with end-to-end anastomosis, or after a straight coloanal procedure, bowel frequency is unpredictable. Function may be improved by construction of a reservoir from the terminal part of the colon. This is made as a J-construction. The resulting coloanal anastomosis will be side to end and can be made either by stapling or by hand-sewing.
- *Defunctioning the anastomosis*: When the intestinal continuity is restored and there is an ultra-low or coloanal anastomosis, formation of a covering ileostomy is necessary. The authors prefer to use a split ileostomy which is matured upstream of both the coloanal anastomosis and the small bowel anastomosis which has been created following ileal conduit formation. This can result in an ileostomy that is quite high in the ileum and can be quite a challenge for the patient to manage. The split ileostomy is closed when patients have recovered from surgery and completed any adjuvant treatments. A water-soluble enema and a distal loopogram, from the efferent limb of the split ileostomy, should be performed to ensure that both the coloanal and small bowel anastomoses have healed without persistent leak or stricturing.

Urinary Tract Reconstruction

Following exenterative surgery, urinary reconstruction is often required and the options for reconstruction are reviewed in this section. Options for reconstruction are influenced by the resection required, neoadjuvant treatment, patient comorbidities, prognosis, and surgeon preference.

Ureteric Reimplantation

If only a pelvic sidewall resection is required, and the bladder is not removed but the ureter is resected, a ureteric reimplantation may be required. If there is enough ureteric length and the bladder is mobile enough, a simple reimplant can be performed. The bladder is commonly mobilized to give extra length to provide a tension-free anastomosis, and the ureter is tunneled through the bladder to reduce the risk of reflux. The ureter is sutured using a dissolvable suture to prevent future stone formation on the suture.

If by simple mobilization of the bladder the anastomosis would be under tension, then other techniques can be used to reduce the tension. Once the bladder is mobilized it can be sutured onto psoas (psoas hitch) on the side reimplantation is required. This holds the bladder up to decrease any tension on the anastomosis. If this still does not allow for a tension-free anastomosis, then a flap can be performed to give extra length. A Boari flap involves mobilizing the bladder and making an oblique incision of the anterior wall. The cranial end is sutured onto psoas and the ureter tunneled through the posterior bladder. The bladder is then closed in the opposite direction to give the extra length required.

Urinary Diversion, Conduit, and Uretostomy

If the bladder cannot be spared, then ureteric implantation into the bowel/neobladder is required. Reconstructing a neobladder in the pelvis and anastomosis to the urethra following pelvic exenteration is not advised. These patients have commonly had pelvic radiotherapy; therefore their wound healing is compromised, and they may have had significant intraoperative blood loss through a long surgical procedure. Common urinary diversions would include an ileal conduit, colonic conduit, and wet colostomy. If ureteric anastomosis is not advisable into a conduit, then the ureters can be brought to the skin as a uretostomy, but this is only performed in exceptional circumstances. A Mitrofanoff continent conduit can also be considered, but this does add extra time to the operation and has the risk of increased complications as there are more anastomoses [1].

For a urinary conduit, the large or small bowel can be used, and commonly an ileal conduit is made on the patient's right side. If there is excess colon, a colonic conduit may be formed, with a bowel stoma on the opposite side. A wet colostomy can be double-barreled with the ureters inserted into the distal limb of the stoma, so the bowel contents only mix with the urine in the stoma bag.

The ureters can also be implanted into the colon as an end colostomy. In this case, urine and stool mix in the colon before exiting into the stoma bag. The main problems with a wet colostomy are the smell as the mixed urine and stool are much more offensive when mixed together. The double-barreled wet colostomy tries to avoid this as the contents only come together in the bag and this has been found to be an acceptable alternative to a conduit [2].

For a continent conduit, a neobladder is made using the cecum and small bowel, much like forming a J- or W-pouch to allow enough volume to store urine. The joins are usually hand-sewn to prevent stone formation on metal staples. Once the pouch is formed, if the appendix is still in situ it can be tunneled up to the skin and opened to allow entry into the neopouch. This can be catheterized to allow emptying of the pouch when required. If the appendix is not available, the ileum can be fashioned into a small appendix-sized tube and tunneled up to the skin surface. The ureters are then sutured into the neobladder. Implantation of the ureters into the conduit or stoma can be performed individually with them entering the conduit at separate sites. The alternative is to anastomose the ureters together first and have one single anastomosis with the conduit.

Urological reconstruction following pelvic exenteration is associated with significant complications. Complications occur in 59% [3] of patients following pelvic exenteration, and this is higher for those patients having recurrent surgery. Urinary leak occurs in 16%, with nearly half occurring within the first month. An R2 resection, more complex surgery, and cardiovascular comorbidities are associated with increased leak risk. If a leak occurs there was understandably a longer length of stay [4]. (See Chapter 16 for more details)

Reconstruction of Perineum

The perineal defect following resection of an advanced or recurrent pelvic malignancy can be considerable, with loss of not only soft tissue but also bony structures. The vast majority of patients will have received chemoradiotherapy treatment before surgery, and therefore getting the perineal wound to heal is a great challenge for the surgeon, and remains one of the major causes of postoperative morbidity in both the short and long term (Figure 17.1). Primary closure of the defect is often not possible, and there is evidence that a flap reduces perineal wound complications. The principles of the flap are to provide adequate coverage with healthy tissue that has good potential healing of both donor and recipient sites and which avoids long-term

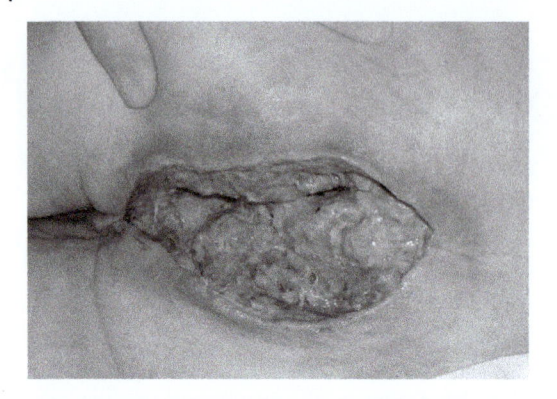

Figure 17.1 Dehiscence of an irradiated perineal wound. *Source:* Dimitrios Patsouras, Alexis Schizas, and Mark George.

problems, including delayed wound healing, perineal sinuses, and/or herniation [5]. The options for reconstruction vary depending on the size of the defect – with smaller defects following extralevator excision of the rectum suitable for either mesh or a local/pedicle flap, and larger defects following sacrectomy or penectomy potentially requiring multiple flaps.

Omentum

The omentum can be mobilized to fill dead space in the pelvis. It is, however, very variable in its size and length and in the authors' opinion cannot be relied upon for perineal reconstruction. It has been reported to reduce overall major abdominal complications when compared with patients who do not have the omentum transposed to the pelvis [6].

Mesh

The use of biological mesh for perineal reconstruction is a simple method of perineal defect closure. It is quicker than flap reconstruction and can be performed by the colorectal surgeon rather than requiring plastic surgery involvement. While it can provide support to prevent perineal herniation, it does not fill the dead space in an empty pelvis. It is sufficient for smaller perineal wounds such as extralevator abdomino-perineal excision (APE) but not for larger defects [7].

Pedicle Flaps

There are three pedicle flaps which have mainly been used for perineal reconstruction: rectus abdominis, gracilis, and anterior thigh flaps.

The rectus abdominis flap has been the most commonly used over the years. The muscle is disconnected superiorly and mobilized off the posterior rectus sheath to run on the inferior epigastric vessels. The overlying skin and fat are included on the flap and these can be taken vertically (vertical rectus abdominal muscle (VRAM)) or obliquely (ORAM) [8, 9]. The pedicle flap is then taken down to the pelvis and inserted to fill the perineal defect. This flap provides excellent coverage of the perineal defect following extralevator APE and can also facilitate posterior vaginal wall reconstruction [10] (Figure 17.2). However, VRAM flap has a failure rate of up to 12.5%, due to flap necrosis from compromised blood supply. The donor site of the anterior abdominal wall may require a mesh reconstruction, and despite this many patients will have significant abdominal wall weakness. If both a urostomy and a colostomy are being formed, then one of the ostomies will come through the donor site, with the added risk of parastomal herniation. Technical modification to improve VRAM outcomes have been studied; the fascia-sparing VRAM flap, component separation of donor-site closure, mesh reconstruction, and omental flap with VRAM have all be reported with varying success [11].

Gracilis flaps can be raised and these run off perforator vessels from the deep femoral artery. The flap can be passed across the inner groin crease to be inserted into the perineal defect. A unilateral gracilis flap can fill most perineal defects. Neovaginal reconstruction is possible if bilateral flaps are raised where total vaginectomy has been performed. If double ostomies have been raised, then use of the gracilis allows both stomas to pass through

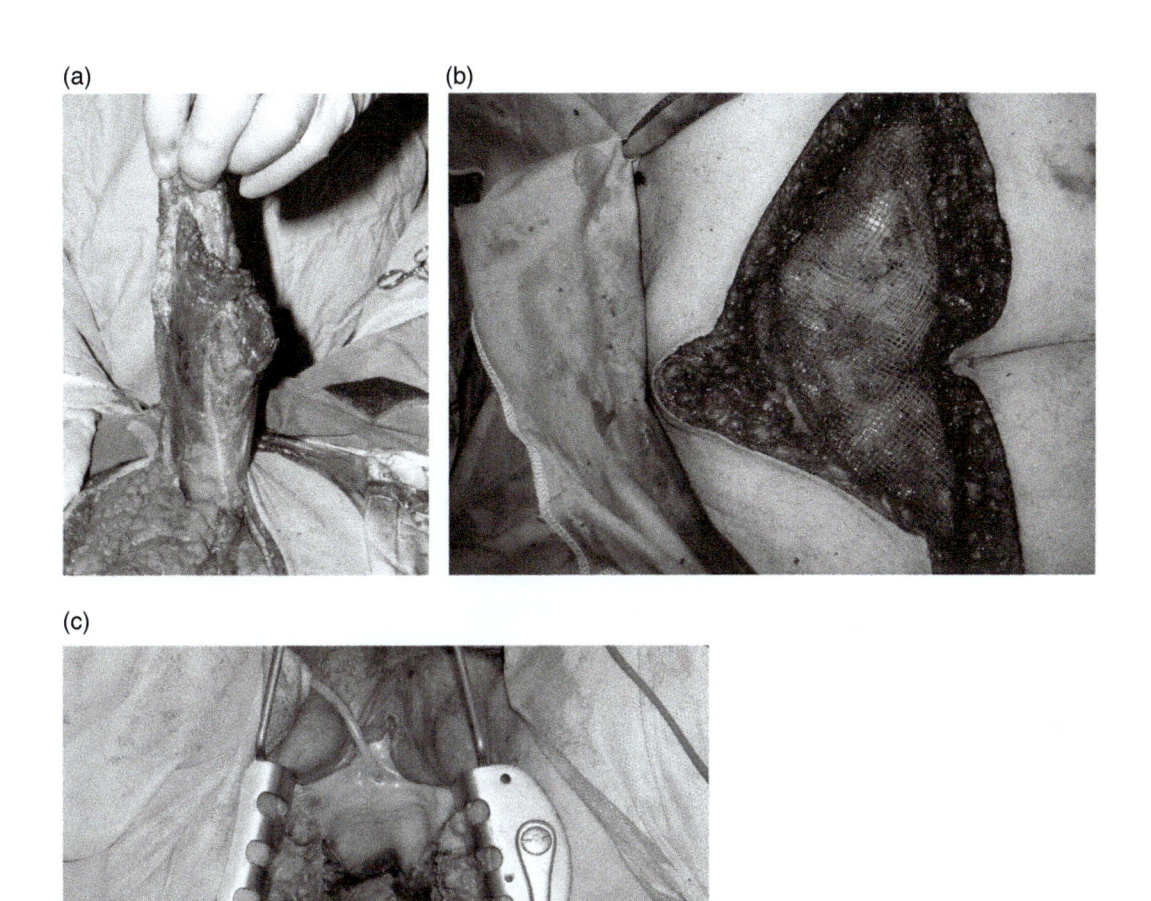

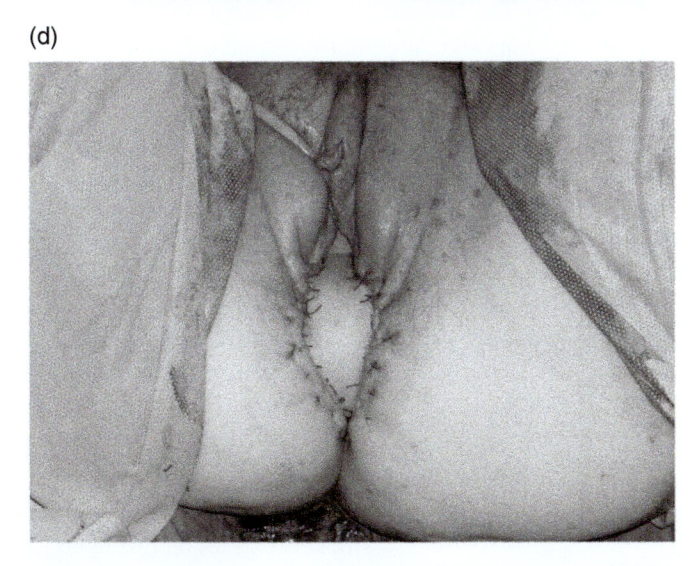

Figure 17.2 (a,b) Vertical rectus muscle flap raised and running on the inferior epigastric artery. with mesh reconstruction of the abdominal wall donor site. (c,d) VRAM with posterior vaginal wall reconstructed following APE with posterior vaginectomy. *Source:* Dimitrios Patsouras, Alexis Schizas, and Mark George.

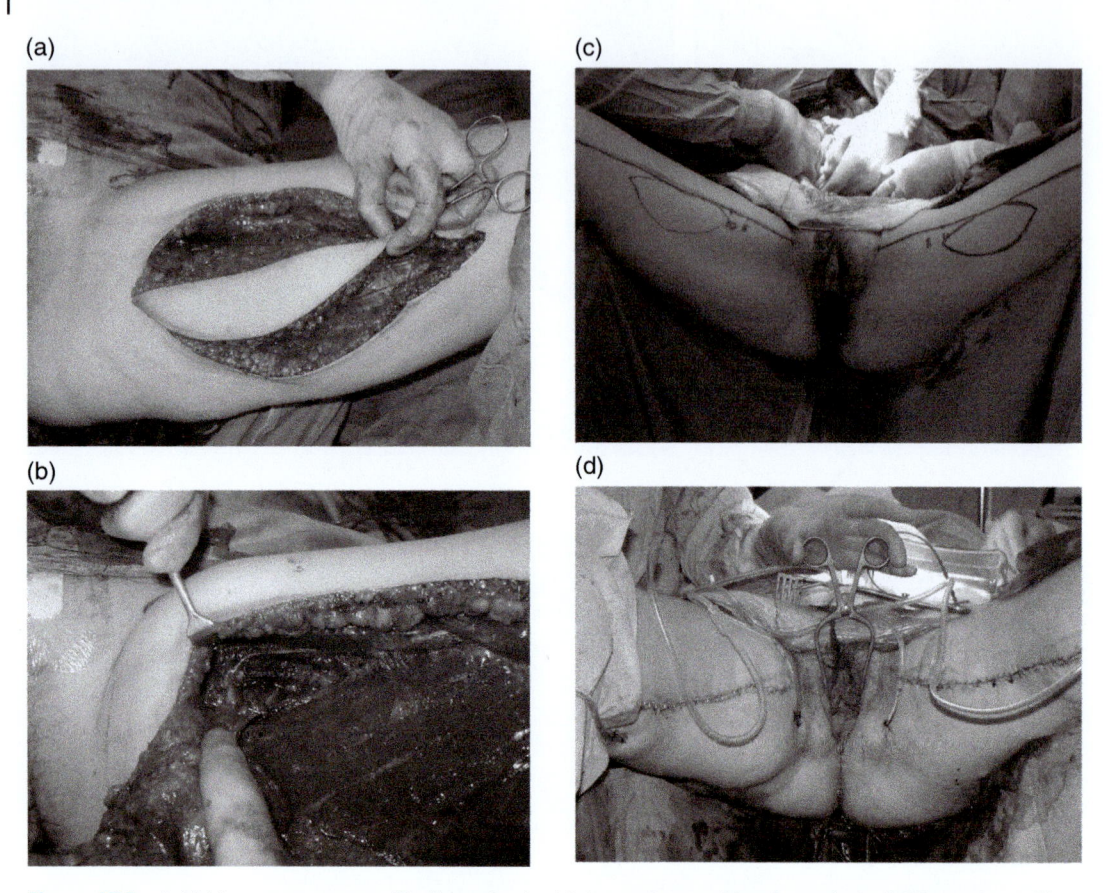

Figure 17.3 (a,b) Myocutaneous gracilis flap raised with its perforator blood supply. (c,d) Bilateral gracilis flaps with neovaginal reconstruction. *Source:* Dimitrios Patsouras, Alexis Schizas, and Mark George.

intact rectus muscle with the benefit of fewer parastomal hernias. Both donor and recipient site complications are similar to VRAM flaps [12, 13] (Figure 17.3).

The anterolateral thigh flap runs off perforators from the descending branch of the lateral femoral circumflex artery and is very versatile, with low donor site morbidity. In the authors' experience it is the flap of choice for suprapubic defects and is often used with other flaps such as inferior gluteal perforator (IGAP) flaps to give tissue coverage following extensive perineal tissue loss following exenteration with penectomy [14] (Figure 17.4).

Fasciocutaneous Flaps

With an increasing number of laparoscopic APE operations being performed, the VRAM flap is not the ideal choice as this flap involves a large abdominal incision. The use of local perforator flaps to reconstruct the perineum provides a possible solution to allow a laparoscopic approach from above with a perineal excision and subsequent local reconstruction. The IGAP is commonly used. The flap is raised off the gluteal muscle and can be moved medially into the pelvis. This flap can be unilateral for smaller defects or bilateral for larger defects [15] (Figure 17.5). A neovagina reconstruction is also possible, although the authors have seen a number of perineal hernia following this type of reconstruction and therefore do recommend using a mesh as well as the IGAP flap to try to reduce this. Overall, the flap is very robust, with some series reporting no flap necrosis. However, patients do find it uncomfortable to sit for prolonged periods of time

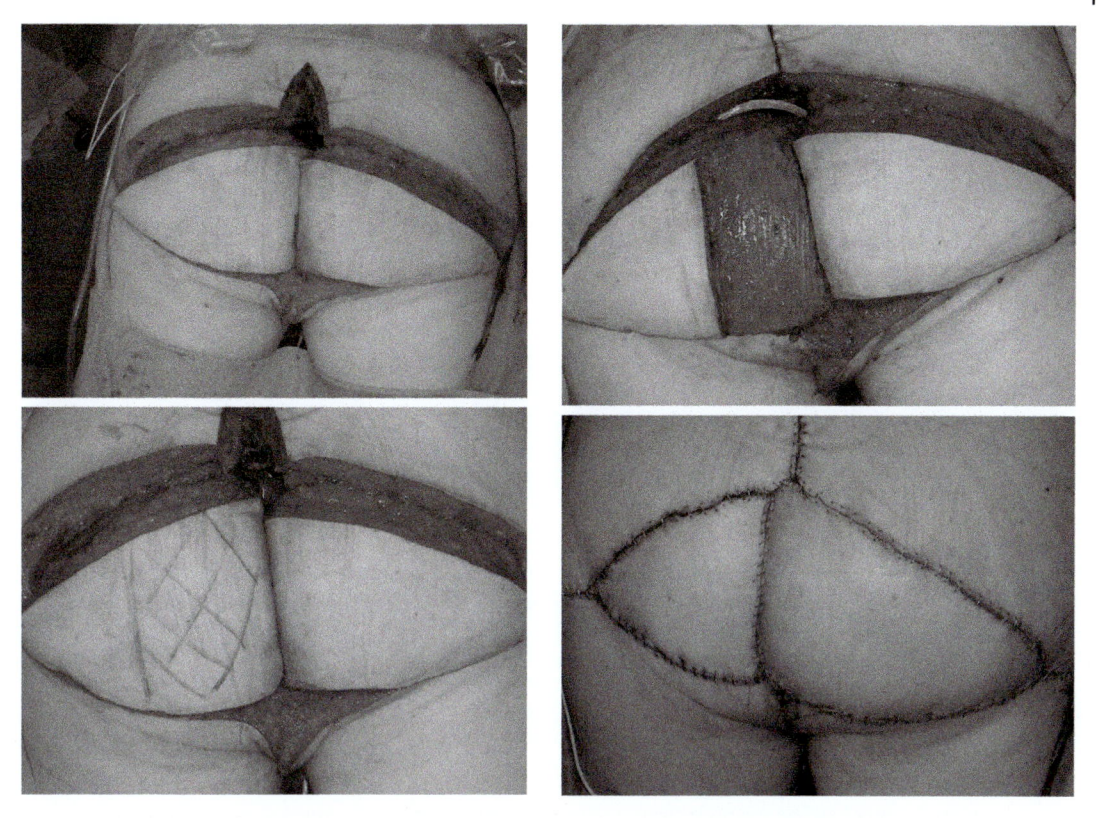

Figure 17.4 Bilateral inferior gluteal artery perforator flaps. Area to be de-epithelialized is marked, then the de-epithelization with this flap is moved into the pelvic cavity, giving the final result.

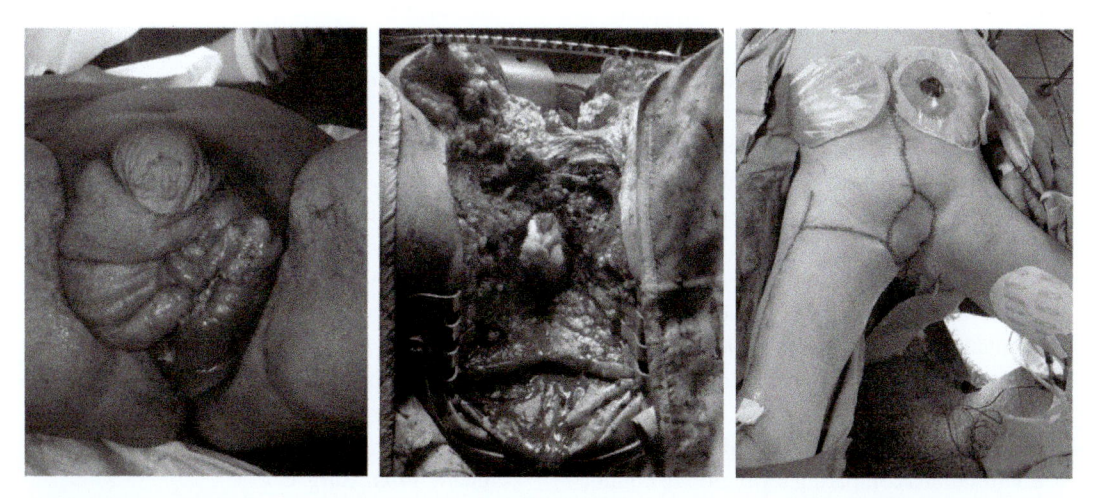

Figure 17.5 Recurrent anal SCC with urethro-perineal fistulation. Pelvic exenteration with penectomy. Reconstruction performed with anterolateral thigh flap and IGAPs. *Source:* Dimitrios Patsouras, Alexis Schizas, and Mark George.

after surgery for many months especially when bilateral flaps have been used.

Myocutaneous Flaps and Free Flaps

Gluteus maximus flaps have been used following ELAPE with varying success. However, whilst the majority of perineal wounds are healed at one year, 41.5% of patients suffered perineal wound complications [16]. Alternatively, free flaps have been reported when other options are not feasible. Latissimus dorsi has been used with good success but has only been reported in limited series [17]. The one major downside of free flaps is the considerable additional time added to an already long operation. Therefore patient selection is key.

Summary Box

- Restoration of bowel continuity may be possible. Functional outcome must be discussed with the patient preoperatively.
- The type of urinary reconstruction should be discussed with the patient preoperatively, particularly if a continent urostomy is being considered.
- Due to preoperative radiotherapy, all perineal wounds should be considered for flap reconstruction.

References

1 Forner, D.M. and Lampe, B. (2011). Ileal conduit and continent ileocecal pouch for patients undergoing pelvic exenteration: comparison of complications and quality of life. *Int. J. Gynecol. Cancer* 21 (2): 403–408.

2 Gan, J. and Hamid, R. (2017). Literature review: double-barrelled wet colostomy (one stoma) versus Ileal conduit with colostomy (two stomas). *Urol. Int.* 98 (3): 249–254.

3 Brown, K.G., Solomon, M.J., Latif, E.R. et al. (2017 Mar). Urological complications after cystectomy as part of pelvic exenteration are higher than that after cystectomy for primary bladder malignancy. *J. Surg. Oncol.* 115 (3): 307–311.

Urological reconstruction following exenteration for advanced pelvic malignancy should be undertaken by a dedicated urology team to help minimize complications.

4 Teixeira, S.C., Ferenschild, F.T., Solomon, M.J. et al. (2012 Apr). Urological leaks after pelvic exenterations comparing formation of colonic and ileal conduits. *Eur. J. Surg. Oncol.* 38 (4): 361–366.

5 Devulapalli, C., Jia Wei, A.T., DiBiagio, J.R. et al. (2016 May). Primary versus flap closure of perineal defects following oncologic resection: a systematic review and meta-analysis. *Plast. Reconstr. Surg* 137 (5): 1602–1613.

Primary closure is associated with twice the perineal wound complication rate compared with flap closure.

6 Hultman, C.S., Sherrill, M.A., Halvorson, E.G. et al. (2010). Utility of the omentum in pelvic floor reconstruction following resection of anorectal malignancy: patient selection, technical caveats, and clinical outcomes. *Ann. Plast. Surg.* 64 (5): 559–562.

7 Alam, N.N., Narang, S.K., Köckerling, F. et al. (2016). Biologic mesh reconstruction of the pelvic floor after Extralevator abdominoperineal excision: a systematic review. *Front. Surg* 3: 9.

8 Chan, S., Miller, M., Ng, R. et al. (2010). Use of myocutaneous flaps for perineal closure following abdominoperineal excision of the rectum for adenocarcinoma. *Colorectal Dis.* 12 (6): 555–560.

9 Abbott, D.E., Halverson, A.L., Wayne, J.D. et al. (2008). The oblique rectus abdominal myocutaneous flap for complex pelvic wound reconstruction. *Dis. Colon Rectum* 51 (8): 1237–1241.

10 Horch, R.E., Hohenberger, W., Eweida, A. et al. (2014). A hundred patients with vertical rectus abdominis myocutaneous (VRAM) flap for pelvic reconstruction after total pelvic exenteration. *Int. J. Color. Dis.* 29 (7): 813–823.

11 Campbell, C.A. and Butler, C.E. (2011). Use of adjuvant techniques improves surgical outcomes of complex vertical rectus abdominis myocutaneous flap reconstructions of pelvic cancer defects. *Plast. Reconstr. Surg.* 128 (2): 447–458.

12 Singh, M., Kinsley, S., Huang, A. et al. (2016). Gracilis flap reconstruction of the perineum: an outcomes analysis. *J. Am. Coll. Surg.* 223 (4): 602–610.

13 Chong, T.W., Balch, G.C., Kehoe, S.M. et al. (2015). Reconstruction of large perineal and pelvic wounds using Gracilis muscle flaps. *Ann. Surg. Oncol.* 22 (11): 3738–3744.

14 Wong, S., Garvey, P., Skibber, J., and Yu, P. (2009). Reconstruction of pelvic exenteration defects with anterolateral thigh-vastus lateralis muscle flaps. *Plast. Reconstr. Surg.* 124 (4): 1177–1185.

15 Hainsworth, A., Al Akash, M., Roblin, P. et al. (2012 Apr). Perineal reconstruction after abdominoperineal excision using inferior gluteal artery perforator flaps. *Br. J. Surg.* 99 (4): 584–588.
IGAP flap has proven to be a very reliable flap for perineal reconstruction with few complications.

16 Anderin, C., Martling, A., Lagergren, J. et al. (2012). Short-term outcome after gluteus maximus myocutaneous flap reconstruction of the pelvic floor following extra-levator abdominoperineal excision of the rectum. *Colorectal Dis.* 14 (9): 1060–1064.

17 Abdou, A.H., Li, L., Khatib-Chahidi, K. et al. (2016). Free latissimus dorsi myocutaneous flap for pelvic floor reconstruction following pelvic exenteration. *Int. J. Color. Dis.* 31 (2): 385–391.

18

Minimizing Morbidity from Pelvic Exenteration

Meara Dean[1], Alex Colquhoun[1], Peter Featherstone[2], Nicola S. Fearnhead[1], and R. Justin Davies[1]

[1] *Department of Surgery, Cambridge University Hospitals NHS Foundation Trust, Cambridge, UK*
[2] *Department of Intensive Care Medicine and Anaesthesia, Cambridge University Hospitals NHS Foundation Trust, Cambridge, UK*

Background

Pelvic exenteration is associated with major psychological, psychosexual, physiological, and functional implications for patients. A multidisciplinary team approach is important to guide patient selection and management, and surgery should be performed at specialist centers that have the resources to provide the complex care required. Many surgical techniques are used in exenteration surgery, requiring the expertise of a range of specialists including colorectal surgery, urology, gynecological oncology, reconstructive plastic surgery, interventional radiology, orthopedics, and vascular surgery, all supported by highly specialized perioperative and nursing care teams to minimize the impact of the surgical insult and potential morbidity for the patient. Careful planning is vital at each stage of the patient's management in order to minimize risk. This chapter outlines key risk reduction considerations in intra- and postoperative phases of care.

Knowing the Risks

Advances in modern surgical practice have widened the indications for pelvic exenteration, with recent case series quoting acceptable in-hospital mortality (1–3%) comparable to major colorectal resection. This contrasts with persistently high rates of morbidity (34–80%) [1–4]. Morbidity and mortality increase with more radical procedures, such as en-bloc sacral resection [5].

Although potentially morbid, pelvic exenteration is often the only curative option available to patients with locally advanced or recurrent pelvic malignancy. Surgical-related morbidity needs to be weighed against the considerable risk of morbidity caused by the cancer itself. Patients may experience intractable pain from invasion of adjacent nerves, muscles, or bone or symptomatic invasion or obstruction of the urological or gastrointestinal systems, sexual dysfunction, and functional consequences of neoadjuvant treatments.

Postoperative quality of life (QoL) is a fundamental outcome measure in this patient group. Baseline QoL is the strongest predictor of postoperative QoL [6]. Factors associated with reduced postoperative QoL include female sex, total pelvic exenteration, and positive surgical resection margins [6, 7]. When compared to non-operative patients, QoL has been shown to improve rapidly in the early postoperative period, and at nine months patient-reported postoperative outcomes are comparable with those who do not have surgery, after which there

Surgical Management of Advanced Pelvic Cancer, First Edition.
Edited by Michael E. Kelly and Desmond C. Winter.
© 2022 John Wiley & Sons Ltd. Published 2022 by John Wiley & Sons Ltd.

is a decline in QoL and patient-reported outcomes for patients who do not have surgery [8].

Units performing exenteration surgery should monitor their clinical outcomes and ideally QoL outcomes to facilitate quality improvement initiatives and the identification of adverse outcomes, with learning and feedback to all team members. Most outcome data in the literature are from single-center series; however, a more recent international collaboration has reported on the outcomes for a large multi-center patient cohort [9]. This has been useful to identify the factors associated with improved outcomes, with data confirming the importance of a clear resection margin on disease-free and overall survival.

Intraoperative Management

General Considerations

Surgical Safety Checklist
Given the broad range and large number of intraoperative considerations, it may be beneficial to use a perioperative checklist (Table 18.1) to ensure all points are addressed adequately.

Anesthesia
Anesthesia for pelvic exenteration begins with thorough preoperative assessment, including explanation of the risks associated with general anesthesia and the insertion of invasive arterial and central venous lines, as well as describing the options available for postoperative pain relief. Although epidural analgesia often proves effective in this patient cohort, the likelihood of providing adequate sensory blockade across all potential wound sites should be balanced alongside the standard risks associated with this technique.

Intravenous induction is followed by maintenance with a volatile anesthetic agent in oxygen/air plus infusions of remifentanil and muscle relaxant. Both depth of anesthesia and degree of neuromuscular blockade should be monitored intraoperatively. A standard cuffed endotracheal tube is adequate in cases that do not require prone positioning (where an armored tube becomes necessary). Lung-protective ventilation strategies have proven beneficial in patients undergoing major surgery and are recommended. Insertion of a nasopharyngeal temperature probe allows continuous temperature monitoring, and an under-body warming mattress and tube-shaped forced air warmer prevent hypothermia. Blood glucose should be checked regularly and maintained between 6 and 10 mmol/l.

Intraoperative gastric drainage and large-bore intravenous access are mandatory. Primed equipment for rapid transfusion, e.g. the Belmont Rapid Infuser, should be set up at the outset. Central venous and intra-arterial blood pressures are monitored continuously. Dynamic indices of fluid responsiveness may also be useful in guiding fluid replacement. Near-patient blood gas analysis and thromboelastography facilitate rapid assessment of biochemical and hematological parameters.

Venous Thromboembolism Prophylaxis
Sequential calf compression devices are applied, although opinion is divided on additional use of thromboembolic prophylactic stockings. As hemorrhage and attendant coagulopathy may result in deferred administration of chemical venous thromboembolic (VTE) prophylaxis with low molecular weight heparin beyond the recommended 12 hours of surgery, calf compression is particularly important in this patient group. Recent deep venous thrombosis should also raise the possibility of needing preoperative inferior vena cava (IVC) filter placement.

Patient Positioning
Patients are positioned in the Lloyd-Davies position, with attention to padding of pressure areas and the patient's eyes. The gel mat may be folded on itself to elevate the pelvis if posterior access or sacrectomy is required. Minimizing lumbar lordosis with anterior

Table 18.1 Surgical checklist for pelvic exenteration.

Pelvic exenteration	Day-of-surgery checklist
Discussion at team brief Confirmation: • Consent form signed • Stoma siting completed • Availability of high-dependency bed • Allergies Operative plan: • Outline and timing of key stages • Anticipated position changes • Teams involved • Optimization strategy and breaks Patient safety: • Calf compression devices • Venous thromboembolism prophylaxis • Antibiotic and antifungal prophylaxis • Administration of tranexamic acid • Pressure area protection • Patient warming equipment Discuss transfusion planning: • Valid group and hold • Blood cross-matched • Potential for massive transfusion protocol • Rapid infusion equipment available • Coagulation monitoring (thromboelastography) Well legs planning: • Matching leg stirrups to size of patient • Timing restrictions for lower limb elevation • Timetable for knee flexion • Mean arterial pressure during limb elevation Anesthetic plan: • Intubation requirements • Lines and access • Postoperative analgesia • Special concerns Surgical equipment: • Instrument sets • Energy devices • Specialty team requirements • Disposables • Sutures • Hemostatic agents • Stoma appliances Imaging: • Imaging available • Imaging review prior to surgery	*Confirmation prior to skin incision* Prophylaxis: • Antibiotics +/− antifungals administered • Calf compression • Tranexamic acid administered • Rectal washout Monitoring: • Anesthetic monitoring • Adequate intravenous access • Blood glucose monitoring • Gastric drainage • Urinary catheterization Positioning: • Eye protection • Upper limbs padded in neutral position • Hand protection • Legs comfortable at hips and knees • Warming equipment Equipment check: • Rapid infusers • Energy devices • Suction • Surgical requirements *On completion of procedure* Safety checks: • Skin integrity • Lower limb perfusion • Check for compartment syndrome Surgical sign out: • Swab and instrument counts correct • Pathology specimen labels and requests Communication: • Update next of kin Handover of postoperative care plan: • Postoperative pain relief • Anesthetic concerns • Antibiotic prophylaxis • Venous thromboembolism prophylaxis • Patient positioning and mobilization plans • Drain and wound management • Stent flushes • Flap observations • Nutritional intake • Physiotherapy

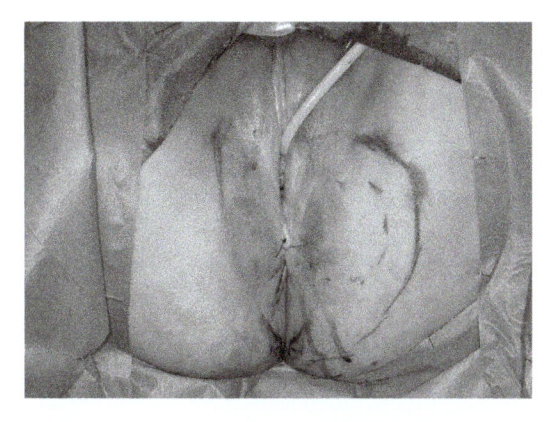

Figure 18.1 Preoperative perineum setup, with skin marking to indicate intended resection margins. *Source:* Meara Dean, Alex Colquhoun, Peter Featherstone, Nicola S. Fearnhead, and R. Justin Davies.

pelvic tilt also aids in ensuring adequate exposure of the perineum (Figure 18.1).

Intermittent pneumatic calf compression is applied, with feet positioned so the heel fits well into the heel of the stirrup, ensuring no pressure is placed on the calf or the region of the peroneal nerve, as this may lead to neuropraxia and/or compartment syndrome. Lower limbs should be rechecked during the operation to ensure they have not moved out of the stirrups, that there is no pressure, that knees remain flexed, and that calves are soft. Prolonged hip flexion can cause neuropraxia, particularly of the peroneal or obturator nerve, so the legs should be moved and lowered intermittently during the operation. Times for leg repositioning should be monitored, regulated to avoid overlong periods of potential poor perfusion, and recorded [10]. Maintaining lower limb perfusion with adequate mean arterial pressure during periods of elevation is also essential to avoid compartment syndrome.

Perioperative Surgical Site Infection Bundle

Prophylactic antibiotics are administered at induction and at appropriate time intervals throughout the procedure. Consideration to timing and antibiotic pharmacokinetics is important, with repeated doses provided to ensure adequate levels of circulating antibiotic prophylaxis. An antifungal should be administered if the vagina is opened during pelvic exenteration surgery.

Abdominal skin is prepared prior to skin incision using an aqueous or alcohol-based preparation. Pooling of alcohol-based preparation should be avoided and the solution should be allowed to dry by evaporation. The abdominal wound may be protected by using packs or retraction systems such as the Alexis wound protector. The OmniTract is an alternative which provides adjustable fixed retraction. When retraction is not required, pressure on the wound should be released to avoid tissue trauma and ischemia. The perineal region should be prepared using an aqueous preparation solution as it is difficult to avoid pooling in this area. The anus may be sutured closed to minimize contamination during dissection. It is useful to staple the drapes to the perineal region to keep them in place, ensuring all staples are removed on completion.

Urinary Catheters

A large-caliber urinary catheter with thermal probe is inserted using aseptic technique for metered urine collection. Selective preoperative retrograde ureteric stent placement may facilitate ureteric protection where the ureters are at particular risk of injury due to bulky tumors, reoperative surgery, and previous radiotherapy.

Team Communication

Clear, concise, and continuous communication between surgical and anesthetic teams is essential for safe exenterative surgery. An interactive working environment ensures that the patient remains in optimal physiological condition throughout, with planned breaks in surgery to ensure attention to optimization of patient position, ventilation, metabolic status, and clotting disturbances. The operative plan should be constantly reassessed and discussed.

Surgical Considerations

Pelvic cancer surgery requires indepth knowledge of complex pelvic anatomy in order to prevent complications. Distortion of normal anatomy may occur in the irradiated pelvis or in cases of previous surgery or recurrent cancer. A wise approach is to circumnavigate areas of difficulty and constantly re-evaluate progress.

The aim is to perform en-bloc removal to achieve a clear resection margin (R0) whilst minimizing complications. Clear resection margins are the most important predictor of long-term survival [11], and uninvolved structures, e.g. the bladder, prostate, or sacrum, may need to be resected en bloc with the specimen either to ensure an adequate margin or to allow a good functional outcome. An individualized approach is necessary depending on the location of the tumor and involved organs, with a clear preoperative plan.

Pelvic exenteration is most commonly performed via an open approach for most cases; however, laparoscopic, robotic, and trans-anal approaches have also been described in highly selected patients [12]. Surgical techniques such as pelvic sidewall resection, en-bloc sacrectomy, and pubic bone resection may be required to achieve clear margins and have been associated with improved survival [13].

Major Hemorrhage

Major hemorrhage is extensively covered in Chapter 19. However, with an increased trend to perform more radical resections, with resultant longer operative times and greater intraoperative blood loss, good preoperative planning can minimize the risk of substantial blood loss.

Preoperative Considerations

Preoperatively the surgeon should consider the patient and disease factors that result in precipitating blood loss. Radiological clues to suggest vessel involvement include cicatrization of the vessels and vascular invasion. The surgeon should discuss the likelihood and management of intraoperative blood administration with the perioperative team during briefing. Blood products should be administered as necessary within a restrictive targeted transfusion policy with permissive anemia in the stable patient.

Prophylactic tranexamic acid should be administered to patients preoperatively if blood loss is expected to exceed moderate blood loss (> 500 ml). The use of tranexamic acid in this setting has been associated with reduction in mortality in meta-analysis [14]. It has a good safety profile, is low cost, and is easy to administer.

Massive transfusion protocol should be followed in the event of major hemorrhage. Staff should have identified supportive roles in communicating with hematology and the blood bank, transporting blood products, and conducting urgent blood tests. Near-patient thromboelastography testing provides "real-time" data to guide blood component replacement.

Intraoperative Considerations

Bleeding may arise from named major vessels, presacral veins, perforating veins, and divided muscles. Major arteries may be pre-emptively isolated and controlled with vascular slings as required (Figure 18.2). Managing intraoperative major hemorrhage requires a team approach. Immediate control with direct pressure using a finger, pledget, or targeted packing should occur while simultaneously advising the anesthetic and scrub team of the situation and the need for any additional equipment, blood products, or staff such as additional surgical expertise. Additional equipment may include vascular instruments or sutures, extra suction devices, retractors to maximize exposure, and extra lighting [15].

Definitive control of pelvic bleeding depends on the type of injury. Injury to a common iliac or internal iliac artery or vein is obvious and massive. After immediate packing and optimization of exposure, the packing is slowly removed to determine the site and nature of the injury. If arterial bleeding is identified, the vessel should be mobilized above and below, and the vessel looped or clamped. The injury is then repaired using a fine vascular suture or the vessel ligated if required. Venous bleeding is controlled with proximal and distal pressure control and the defect repaired with non-absorbable monofilament suture. The internal iliac or its tributaries

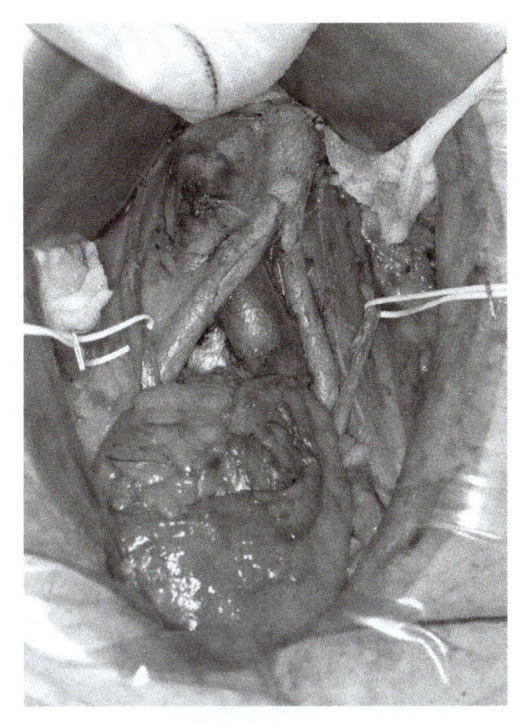

Figure 18.2 Exposure of the aortic bifurcation and common iliac confluence. *Source:* Meara Dean, Alex Colquhoun, Peter Featherstone, Nicola S. Fearnhead, and R. Justin Davies.

can be ligated to control major hemorrhage. Superficial venous bleeding can be controlled using electrocautery or argon beam coagulation (APC). APC can also be safely used over the IVC and iliac veins.

Presacral or periosteal bleeding may require a range of techniques to obtain control. Interval packing with swabs or direct pressure can be particularly useful while the presacral plane is developed further to allow access [16, 17]. Descriptions of surgical techniques to control bleeding or use of hemostatic agents are described elsewhere (Chapter 18).

However, major hemorrhage during pelvic dissection can rapidly lead to a life-threatening situation. If a patient is hemodynamically unstable, leaving pelvic packing in place for 24–48 hours is likely to be the most appropriate management to reduced morbidity and ensure oncological integrity of the procedure. Separation of abdominal and pelvic compartments with plastic wound retrieval bags and catheterization of ureters with feeding tubes may be considered in this situation. Pelvic packing allows correction and restoration of blood volume, coagulopathy, metabolic status, and temperature. On return to theater, packs are removed and hemostasis ensured, with appropriate adjuncts as necessary.

There are occasional circumstances where the exenterative surgeon needs to be aware that pelvic packing may not adequately control hemorrhage. This situation only occurs with venous bleeding arising at or outside the pelvic brim, where damage-control procedures may be necessary, such as ligation of the IVC or femoral cutdown.

Urological Surgical Considerations

Once ureters are transected, pediatric feeding tubes may be inserted to drain the ureters (Figure 18.3) to prevent obstructive nephropathy and resultant electrolyte imbalance. If only a short period of time is likely prior to reconstruction, then the ureters may simply be clipped. If tumor is involving the uroepithelium, avoiding urine spillage in the surgical field is essential.

En-bloc cystectomy usually requires anterior dissection along the retropubic space of Retzius along the periosteum of the pubic bone. In patients who require a more radical excision of the anterior pelvic soft tissue, an alternative technique can be used that allows excision of

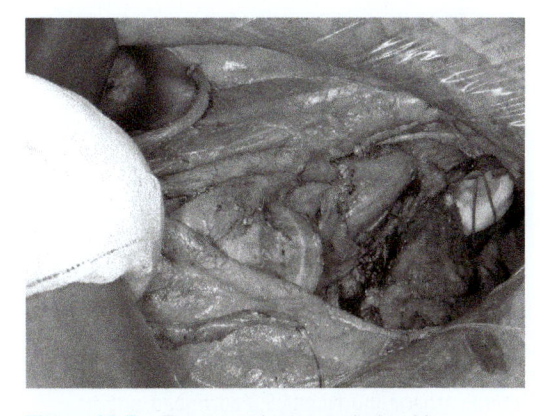

Figure 18.3 Transected ureters drained by pediatric feeding tubes. *Source:* Meara Dean, Alex Colquhoun, Peter Featherstone, Nicola S. Fearnhead, and R. Justin Davies.

the urogenital diaphragm, membranous urethra, and base of the penile urethra [18]. If there is concern regarding direct tumor infiltration or abutting of the public symphysis or inferior public rami, en-bloc pubic bone resection may be performed [19].

Managing the Empty Pelvis

After en-bloc resection of the pelvic organs the empty pelvic cavity may potentially fill with small intestine (Figure 18.4), leading to potential complications including small bowel obstruction and perineal herniation. If local recurrence occurs in this area, the small bowel may become involved, resulting in enterocutaneous fistula.

Options to fill the pelvic cavity include an omental pedicled flap, cecal mobilization, myocutaneous reconstructive flaps, biological mesh to separate the true pelvis from the abdominal cavity, and skin expanders and implants more commonly used in mammary reconstruction [20–23]. These techniques aim to displace the small intestine above the sacral promontory, and so allow early targeted postoperative re-irradiation where preoperative risk of enteritis was deemed unacceptably high due to interposed small bowel in the radiation field. Keeping small bowel loops out of the pelvis and away from the perineal bed reduces the risk of formation of obstruction, radiation injury, and enteroperineal fistulas. Small case series have shown that the use of mammary implants is well tolerated and can reduce rates of readmission due to early and late complications [24]. Tissue expanders have also been used to treat perineal hernias post exenteration [25].

Stoma Formation

Preoperative stoma marking is the first step to avoid a dysfunctional stoma, as a poorly placed stoma is more prone to hernia, prolapse, leaking, skin excoriation, sepsis, and difficulties with device placement. The ideal position is within the rectus abdominis muscle, in an area of flat skin, at a height that is visible and accessible to the patient. The position is marked with the patient supine, and then checked with the patient sitting and standing. This is particularly important in obese patients. Attention should be paid to the siting of the stoma in relation to drains and potential skin flaps. Multiple stomas require particularly careful siting.

Although often the last stage of a long operation, attention should be focused on performing technically well-constructed stoma(s). The skin edges and fascia should be grasped to align the skin with the abdominal wall. A stoma aperture should be created that matches the size of the bowel with its mesentery. The aperture should not be too tight, which can lead to postoperative bowel obstruction or stoma ischemia, or too loose which can lead to prolapse or herniation. Care should be taken not to injure the inferior epigastric vessels, as this potentially increases risk of subsequent parastomal herniation. The undersurface of the defect should be inspected for bleeding. If practicable, omental graft should be passed lateral to a left-sided colostomy to obliterate the lateral space. The bowel should be delivered in a tension-free manner to minimize the complication of stoma retraction and allow adequate

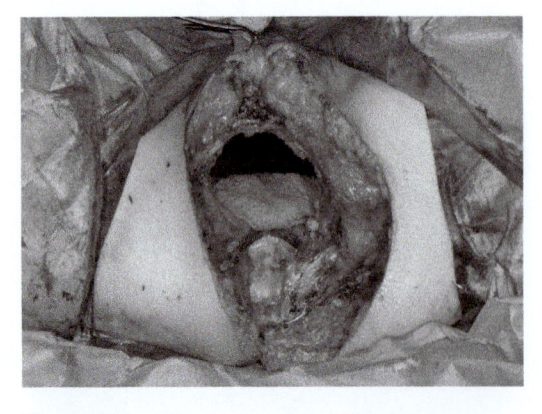

Figure 18.4 The empty pelvis following total exenteration with partial sacrectomy and sidewall dissection. Source: Meara Dean, Alex Colquhoun, Peter Featherstone, Nicola S. Fearnhead, and R. Justin Davies.

mucocutaneous apposition. A clear appliance should be applied to allow postoperative assessment of perfusion.

Postoperative Management

Critical Care

Exenterative surgery usually involves long operating times and the potential for major blood loss and physiological compromise. Postoperatively, patients should be managed in an Intensive Care or Higher Dependency Care setting. Epidural use is common in this setting, with plain epidural often being supplemented with opiate-based patient-controlled analgesia (PCA).

Venous Thromboembolic Prophylaxis

Sequential calf compression devices or compression stockings are continued along with chemical VTE prophylaxis, ideally starting within 12 hours of surgery. Extended thromboembolic prophylaxis for 28 days is advised due to the high rate of VTE in this patient cohort [26]. In some cases, the risk of hemorrhage will need to be balanced against the risk of VTE.

Enhanced Recovery after Surgery

Enhanced recovery after surgery (ERAS) programs have been validated in the elective colorectal setting [27], with benefits of reduced length of hospital stay, perioperative morbidity and mortality, and healthcare costs [28], and improved patient satisfaction [29]. These benefits have been described in both open and laparoscopic colorectal surgery [30]. ERAS protocols were based on established practice guidelines and evidence-based literature. Varied interventions are usually provided in a "bundle," commencing in the weeks before elective surgery, and continuing intraoperatively and in the postoperative period [31].

Aspects of ERAS programs that are particularly important for patients undergoing exenteration are postoperative physiotherapy and pain management. Physiotherapy is required from the first postoperative day to assist with chest physiotherapy, patient positioning, and mobilization at the earliest opportunity. Multimodal pain management is the preferred approach, with the use of regional, antineuropathic agents and opiate-sparing techniques [32].

Postoperative Complications

Early Complications

Early diagnosis and management of postoperative complications is important to minimize morbidity and improve patient outcomes. Acute postoperative complications are mostly related to the enormity of the physiological insult, and include cardiovascular compromise, metabolic derangement, coagulopathy, and renal impairment due to third space losses. Major postoperative complications are common and will inevitably prolong hospitalization [33]. Given the individualization of surgical procedure, the surgical team needs to communicate specific anticipated risks with the critical care team.

Cardiopulmonary complications
These patients are at high risk of cardiac events, pulmonary embolism, and adult respiratory distress syndrome (ARDS). Clinicians should monitor symptoms and have a low threshold to investigate with relevant blood tests and imaging.

Postoperative Bleeding
Hemoglobin should be monitored postoperatively. If there was major blood loss intraoperatively, the hematology team should be consulted and additional blood tests performed including platelet count, clotting profile, and calcium.

Surgical Site Infection

Wound infection is a common surgical complication, as most patients have cancer and have had radiotherapy to the operative field. Wounds should be frequently inspected and consideration given to vacuum-assisted closure dressings over wounds. Some groups have adopted the policy of five days of prophylactic intravenous antibiotics following surgery [34]. Deep pelvic collection within the empty pelvis is common. It is best diagnosed with postoperative cross-sectional imaging and managed with radiologically guided percutaneous drainage.

Flap Complications

Early complications of the myocutaneous flaps include necrosis, hematoma/seroma, and dehiscence. Attention to patient positioning is vital to preventing flap complications, with attention to offloading pressure on the flap and closing flaps over drains.

Prolonged ileus

Due to long operating times patients are at high risk of developing postoperative ileus. It is reasonable to consider early total parenteral nutrition (TPN) until diet is established.

Renal impairment

Renal function should be monitored postoperatively. Nephrotoxic medication should be withheld in the early postoperative period.

Urinary Leak

Ureteric stents placed via an ileal conduit will require regular flushes to ensure patency. Drains are left in the empty pelvis. The drain fluid creatinine should be checked postoperatively and the anastomosis assessed with stentogram prior to stent removal.

Stoma

Stoma(s) should be inspected postoperatively to ensure viability. The stoma often appears edematous and protruding in the initial days postoperatively. If stoma retraction occurs, early use of a convex pouching system may be beneficial.

Long-Term Complications

Minimization of long-term functional morbidity requires ongoing input from both surgeons and specialist nurses to proactively identify and address functional deficits during follow-up. Surveillance for recurrent cancer is discussed elsewhere; however, it is important to consider, as patients may present with non-specific symptoms initially.

Chronic Pain

Postoperatively patients have high levels of chronic pain, with rates of 70% quoted in the literature three years after exenteration [35]. Minimizing chronic postoperative pain starts with adequate management of perioperative pain.

Bowel Obstruction

Where possible, postexenteration bowel obstruction should be managed conservatively. Reoperation after exenteration is extremely difficult and will often lead to further morbidity.

Urological

Potential long-term urological complications include recurrent urinary tract infections, parastomal hernia, hydronephrosis, and ureteroileal stricture. Renal function will require long-term surveillance with annual investigations following ureteric diversion.

Sexual Function

Sexual dysfunction is a significant problem postoperatively, with difficulty in achieving orgasm and issues with body image common in both sexes [36]. Assessing sexual function may require targeted questioning to identify potentially remediable problems that the patient may not volunteer. Patients with sexual dysfunction should be referred for specialist assessment and treatment. Assessment should be performed using validated tools such as the International Index of Erectile Function (IIEF) and the Female Sexual Function Index (FISI).

In men, sexual dysfunction usually consists of erectile dysfunction and retrograde ejaculation. In females, problems with vaginal lubrication, dyspareunia, and lack of arousal are more common. Premenopausal women should be counseled as to the effects of inducing menopause. Risk factors for the development of sexual dysfunction include nerve damage, significant blood loss, preoperative radiotherapy, anastomotic leak, and the presence of a stoma [37].

For patients requiring exenteration with removal of the female reproductive organs, vaginal reconstruction with plastic surgery is a possible option. Preoperative counseling with the patient and their partner in respect to options for sexual function is important. The most common method for reconstruction is with myocutaneous skin flaps, such as gracilis or rectus abdominis. An alternative method uses a colonic conduit. A realistic explanation of the functional outcomes of the neovagina is a vital part of patient counseling before surgery.

Incisional, Perineal, and Parastomal Hernia

Patients should be educated regarding the risk of developing incisional and parastomal hernias. The stoma and abdominal and perineal wounds should be examined during postoperative visits. If symptomatic and adversely affecting QoL, patients should be referred for surgical repair.

Mental Health

Pelvic exenteration surgery requires a prolonged recovery time. Patients must cope with postoperative pain and fatigue, and uncertainty regarding their oncological outcome. They also need to adjust to an altered body imagine, with postoperative low body image commonly reported [38]. This is an understudied area; however, a recent study has shown that 44% of patients report some level of depression three years on from exenteration surgery [39]. Local practice involves psychological support via the liaison psychiatry counseling service.

Summary Box

- Pelvic exenteration surgery may be performed with low mortality rates in specialist multidisciplinary centers, but overall morbidity is high.
- Steps to reduce morbidity should be employed throughout the patient journey.
- A day-of-surgery safety checklist to address key anesthetic and surgical risk reduction strategies is useful.
- Early identification and treatment of postoperative complications helps minimize morbidity.
- Maintaining databases and performing regular audit are vital to assess outcomes and ensure high-quality care.

References

1 Gannon, C.J., Zager, J.S., Chang, G.J. et al. (2007). Pelvic exenteration affords safe and durable treatment for locally advanced rectal carcinoma. *Ann. Surg. Oncol.* 14: 1870–1877.

2 Law, W.L., Chu, K.W., and Choi, H.K. (2000). Total pelvic exenteration for locally advanced rectal cancer. *J. Am. Coll. Surg.* 190: 78–83.

3 Ferenschild, F.T., Varmaas, M., Verhoef, C. et al. (2009). Total pelvic exenteration for locally advanced rectal cancer. *World J. Surg.* 33: 1502–1508.

4 Vermaas, M., Ferenschild, F.T.J., Verhoef, C. et al. (2007). Total pelvic exenteraiton for primary locally advanced and locally recurrent rectal cancer. *Eur. J. Surg. Oncol.* 33: 452–458.

5 Melton, G.B., Paty, P.B., Boland, P.J. et al. (2006). Sacral resection for recurrent rectal cancer: analysis of morbidity and treatment results. *Dis. Colon Rectum* 49: 1009–1107.

6 Rausa, E., Kelly, M.E., Bonavina, L. et al. (2017). A systematic review examining the quality of life following pelvic exenteration for locally advanced and recurrent rectal cancer. *Colorectal Dis.* 19 (5): 430–436.

7 Dis Colon Rectum 2015 Aug;58(8):753-61. doi: 10.1097/DCR.0000000000000403. Effect of Surgery on Health-Related Quality of Life of Patients With Locally Recurrent Rectal Cancer Gianluca Pellino 1 , Guido Sciaudone, Giuseppe Candilio, Francesco Selvaggi

8 Young, J.M., Badgery-Parker, T., Masya, L.M. et al. (2014). Quality of life and other patient reported outcomes following exenteration for pelvic malignancy. *Br. J. Surg.* 101 (3): 277–287.

9 PelvEx Collaborative (2019). Surgical and survival outcomes following pelvic exenteration for locally advanced primary rectal cancer: results from an international collaboration. *Ann. Surg.* 269 (2): 315–321.

10 Gill, M., Fligelstone, L., Keating, J. et al. (2019). Avoiding, diagnosing and treating well leg compartment syndrome after pelvic surgery. *Br. J. Surg.* 106: 1156–1166.

11 Bhangu, A., Ali, S.M., Darzi, A. et al. (2012). Meta-analysis of survival based on resection margin status following surgery for recurrent rectal cancer. *Colorectal Dis.* 14 (12): 1457–1466.

12 PelvEx Collaborative (2018). Minimally invasive surgery techniques in pelvic exenteration: a systematic and meta-analysis review. *Surg. Endosc.* 32 (12): 4707–4715.

13 PelvEx Collaborative (2018). Factors affecting outcomes following pelvic exenteration for locally recurrent rectal cancer. *Br. J. Surg* 105: 650–657.

14 NICE (2015). *Blood transfusion. NICE Guideline NG24*. London: NICE.

15 Beyond TME Collaborative (2013). Consensus statement on the multidisciplinary management of patients with recurrent and primary rectal cancer beyond the total mesorectal excision planes. *Br. J. Surg.* 100 (8): 1009–1014.

16 Jiang, J., Li, X., Wang, Y. et al. (2013). Circular suture ligation of presacral venous plexus to control presacral bleeding during rectal mobilization. *J. Gastrointest. Surg.* 17 (2): 416–420.

17 Harrison, J.L., Hooks, V.H., Pearl, R.K. et al. (2003). Muscle fragment welding for control of massive presacral venous bleeding during rectal mobilization. *Dis. Colon Rectum* 46 (8): 1115–1117.

18 Solomon, M.J., Austin, K.K., Masya, L., and Lee, P. (2015). Pubic bone excision and perineal urethrectomy for radical anterior compartment excision during pelvic exenteration. *Dis. Colon Rectum* 58: 1114–1119.

19 Austin, K.K., Herd, A.J., Solomon, M.J. et al. (2016). Outcomes of pelvic exenteration with en bloc partial or complete pubic bone excision for locally advanced primary or recurrent pelvic cancer. *Dis. Colon Rectum* 59: 831–835.

20 Sugarbaker, P.H. (1983). Intrapelvic prothesis to prevent injury of the small intestine with high dosage pelvic irradiation. *Surg. Gynecol. Obstet* 157: 269–271.

21 Sezeur, A., Abbou, C., Chopin, D. et al. (1989). Protection of the small intestine against irradiation by means of a removable adapted prosthesis. *Dig. Surg.* 6: 83–85.

22 Tuecha, J.J., Chaudronb, V., Thomab, V. et al. (2004). Prevention of radiation enteritis by intrapelvic breast prosthesis. *Eur. J. Surg. Oncol* 30: 900–904.

23 Burnett, A.F., Coe, F.L., Klement, V. et al. (2000). The use of pelvic displacement prosthesis to exclude the small intestine from the radiation field following radical hysterectomy. *Gynecol. Oncol.* 79: 438–443.

24 Valle, M., Federici, O., Ialongo, P. et al. (2011). Prevention of complications following pelvic exenteration with the use of mammary implants in the pelvic cavity:

technique and results of 28 cases. *J. Surg. Oncol.* 103 (1): 34–38.

25 Ali, J.M., Stabler, A., Hall, N.R. et al. (Hernia 2013). Tissue expanders: early experience of a novel treatment option for perineal herniation. 17 (4): 545–549.

26 NICE (2018). Venous thromboembolism in over 16s: reducing the risk of hospital acquired deep vein thrombosis or pulmonary embolism. NICE Guideline NG89. London: NICE.

27 Kehlet, H. and Wilmore, D.W. (2002). Multimodal strategies to improve surgical outcome. *Am. J. Surg.* 183: 630–641.

28 Hjort Jakobsen, D., Sonne, E., Basse, L. et al. (2002). Convalescence after colonic resection with fast track versus conventional care. *Scand. J. Surg.* 93: 24–28.

29 Thiele, R.H., Rea, K.M., Turrentine, F.E. et al. (2015). Standardization of care: impact of an enhanced recovery protocol on length of stay, complications, and direct costs after colorectal surgery. *J. Am. Coll. Surg.* 220: 430–443.

30 Currie, A.C., Malietzis, G., Jenkins, J.T. et al. (2016). Network meta-analysis of protocol driven care and laparoscopic surgery for colorectal cancer. *Br. J. Surg.* 103: 1783–1794.

31 Nygren, J., Thacker, J., Carli, F. et al. (2012). Guidelines for perioperative care in elective rectal/pelvic surgery: enhanced recovery after surgery society recommendations. *Clin. Nutr.* 31: 801–806.

32 Lim, J.S., Koh, C.E., Liu, H. et al. (2018). The orice we pay for radical curative pelvic exenterations: prevalence and management of pain. *Dis. Colon Rectum* 61 (3): 314–319.

33 Bhangu, A., Ali, S.M., Brown, G. et al. (2014). Indications and outcome of pelvic exenteration for locally advanced primary and recurrent rectal cancer. *Ann. Surg.* 259 (2): 315–322.

34 Koh, C.E., Solomon, M.J., Brown, K.G. et al. (2017). The evolution of pelvic exenteration practice at a single center: lessons learned from over 500 cases. *Dis. Colon Rectum* 60 (6): 627–635.

35 Young, J., Solomon, M., Steffens, D., and Koh, C. (2018). Long term consequences of exenterative surgery for people with pelvic cancer. *J. Clin. Onc.* 36 (7): 118.

36 Hendren, S., O'onnor, B., Liu, M. et al. (2005). Prevalence of male and female sexual dysfunction is high following surgery for rectal cancer. *Ann. Surg.* 242: 212–223.

37 Lange, M., Marijnen, C., Maas, C. et al. (2009). Risk factors for sexual dysfunction after rectal cancer treatment. *Eur. J. Cancer* 45: 1578–1588.

38 Armbruster, S.D., Sun, C.C., Westin, S.N. et al. (2018). Prospective assessment of patient reported outcomes in gynecologic cancer patients before and after pelvic exenteration. *Gynecol. Oncol.* 149 (3): 484–490.

39 Young, J., Solomon, M., Steffens, D., and Koh, C. (2018). Long term consequences of exenterative surgery for people with pelvic cancer. *J. Clin. Oncol.* 36 (7): 118.

19

Crisis Management

Henrik Kidmose Christensen, Mette Møller Sørensen, and Victor Jilbert Verwaal

Department of Surgery, Aarhus University Hospital, Denmark

Background

Tumor resection of advanced pelvic and recurrence pelvic cancers is highly challenging, because the resections often are performed outside the standard surgical resections planes, and therefore are associated with considerable morbidity and mortality. Primary advanced tumors are typically adherent to or invading adjacent organs or fascia within the pelvis, while recurrent tumors occur outside normal anatomical planes due to prior cancer resection.

To obtain clear margins, extended multivisceral resections are required [1]. Both the patient and the surgeon must accept an increased risk of complications such as hemorrhage, unintended organ injury, neuropraxia, and issues like abdominal compartment syndrome [2].

Prior to Surgery

Preoperative evaluation and education of patients is the most important aspect in preparing patients for the treatment of advanced cancers. When planning the operative strategy, risk evaluation should be taken into account, as the complication risk is much higher in extensive surgical resections and should be balanced against the possible survival gain [3, 4]. Knowledge of tumor anatomy is vital to tailor each resection to the specific patient [5]. Preoperative imaging is important when planning the surgical procedure (Figure 19.1). Magnetic resonance imaging (MRI) provides the best assessment of tumor involvement of nearby organs and structures. Some advocate Advanced Multimodality Image Guided Operating (AMIGO) when planning the surgical procedure. This is a state-of-the-art medical and surgical research environment that houses a complete array of advanced imaging equipment and interventional surgical systems [6]. Knowledge of normal anatomy combined with improved imaging modalities (computed tomography (CT) and MRI) and new technology (3D printing) give the best-possible preparation to clarify the tumor specifics, including involved vasculature and nerves, and can help plan reconstruction. If major vessels are involved such as the external iliac artery, it may be better to plan a graft or perform an axillo-femoral bypass or a femoro-femoral bypass as a prior procedure before undertaking the definitive resection.

In one study of 377 patients undergoing pelvic exenteration it was noted that 57% of patients had a complication, and bleeding requiring a transfusion arose in 1/3 of the patients [7]. Intraoperative bleeding is a major issue when performing a major resection in the confines of a narrow pelvis. Therefore preoperative transfusion considerations are needed if substantial blood loss is likely.

Surgical Management of Advanced Pelvic Cancer, First Edition.
Edited by Michael E. Kelly and Desmond C. Winter.
© 2022 John Wiley & Sons Ltd. Published 2022 by John Wiley & Sons Ltd.

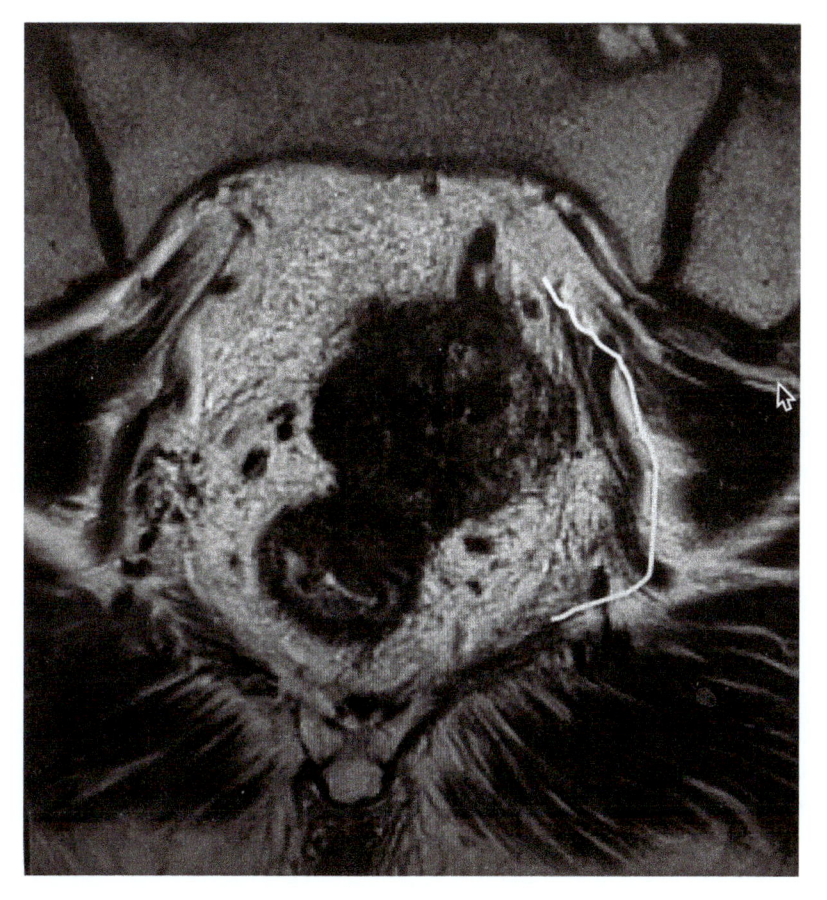

Figure 19.1 MRI used for planning surgery at the pelvic side wall.

Anesthetic involvement needing pre-and intraoperative plans is vital. Cessation of new non-vitamin K oral anticoagulants (NOACs) or other pharmacological agents needs to be carefully planned to balance the risk of arterial thrombus or venous thromboembolism [8].

Intraoperative Management

Hemorrhage Control

It is best to begin the pelvic dissection in a plane free of adhesions, in an area away from the tumor where possible [9–11]. Early identification and control of key vessels and structures is imperative. Intraoperatively, the tactile sense of the surgeon is useful to distinguish between soft normal tissue and tumor-involved tissue (which is often fibrotic and hard). Sometimes it can be difficult (impossible) to distinguish tumor from radiotherapy-related fibrosis or scar tissue. Aggressive resection of adherent structures is often required to avoid compromising the surgical margin.

Anatomical variation regarding the veins in the pelvis is a potential challenge during removal of the tumor. Surgical clips are useful but can fall off during further dissection. Alternatively, electrothermal bipolar vessel sealing (EBVS) has revolutionized pelvic surgery and can seal blood vessels up to 7 mm in diameter [12]. Sometimes, temporary sealing can improve the ability to remove the tumor before final closure of the vessels definitively (suture ligation), especially when dealing with the pelvic sidewall.

New hemostatic patches are available with different coagulation features. Veriset™ has three human components that promote hemostasis [13]. Starsil® is a plant-derived polysaccharide hemostatic powder that can be used as an alternative to bone-wax when bleeding occurs after sacrectomy [14]. Floseal™ is an agent that contains high concentration of human thrombin, converting fibrinogen into fibrin monomers, and accelerates clot formation [15]. Surgiflo® provides a gelatin–thrombin hemostatic matrix for platelet adherence [16]. Alternatively, Tachosil® is a fibrin sealant patch that promotes hemostasis by triggering the last stage of the coagulation cascade to create a fibrin clot [17]. Personal experience and preference dictate which products to use, but in general most of these patches are best on bigger surfaces with continuous ooze. In addition, these products are a supplement to conventional hemostatic methods.

For major hemorrhage, packing of the pelvis with surgical swabs/packs remains the fundamental management strategy. The resection may be abandoned, packs may be left in situ, and it is possible for reevaluation in theater 24–48 hours later when the patient is hemodynamically stable. Resuscitative endovascular balloon occlusion of the aorta is a technique for temporary stabilization of patients with non-compressible torso hemorrhage, but there is limited evidence regarding its role in major pelvic surgery [18]. In addition, there are studies examining the use of recombinant factor VIIa (NovoSeven®RT) in uncontrolled hemorrhage [19].

Postoperative Hemorrhage

Significant blood loss in the early postoperative phase is infrequent. It usually results in a patient returning to the operating room for exploration. Typical causes include a slipped ligature or dislodgement of a diathermy coagulum as blood pressure recovers from the anesthesia.

Late secondary hemorrhage is rare and typically occurs seven to ten days after surgery. This can be due to an infective collection, pressure effect from a surgical drain eroding an adjacent blood vessel, or ruptured mycotic pseudo-aneurysm. Interventional radiological embolization has significantly improved the management of secondary hemorrhage.

Nerve Damage

One of the most substantial side effects of advanced pelvic surgery is functional impairment due to nerve damage after a further successful resection. Nerve injury occurs in approximately 2% of all pelvic surgery and is more frequent in pelvic exenteration [20]. In principle, there are two categories that result in a nerve injury. The first category includes intended nerve resection to achieve clear margins. The sciatic, femoral, and obturator nerves are the most common nerves to be sacrificed. The second category of nerve injury is due to an unintended iatrogenic cause. There are three ways this typically occurs: transection injury, entrapment of the nerve, or compression/stretching injury. Transection results in immediate functional loss [21]. Entrapment of nerves occurs when nerves are caught in a suture or supporting mash. This can be associated with chronic pain and can be difficult to manage [22]. Compression or overstretching of the nerve gives mostly functional loss due to ischemia or compression of the vasa nervorum. The most common cause of this injury is due to instrumental retraction. The overwhelming majority of compression or retractor injuries are self-resolving. In very select cases a repair of the damaged nerve may be need to improve functional status. Proper positioning of the patient is the key to prevention of nerve injury [23]. Prolonged duration of the Trendelenburg position and lithotomy position should be avoided in long operations. If necessary the patient should be put back in the supine position, with the legs down for a period. Care should be given to the placement of retractors. Avoiding deep imprecise sutures for bleeding or excessive electrocauterization is also paramount.

Obturator Nerve

The obturator nerve, which starts at the root of L4 and enters the medial side of the psoas muscle, follows the sidewall along the second branch of the internal iliac artery. It is at risk when the tumor or metastasis involves the lateral pelvic wall [24, 25]. An injury will result in weakness of the adductor muscles. Remarkably, walking is not very affected by transection, but more advanced movement can be impaired.

Femoral Nerve

The femoral nerve lies on the dorsal and distal aspect of the psoas muscle (lateral side). It starts at the root of L4 and tracts follow the femoral artery. This nerve is at risk when resecting part or all of the psoas. Injuries are more commonly secondary to self-retaining retractors especially in patients who are thin and have a narrow pelvis [25, 26]. Most compression injuries are self-resolving; however, significant injuries can result in weakness of hip flexion and knee extension. This is a significant deformity, reducing mobility including sitting down, standing up from sitting, and difficulty in going up/down stairs. Physiotherapy and/or a knee-brace may help; in select cases, microsurgical replacement of the nerve can lead to function recovery.

Sciatic Nerve

The sciatic nerve is formed from a collection of fibers involving L4–S3 roots. The fiber unites to form a single nerve in front of the piriformis muscle, and passes through the greater sciatic foramen to exit the pelvis. Inadvertent injury caused by transection results in foot drop and some lower limb weakness/paresis. With good ankle and foot splinting/prothesis and extensive physiotherapy, it may be possible to restore some ambulation.

Sacralplexus

Unintended injury to the sacral plexus roots (S1–S4) mostly results from deep suturing in the dorsal pelvic wall and floor or in sacral bone resection [27]. Alternatively, compression by collection/abscess can cause compression of the distal aspect of the nerve. Most symptoms start shortly after the operation and vary from pain to rectal, urinary, or sexual dysfunction. Removal of the suture can relieve the symptoms or another option is injection with a gamma-aminobutyric acid (GABA) antagonist. When the symptoms are due to an infection/collection, drainage will resolve symptoms in most cases [28].

Injury to Bowel or Urinary Tract

Injury to the bowel can occur during dissection of adhesions from prior surgery, or due to inadvertent use of retractors or diathermy. Intestinal injury often involves the small bowel and can vary from small serosal tears to full-thickness laceration to the bowel or mesentery. Early identification and management avoids delayed complications.

Iatrogenic ureteral injury during pelvic surgery is well described, even as surgical techniques have improved. In severe incidences, preoperative ureteral stenting (including lighted stents) may be used. However, prophylactic stenting is not complication-free and routine use is controversial. Accurate identification of the ureters is a vital step in prevention of iatrogenic ureteral injuries. However, distortion of normal anatomy by large pelvic masses, prior surgery, or irradiation therapy can increase risk of injury. If there is concern about a ureteral injury, early check of drain creatinine level plus dedicated radiological imaging are essential for early identification. A delayed recognition of ureteral injuries may require temporary urinary diversion via a percutaneous nephrostomy prior to definitive surgical repair. In select cases, immediate ureteral reconstruction in the postoperative period can be achieved, but postoperative tissue edema and inflammation can render definite management difficult.

Postoperative Management

Abdominal Compartment

Abdominal compartment syndrome can occur after major abdominal/pelvic surgery [29, 30]. One of the most common etiological factors is massive infusion of crystalloid fluids during the intraoperative period [31, 32]. A physiological consequence of this is reduced venous return, impairing cardiac output, resulting in impaired renal function due to reactive vasoconstriction via activation of the renin-angiotensin system. In addition, there is reduced intestinal perfusion due to lower mesenteric blood flow and impairment of the liver's ability to clear lactate. The management of abdominal compartment syndrome often requires surgical decompression by opening of the abdominal wound. This can result in issues with wound closure, incisional hernia, loss of reconstructive flaps, and delayed recovery [33].

Delayed Presentation of Bowel or Urinary Tract Injury

Inadvertent enterotomy is a dangerous complication, with considerable morbidity and/or mortality. Any patient with signs of deterioration, features of peritonitis, sepsis, or increased abdominal pain after pelvic exenteration must be investigated promptly. Studies have shown a 20% incidence of inadvertent enterotomy in patients who had a repeat laparotomy, especially where dividing of adhesions was required [34, 35].

Early intervention is needed to limit morbidity, typically with the creation of a proximal stoma [36]. In cases where stoma formation is impossible due to severe adhesions, carcinomatosis, obesity, postoperative inflammation, shortening of the mesentery, or a frozen abdomen/pelvis the surgeon is left with less-optimal choices. In these cases, placement of a Foley catheter as a controlled enterostomy or fistula is an option [4]. The balloon is inflated with 3 ml of saline and a purse-string suture of absorbable material is placed around the perforation. The defect is then anchored to the anterior abdominal wall with absorbable sutures. The catheter is fixed so that the balloon exerts gentle pressure to the area, to help promote a controlled fistula tract [37].

Massive Transfusion

Massive blood transfusion is defined as replacement of a patient's total blood volume within a 24-hour period. Consequences of massive blood transfusion are dependent on early restoration of changes in body biochemistry, such as hypocalcemia, hypomagnesemia, and hypokalemia. In addition, coagulopathy and hypothermia most be corrected. Blood transfusion is also associated with higher risk of venous thromboembolism in multitransfused trauma patients or those with advanced cancer [38]. Rare complications of massive transfusion includes lower extremity compartment syndrome and myocardial infarction.

Summary Box

- Both the patient and the surgeon must be aware an increased risk of complications with pelvic exenterative surgery, including massive hemorrhage, unintended organ injury, neuropraxia, and/or abdominal compartment syndrome.
- Optimal preoperative imaging is essential prior to advanced pelvic surgery.
- Multivisceral resection often outside normal surgical planes is associated with a higher rate of complications and careful intraoperative strategies must be established to deal with complications.
- Patients must be counseled and well informed of possible issues and be made aware of potential long-term sequela.

References

1 Yeo, H.L. and Paty, P.B. (2014). Management of recurrent rectal cancer: practical insights in planning and surgical intervention. *J. Surg. Oncol.* 109: 47–52.

2 Musters, G.D., Buskens, C.J., Bemelman, W.A., and Tanis, P.J. (2014). Perineal wound healing after abdominoperineal resection for rectal cancer: a systemic review and meta-analysis. *Dis. Colon Rectum* 57: 1129–1139.

3 Nielsen MB (2012). Outcome following intended curative treatment of locally recurrent rectal cancer. PhD thesis. Aarhus University, Denmark.

4 Iversen, L.H., Nørgaard, M., Jacobsen, J. et al. (2009). The impact of comorbidity on survival of Danish colorectal cancer patients from 1995–2006 – a population-based cohort study. *Dis. Colon Rectum* 52: 71–78.

5 Skandalakis, J.E., Kingsnorth, A.N., Colborn, G.L. et al. (2004). Large intestine and anorectum. In: *Surgical Anatomy* (ed. P.N. Skandalakis), 904–907. Athens: Paschalis Medical Publications.

6 Tempany, C.M.C., Jagadeesan, J., Kapur, T. et al. (2015). Multimodal imaging for improved diagnosis and treatment of cancers. *Cancer* 121: 817–827.

7 Speicher, P.J., Turley, R.S., Sloane, J.L. et al. (2014). Pelvic exenteration for the treatment of locally advanced colorectal and bladder malagnancies in the modern era. *J. Gastrointest. Surg.* 18: 782–788.

8 Verma, A., Ha, A.C.T., Rutka, J.T., and Verma, S. (2018). What surgeons should know about non-vitamin K oral anticoagulants. A review. *JAMA Surg.* 153: 577–585.

9 Solomon, M.J., Brown, K.G.M., Koh, C.E. et al. (2015). Lateral pelvic compartment excision during pelvic excision. *Br. J. Surg.* 102 (17): 1710–1717.

10 Hockel, M. (2008). Laterally extended endopelvic resection (LEER) – principles and practice. *Gynecol. Oncol.* 111: S13–S17.

11 Bouchard, P. and Efron, J. (2010). Management of recurrent rectal cancer. *Ann. Surg. Oncol.* 17: 1343–1356.

12 Milsom, J., Trencheva, K., Monette, S. et al. (2012). Evaluation of the safety, efficacy, and versatility of a new surgical energy device (Thunderbeat) in comparison with harmonic ACE, Ligasure V, and Enseal devices in a porcine model. *J Laparoendosc. Adv. Surg. Tech.* 22: 378–386.

13 Lewis, K.M., Schivic, A., Hedrich, H.-C. et al. (2014). Hemostatic efficacy of a novel PEG-coated collagen pad in clinically relevant animal models. *Int. J. Surg.* 12: 940–944.

14 Schmitz, C. and Sodian, R. (2015). Use of a plant-based polysaccharide hemostat for the treatment of sternal bleeding after median sternotomy. *J. Cardiothorac. Surg.* 10: 59.

15 Nasso, G., Piancone, F., Bonifazi, R. et al. (2009). Prospective, randomized clinical trial of the FloSeal matrix sealant in cardiac surgery. *Ann. Thorac. Surg.* 88: 1520–1526.

16 Price, J.S., Tackett, S., and Patel, V. (2015). Observational evaluation of outcomes and resource utilization from hemostatic matrices in spine surgery. *J. Med. Econ* Jun 1: 1–10.

17 Marano, L. and Di Martino, N. (2016). Efficacy of human fibrinogen-thrombin patch (Tarcosil) clinical application in upper gastrointestinal surgery. *J. Investig. Surg.* 29: 352–358.

18 Sadeghi, M., Nilsson, K.F., Larzon, T. et al. (2018). The use of aortic balloon occlusion in traumatic shock: first report from the ABO trauma registry. *Eur. J. Trauma Emerg. Surg.* 44: 491–501.

19 Kenet, G., Walden, R., Eldad, A., and Martinowitz, U. (1999). Treatment in traumatic bleeding with recombinant factor VIIa. *Lancet* 359: 1879.

20 Cardosi, R.J., Cox, C.S., and Hoffman, M.S. (2002). Postoperative neuropathies after major pelvic surgery. *Obstet. Gynecol.* 100 (2): 240–244.

21 Ducic, I., Moxley, M., and Al-Attar, A. (2006). Algorithm for treatment of postoperative incisional groin pain after cesarean delivery or hysterectomy. *Obstet. Gynecol.* 108: 27–31.

22 Sippo, W.C. and Gomec, A.C. (1987). Nerve-entrapment syndromes from lower abdominal surgery. *J. Fam. Pract.* 25: 585–587.

23 Chan, J.K. and Manetts, A. (202). Prevention of femoral nerve injuries in gynecologic surgery. *Am. J. Obstet. Gynecol.* 186: 1–7.

24 Corona, R., De Cicco, C., Schonman, R. et al. (2008). Tension-free vaginal tapes and pelvic nerve neuropathy. *J. Minim. Invasive Gynecol.* 15: 262–267.

25 Irvin, W., Andersen, W., Taylor, P., and Rice, L. (2004). Minimizing the risk of neurologic injury in gynecologic surgery. *Obstet. Gynecol.* 103: 374–382.

26 Noldus, J., Graefen, M., and Huland, H. (2002). Major postoperative complications secondary to use of the Bookwalter self-retaining retractor. *Urology* 60: 964–967.

27 Flynn, M.K., Weidner, A.C., and Amundsen, C.L. (2006). Sensory nerve injury after uterosacral ligament suspension. *Am. J. Obstet. Gynecol.* 195: 1869–1872.

28 Wang, R. (2007). Penile rehabilitation after radical prostatectomy: where do we stand and where are we going? *J. Sex. Med.* 4: 1085–1097.

29 Morken, J. and West, M.A. (2001). Abdominal compartment syndrome in the intensive care unit. *Curr. Opin. Crit. Care* 7: 268–274.

30 Saggi, B.H., Sugerman, H.J., Ivatury, R.R., and Bloomfield, G.L. (1998). Abdominal compartment syndrome. *J. Trauma* 45: 597–609.

31 Holodinsky, J.K., Roberts, D.J., Ball, C.G. et al. (2013). Risk factors for intra-abdominal hypertension and abdominal compartment syndrome among adult intensive care unit patients: a systematic review and meta-analysis. *Crit. Care* 17: R249.

32 Malbrain, M.L., Cheatham, M.L., Kirkpatrick, A. et al. (2006). Results from the international conference of experts on intra-abdominal hypertension and abdominal compartment syndrome. I. Definitions. *Intensive Care Med.* 32: 1722–1732.

33 Kirkpatrick, A.W., Roberts, D.J., De Waele, J. et al. (2013). Intra-abdominal hypertension and the abdominal compartment syndrome: updates, consensus, definitions and clinical practice guidelines from the World Society of the Abdominal Compartment Syndrome. *Intensive Care Med.* 39: 1190–1206.

34 Krabben, A.A. (2000). Morbidity and mortality of inadvertent enterotomy during adhesiotomy. *Br. J. Surg.* 87 (4): 467–471.

35 Van Goor, H. (2007). Consequenses and complications of peritoneal adhesions. *Colorectal Dis.* 9 (Suppl 2): 25–34.

36 Schein, M. (1999). Postoperative small bowel leak. *Br. J. Surg.* 86: 979–980.

37 Tøttrup, A. (2010). Foley catheter enterostomy for postoperative bowel perforation: an effective source control. *World J. Surg.* 34: 2752–2754.

38 Goel, R., Patel, E.U., Cushing, M.M. et al. (2018). Association of perioperative red blood cell transfusions with venous thromboembolism in a North American Registry. *JAMA Surg.* 153 (9): 826–833.

20

Quality of Life and Patient-Reported Outcome Measures Following Pelvic Exenteration

Daniel Steffens[1], Cherry Koh[1,2,3,4], and Michael Solomon[1,2,3,4]

[1] *Surgical Outcomes Research Centre (SOuRCe), Royal Prince Alfred Hospital, Sydney, New South Wales, Australia*
[2] *RPA Institute of Academic Surgery, Royal Prince Alfred Hospital, Sydney, New South Wales, Australia*
[3] *Department of Colorectal Surgery, Royal Prince Alfred Hospital, Sydney, New South Wales, Australia*
[4] *Discipline of Surgery, Central Clinical School, Sydney Medical School, University of Sydney, Sydney, New South Wales, Australia*

Background

Advanced cancers of the pelvis are morbid cancers. At the time of presentation, most patients are highly symptomatic [1]. The high symptom burden is likely at least in part to be accountable for the poor quality of life of these patients at diagnosis [2]. Surgical treatment of these advanced cancers involves radical resection of all contiguously involved pelvic structures, which generally includes resection of the rectum and the genitourinary organs but may also extend to include major neurovascular structures of the pelvis or the bony pelvis itself. Because of the complexity of these operations, postoperative recovery is usually prolonged and operative morbidity is high. Furthermore, the radical re-resection, coupled with prior radiotherapy can have long-term functional consequences for the patient such as sexual dysfunction or urinary or fecal incontinence, as well as the need for two stomas. With even more extended resections where major nerve excision is needed, there can be additional implications to lower limb function [3]. All these in turn contribute to adversely affecting the patient's long-term quality of life. Recent studies have also suggested the possibility of persistent pain long after the surgical insult [4, 5]. Not only may pain cause quality of life impediments, but also it has been suggested that pain may influence long-term prognosis [4]. Therefore, while pelvic exenteration may offer a cure, there are definite long-term treatment-related effects for the patient, particularly surrounding function and quality of life.

Quality of Life and Patient-Reported Outcomes Instruments

From an anatomic viewpoint, most functional deficits are predictable based on preoperative imaging and the magnitude of the anticipated resection. Some aspects of patient-reported outcomes, however, are not predictable, such as chronic pain, body-image issues, psychological impacts, or concerns for the future. At present, there is no single validated and standardized tool that adequately captures all relevant aspects of pelvic exenteration. To date, most studies have either combined a number of previously validated tools to report on the outcome of interest, adopted an existing tool to address specific outcomes of clinical interest,

Surgical Management of Advanced Pelvic Cancer, First Edition.
Edited by Michael E. Kelly and Desmond C. Winter.
© 2022 John Wiley & Sons Ltd. Published 2022 by John Wiley & Sons Ltd.

or utilized a non-validated instrument purpose designed for the individual study based on clinical experience. Notwithstanding this, there is now a quality of life instrument specific for patients with locally recurrent rectal cancer that is being developed and validated [6]. The tool has been developed following focus group interviews of expert clinicians and patients diagnosed with locally recurrent rectal cancer which identified two main themes. The two themes identified pertained to health-related quality of life and healthcare services delivery. Within health-related quality of life, several relevant subdomains were identified which included symptoms, sexual function, psychological impact, role, and social functioning, as well as future perspective, while within health services utilization, the subdomains identified included disease management, treatment expectations, and confidence with healthcare professionals [6].

Quality of life assessment instruments and other patient-reported outcome tools commonly used in pelvic exenteration literature are summarized in Table 20.1. As most pelvic exenterations are performed for a malignant indication, most authors have chosen a generic cancer quality of life instrument and its relevant modules to assess the outcomes of interest. The choice of instrument in turn depends on the outcome of interest. The only problem with this approach is the burden of the questionnaires to the patient as the number of instruments increases, which reduces patient compliance if repeated longitudinal measures are intended.

Table 20.1 Common quality of life (QoL) instruments and other health-related quality of life (HRQoL) instruments used in pelvic exenteration studies.

Type of instrument	Domains	Comments
Generic QoL		
SF-36	36-item questionnaire covering eight domains: vitality, physical functioning, bodily pain, general health perception, physical role functioning, emotional role functioning, social role functioning, and mental health. Domains are scored to give two components: a mental health component and a physical health component	Most widely used QoL instrument. There are shorter versions available, e.g. SF12. SF36 scores can be converted into a utility-based score using available statistical packages to calculate cost-effectiveness
AQOL	Four versions with a varying number of items. AQOL 8 has 35 items covering eight domains: independent living, happiness, mental health, coping, relationships, self-worth, pain, and senses	A health-related multi-attribute utility quality of life instrument. Score can be converted to a utility score which permits cost-utility assessment
EQ5D	5-item questionnaire across five domains: mobility, self-care, usual activities, pain/discomfort, and anxiety/depression	Simple to administer. Can be used to calculate QALYs for cost-effectiveness analyses
Cancer-specific		
FACT-G	27-item questionnaire across four domains: physical, social, emotional, and functional well-being	Disease-specific modules complement FACT-G and are available for 20 different cancers
EORTC QLQ-C30	30-item questionnaire covering function, symptoms, and overall quality of life	Disease-specific modules complement QLQ-C30 and are available for 24 different cancers

Table 20.1 (Continued)

Type of instrument	Domains	Comments
Symptom-specific		
Bowel function		
EORTC QLQ-CR29	29-item scale which is to be used as the colorectal cancer subscale in addition to the 30-item QLQ-C30	More comprehensive assessment of bowel function (7 items on stoma, 6 on bowels), urinary [4], and sexual [2] function, as well as gastrointestinal symptoms because of the larger number of items
FACT-C	Total of 36 items which include 27 items from FACT-G. The additional nine items cover abdominal symptoms, bowel function, and stoma care	The "C"-colorectal cancer subscale has only an additional nine items, which simplifies administration and reduces survey burden
Urinary function		
EORTC QLQ-CR29	29-item scale which is to be used as the colorectal cancer subscale in addition to the 30-item QLQ-C30	Contains four questions on urinary function/incontinence
Sexual function		
EORTC QLQ-CR29	29-item scale for colorectal cancer which is to be used as the colorectal cancer subscale in addition to the 30-item QLQ-C30	Contains two questions each for men or women
EORTC QLQ-CX24	24-item subscale designed for cervical cancer to be used in conjunction with QLQ-C30	Contains seven questions about female sexual function. Mostly used in gynecological exenteration literature
EORTC QLQ-EN24	24-item subscale designed for endometrial cancer to be used in conjunction with QLQ-C30	Contains six questions about female sexual function. Mostly used in gynecological exenteration literature
EORTC QLQ-OV-28	28-item subscale designed for ovarian cancer to be used in conjunction with QLQ-C30	Contains four questions about female sexual function. Mostly used in gynecological exenteration literature
EORTC QLQ-PR25	28-item subscale designed for prostate cancer to be used in conjunction with QLQ-C30	Contains six questions about male sexual function
Anxiety/ depression HADS	14-item scale, 7 each for anxiety and depression	Although this has been used previously, the majority of studies will rely on the anxiety/depression questions contained within either FACT or EORTC questionnaires
Pain LANSS	7-item pain scale, specifically for neuropathic pain	Five of the items are part of a bedside questionnaire but the remaining two questions rely on bedside patient assessment
BPI	Long and short forms available. The short form contains 15 items, whereas the long form also asks for other patient-specific information	The short form is most widely utilized
Distress DISTRESS THERMOMETER	A rapid screening tool for psychological distress in cancer patients. Typically 0 to 10 on visual analog scale	Simple, rapid, and effective tool to screen for the presence of distress. However, its use requires validation

(*Continued*)

Table 20.1 (Continued)

Type of instrument	Domains	Comments
Lower limb function		
MSTS	Designed to assess upper and lower limb function in patients with sarcoma. Six items each for upper and lower limbs	Would generally only use upper or lower limb questionnaires depending on the disease
Biagini	6-item questionnaire with two each on motor function, urinary, and bowel function	Non-validated but commonly used instrument in orthopedic literature following sacrectomy

QALY, Quality-adjusted life-year; AQOL, assessment of quality of life; EQ5D, EuroQoL-5D; HADS, Hospital Anxiety and Depression Scale; LANSS, Leeds Assessment of Neuropathic Symptoms and Signs; BPI, Brief Pain Inventory; MSTS, Musculoskeletal Tumor Society Score.

The use of investigator-designed (i.e. non-validated instruments) is also present but this appears to be more common within the orthopedic literature. The use of other validated instruments such as the Modified Obstruction and Defecation Scale (MODS) for bowel function or the International Continence Society (ICS) score for urinary function has also been reported but, once again, mostly within the sarcoma literature. Table 20.2 summarizes the main instruments used within recent quality of life studies in pelvic exenteration patients.

Quality of Life Trajectories Following Pelvic Exenteration

Beyond survival, patients undergoing pelvic exenteration with curative intent for advanced primary or recurrent gynecological and rectal malignancies want to have a minimum acceptable level of quality of life for the extent of their lives. We now describe the quality of life trajectories for patients undergoing pelvic exenteration due to gynecological malignancies (i.e. vaginal, cervical, and uterine cancer), rectal malignancies (i.e. advanced primary or recurrent malignancies), mixed malignancies (i.e. mixed samples, such as rectal, gynecological, and urological malignancies), and palliative exenteration.

Gynecological Malignancies

To date, most of the evidence describing the quality of life trajectories following gynecological malignancies derives from small samples (range, n = 16–62) with short-term follow-up (i.e. up to 12 months postoperative). Most of this evidence is from patients presenting a wide range of gynecological malignancies, including cervical cancer, endometrial cancer, vaginal cancer, ovarian cancer, and uterine cancer [7–15].

Martinez et al. [13] performed a multicenter prospective cohort study with 61 patients evaluating the quality of life at preoperative and then at 1, 3, 6, and 12 months post pelvic exenteration performed with curative intent for gynecological malignancies such as vaginal and cervical cancer (n = 51), uterine cancer (n = 9), and other forms of cancer (n = 1). Quality of life was measured using the EORTC QLQ-C30 (version 3.0) and the EORTC QLQ-OV28 instruments. Only 38% (n = 23) of the patients responded to the last follow-up questionnaire (12 months). Overall, quality of life decreased one month postoperative and reached preoperative level by three months. From 6 to 12 months, quality of life increased above the preoperative scores and remained stable (Figure 20.1a) [13].

All other quality of life measures, such as physical functioning, role functioning,

Table 20.2 Evidence of quality of life (QoL) following pelvic exenteration.

Author, year (country), n	Malignancy (n)	QoL tool	QoL domain	Time point	Main finding
Gynecological malignancies					
Vera, 1981 [29] (USA) n = 19	Recurrent vulvovaginal cancer (n = 1) Recurrent cervical cancer (n = 18)	Open-ended questions	Social Sexual Psychological	Cross-sectional	Patients see their QoL as above-average, in a trend of improvement
Hawighorst et al., 1997 [12] (Germany) n = 28	Recurrent cervical cancer (n = 28)	Cancer Rehabilitation Evaluation System (CARES)	Physical Medical interaction Psychosocial Sexual Marital Global score	Baseline 4 months 12 months	Patients had a significantly better QoL outcome following surgery
Hawighorst et al., 2004 [11] (Germany) n = 62	Recurrent cervical cancer (n = 62)	Cancer Rehabilitation Evaluation System (CARES-SF)	Physical Psychosocial Sexual Medical interaction Marital Global score	Baseline 4 months 12 months	Patients improved QoL within 12 months postoperatively
Forner and Lampe, 2011 [10] (Germany) n = 100	Cervical (n = 54) Endometrial (n = 11) Vulval (n = 20) Vaginal (n = 6) Ovarian (n = 6) Other cancer (n = 3)	Short Form-12 Health Survey Questionnaire (SF-12)	Mental component score Physical component score	Cross-sectional	Overall QoL remains acceptable after pelvic exenteration
Rezk et al., 2013 [14] (USA) n = 16	Endometrial (n = 4) Vaginal (n = 3) Cervical (n = 7) Vulvovaginal (n = 1) Ovarian (n = 1)	European Organization for Research and Treatment of Cancer (EORTC QLQ-C30/QLQ-CR38/ QLQ-BLM30)	Physical function Role function Emotional function Social function Cognitive functions Overall QoL	Baseline 3 months 6 months 12 months	Although patients report some persistent decline in physical function after pelvic exenteration, most adjust well, returning to almost baseline functioning within a year

(*Continued*)

Table 20.2 (Continued)

Author, year (country), n	Malignancy (n)	QoL tool	QoL domain	Time point	Main finding
Ngô et al., 2013 [15] (France) [30] n = 25	Recurrent endometrial cancer (n = 8) Recurrent cervical cancer (n = 17)	European Organization for Research and Treatment of Cancer (EORTC QLQ-C30/ QLQ-CX24)	Physical function Role function Emotional function Social function Cognitive functions Overall QoL	Cross-sectional	Overall QoL was lower than reported in the literature
Dessole et al., 2018 [9] (Italy/Germany) n = 96	Cervical (n = 71) Endometrial (n = 14) Vaginal (n = 4) Vulval (n = 7)	European Organization for Research and Treatment of Cancer (EORTC QLQ-C30/ QLQ-CX24/ QLQ-OV28)	Physical function Role function Emotional function Social function Cognitive functions Overall QoL	Cross-sectional	Pelvic exenteration retains a positive impact on overall QoL
Martinez et al., 2018 [13] (France) n = 61	Vaginal/cervical (n = 51) Uterine (n = 9) Other cancer (n = 1)	European Organization for Research and Treatment of Cancer (EORTC QLQ-C30/ QLQ-OV28)	Physical function Role function Emotional function Social function Cognitive functions Overall QoL	Baseline 1 month 3 months 6 months 12 months	Deterioration of QoL was most significant by 3 months. Overall QoL improved 1 year after surgery
Armbruster et al., 2018 [7] (USA) n = 55	Cervical (n = 22) Uterine (n = 12) Vaginal (n = 11) Vulval (n = 9) Ovarian (n = 1)	Short Form-12 Health Survey (SF-12)	Mental component score Physical component score	Baseline 6 months 12 months	Physical functioning declined, while mental functioning increased slightly in postoperatively
Rectal malignancies					
Guren et al., 2001 [21] (Norway) n = 37	Advanced primary or recurrent rectal – with/ without urostomy (n = 37)	European Organization for Research and Treatment of Cancer (EORTC QLQ-C30/QLQ-CR38/ QLQ-BLM30)	Physical function Role function Emotional function Social function Cognitive functions Overall QoL	Cross-sectional	QoL scores were comparable with the general population

Study	Population	Instrument	Domains	Time points	Key findings
Esnaola et al., 2002 [20] (USA) n = 30	Recurrent rectal (n = 30)	Functional Assessment of Cancer Therapy – Colorectal (FACT-C)	Physical Social/family Emotional Functional	Cross-sectional	After pelvic exenteration, patients reported good QoL
Austin et al., 2010 [16] (Australia) n = 37	Advanced primary rectal (n = 17) Recurrent rectal (n = 20)	Short Form-36 Health Survey Questionnaire (SF-36) Functional Assessment of Cancer Therapy – Colorectal (FACT-C)	Physical component score (SF-36) Mental component score (SF-36) Physical (FACT-C) Social/family (FACT-C) Emotional (FACT-C) Functional (FACT-C) Total score (FACT-C)	Cross-sectional	Overall QoL scores for patients undergoing pelvic exenteration were good, although physical scores were lower and mental scores were higher than the general population.
Beaton et al., 2014 [19] (Australia) n = 31	Recurrent rectal (n = 17) Advanced primary rectal (n = 14)	Functional Assessment of Cancer Therapy – Colorectal (FACT-C)	Total score	Cross-sectional	Mean FACT-C score was 100.7 ± 13.5, indicating good QoL
Pellino et al., 2015 [22] (Italy) n = 30	Recurrent rectal (n = 30)	European Organization for Research and Treatment of Cancer (EORTC QLQ-C30)	Physical function Role function Emotional function Social function Cognitive functions Overall QoL	Baseline 12 months 36 months	Patients with R0 resection demonstrated a prompt and stable recovery of QoL
Choy et al., 2017 [17] (Australia) n = 93	Recurrent rectal (n = 93)	Assessment of Quality of Life (AQOL)	Overall score	Baseline 1 month 3 months 6 months 9 months 12 months	QoL scores initially declined, followed by a recovery period, but mean score did not return to baseline by 12 months

(Continued)

Table 20.2 (Continued)

Author, year (country), n	Malignancy (n)	QoL tool	QoL domain	Time point	Main finding
Radwan et al., 2015 [23] (UK) n = 56	Advanced primary rectal (n = 56)	European Organization for Research and Treatment of Cancer (EORTC QLQ-C30)	Physical function Role function Emotional function Social function Cognitive functions Overall QoL	Baseline 2 weeks 3 months 6 months 12 months 24 months	Patient's recovery baseline QoL within 6 months following pelvic exenteration, improving slightly thereafter
Quyn et al., 2016 [26] (Australia) n = 104	Advanced primary rectal (n = 104)	Short Form-36 Health Survey Questionnaire (SF-36) Functional Assessment of Cancer Therapy - Colorectal (FACT-C)	Physical component score (SF-36) Mental component score (SF-36) Total score (FACT-C)	Baseline Discharge 1 month 3 months 6 months 12 months	QoL improves rapidly after pelvic exenteration and continues to improve over the first year
Mixed malignancies					
Young et al., 2014 [2] (Australia) n = 148	Recurrent rectal (n = 75) Advanced primary rectal (n = 36) Recurrent other (n = 26) Primary other (n = 11)	Short Form-36 Health Survey Questionnaire (SF-36) Functional Assessment of Cancer Therapy - Colorectal (FACT-C)	Physical component score (SF-36) Mental component score (SF-36) Total score (FACT-C)	Baseline 1 month 3 months 6 months 9 months 12 months	QoL improves rapidly after pelvic exenteration surgery
Levy et al., 2016 [25] (Czech Republic) n = 63	Primary rectal (n = 39) Recurrent rectal (n = 15) Rectal/prostate (n = 3) Bladder (n = 2) Anal (n = 2) Cervical (n = 2)	European Organization for Research and Treatment of Cancer (EORTC QLQ-C30/QLQ-CR29)	Physical function Role function Emotional function Social function Cognitive functions	Cross-sectional	Most patients reported a good level of QoL

Roos et al., 2004 [27] (Netherlands) n = 25	Bladder (n = 6) Gynecological (n = 19)	European Organization for Research and Treatment of Cancer (EORTC QLQ-C30/ QLQ-OV28)	Physical function Role function Emotional function Social function Cognitive functions Overall QoL	Cross-sectional	Despite the immense effect of pelvic exenteration on physical, sexual, and social functioning, patients reported similar levels of emotional functioning and general QoL compared to healthy women
Steffens et al., 2018 [28] (Australia) n = 287	Primary rectal (n = 77) Recurrent rectal (n = 119) Primary other (n = 41) Recurrent other (n = 50)	Short Form-36 Health Survey Questionnaire (SF-36) Functional Assessment of Cancer Therapy - Colorectal (FACT-C)	Physical component score (SF-36) Mental component score (SF-36) Total score (FACT-C)	Baseline 6 months 12 months 18 months 24 months 30 months 36 months 48 months 60 months	Overall, QoL returned to baseline within 6 months after pelvic exenteration.

cognitive functioning, and social functioning, followed similar trajectories, declining at one month postoperative and increasing thereafter, except for emotional functioning, which increased during the first six months and remained stable thereafter (Figure 20.2a) [13]. Rezk et al. [14] reported similar results in their prospective study (n = 16). Emotional functioning improved shortly after surgery and significantly improved at 12 months, when compared to baseline.

Armbruster et al. [7] assessed quality of life after pelvic exenteration for a variety of gynecological malignancies, including cervical cancer (n = 22), vaginal cancer (n = 11), uterine cancer (n = 12), vulval cancer (n = 9), and ovarian cancer (n = 1). The short-form 12 Health Survey was used to report on the physical and mental component scores at three time-points (preoperative and 6 and 12 months postoperatively). The physical component score decreased from preoperative to 6 months and remained lower than preoperative by 12 months. The mental component score increased from preoperative to 6 months and remained higher than preoperative by 12 months. Overall, it seems that patients undergoing pelvic exenteration due to gynecological malignancies present an acceptable postoperative quality of life.

Rectal Malignancy

The evidence on quality of life following pelvic exenteration for rectal malignancies has evolved recently, with most significant work conducted by a high-volume pelvic exenteration center in Australia [16–18]. In terms of quality of life trajectories, there are reports in patients presenting with advanced primary rectal malignancies and recurrent rectal malignancies, with most studies following patients up to 12 and 36 months [16–23].

Choy et al. [17] performed a prospective cohort study evaluating quality of life in 117 patients presenting with recurrent rectal malignancy, where 93 underwent pelvic exenteration and 24 did not agree to curative surgery. Quality of life measures were evaluated at preoperative and 1, 3, 6, 9, and 12 months postoperatively using the Assessment of Quality of Life (AQOL) instrument. Quality of life for the recurrent rectal malignancy patients that underwent pelvic exenteration initially declined, followed by a recovery period between 3 and 9 months, but not returning to the preoperative score by 12 months. In contrast, the 24 non-exenteration patients gradually declined their quality of life over the 12 months study period.

Radwan et al. [23] evaluated long-term quality of life trajectories in 56 advanced primary rectal malignancy patients undergoing pelvic exenteration. Quality of life was assessed at preoperative, 2 weeks, 3, 6, 12, and 24 months postoperatively using the EORTC QLQ-C30. Quality of life significantly decreased at 2 weeks postoperative, slightly increasing by 3 months, and improving from preoperative scores by 24 months (Figure 20.1b) [23]. Similarly, Quyn et al. [18] reported quality of life trajectories in 104 patients with locally advanced primary rectal malignancies that underwent pelvic exenteration. Quality of life was assessed using the FACT-C and SF-36 instruments at preoperative and 3, 6, 9, and 12 months postoperatively. Overall, patients have returned to their preoperative quality of life (FACT-C) scores within 3 months postoperatively, increasing slightly from 3 months to 12 months. In addition, the mental and physical component scores (SF-36) decreased in the immediate postoperative period but returned to preoperative levels at 2 months (mental component scores) and 6 months (physical component score). Thereafter, both component scores presented a steady increase up to 12 months.

Patients with advanced primary rectal malignancies experienced a significant decrease in physical functioning, role functioning,

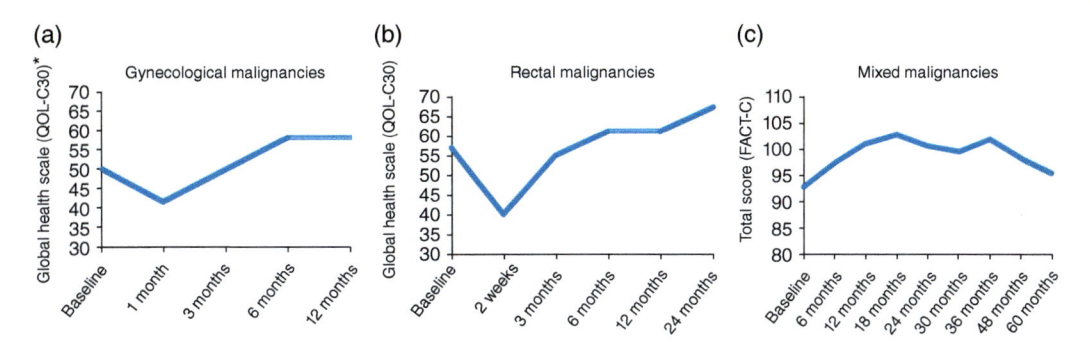

Figure 20.1 Quality of life following pelvic exenteration.
a. *Source:* Redrawn from Martinez A, Filleron T, Rouanet P, Meeus P, Lambaudie E, Classe JM, et al. Prospective Assessment of First-Year Quality of Life After Pelvic Exenteration for Gynecologic Malignancy: A French Multicentric Study. Annals of surgical oncology. 2018;25(2):535-41
b. *Source:* Redrawn from Radwan RW, Codd RJ, Wright M, Fitzsimmons D, Evans MD, Davies M, et al. Quality-of-life outcomes following pelvic exenteration for primary rectal cancer. The British journal of surgery. 2015;102(12):1574-80.
c. *Source:* Redrawn from Steffens D, Solomon MJ, Young JM, Koh C, Venchiarutti RL, Lee P, et al. Prospective cohort study of long-term survival and quality of life following pelvic exenteration. BJS Open. 2018([accepted]):1-8

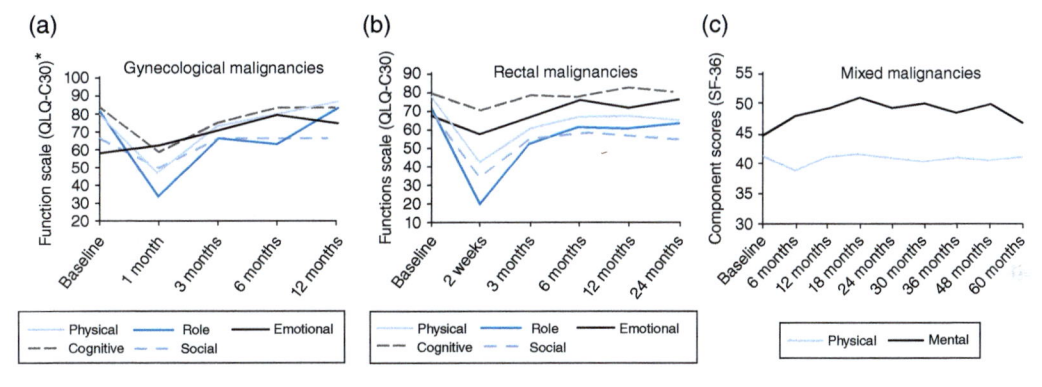

Figure 20.2 Functional, physical, and mental component scores following pelvic exenteration.
a. *Source:* Redrawn from Martinez A, Filleron T, Rouanet P, Meeus P, Lambaudie E, Classe JM, et al. Prospective Assessment of First-Year Quality of Life After Pelvic Exenteration for Gynecologic Malignancy: A French Multicentric Study. Annals of surgical oncology. 2018;25(2):535-41
b. *Source:* Redrawn from Radwan RW, Codd RJ, Wright M, Fitzsimmons D, Evans MD, Davies M, et al. Quality-of-life outcomes following pelvic exenteration for primary rectal cancer. The British journal of surgery. 2015;102(12):1574-80.
c. *Source:* Redrawn from Steffens D, Solomon MJ, Young JM, Koh C, Venchiarutti RL, Lee P, et al. Prospective cohort study of long-term survival and quality of life following pelvic exenteration. BJS Open. 2018([accepted]):1-8

emotional functioning, cognitive functioning, and social functioning during the first few months postoperative [17, 23]. While all functioning scores improved between 2 weeks and 3 months postoperatively, role functioning, physical functioning, and social functioning did not return to preoperative scores within 24 months postoperatively (Figure 20.2b) [23].

Recently, a systematic review investigated quality of life following locally advanced rectal malignancy and local recurrent rectal malignancy [24]. The authors found seven studies (sample size ranged from 30 to 104) investigating quality of life in studies published between 2002 and 2016. In this review it was reported that quality of life following pelvic exenteration for advanced primary or recurrent rectal malignancies improves over the first postoperative year, returning to preoperative status within 2 to 9 months postoperative in the vast majority of the included studies.

Mixed Malignancies

To date, most of the evidence on quality of life trajectories included a sample with mixed malignancies undergoing pelvic exenteration. Such samples reported in the literature included a cohort of patients presenting with advanced primary rectal malignancy, recurrent rectal malignancy, gynecological malignancies, and urological malignancies [2, 25–27].

Steffens et al. [28] reported on the largest prospective cohort of patients described in the literature (287 patients) with the longest follow-up time point (60 months). This included patients presenting with mixed malignancies such as advanced primary rectal malignancy (n = 77), recurrent rectal malignancy (n = 119), advanced primary other malignancies (n = 41), and recurrent other malignancies (n = 50). Quality of life was assessed via the FACT-C and SF-36 instruments and patients were constantly followed from preoperative to 60 months postoperative. The FACT-C total score increased from baseline until 18 months postoperative and remained stable and above preoperative levels within 60 months follow-up (Figure 20.1c) [28]. The mental component score of the SF-36 survey improved up to 18 months postoperative and remained stable thereafter, while the physical component score declined at 6 months postoperative, returning to the preoperative quality of life level by 12 months and remaining stable until the 60 months postoperative follow-up.

Young et al. [2] compared quality of life trajectories over 12 months for patients who did (n = 148) and those who did not (n = 34) undergo pelvic exenteration for mixed malignancies. Quality of life was assessed using the FACT-C and SF-36 instruments and patients were followed at preoperative, predischarge, and 1, 3, 6, 9, and 12 months postoperatively. Quality of life decreased after pelvic exenteration but improved and was comparable to those who did not undergo pelvic exenteration within 1 month postoperatively. After 6 months, patients that underwent pelvic exenteration improved slightly to 12 months, while patients that did not undergo pelvic exenteration declined by the 12 month postoperative measure.

Palliative Exenteration

Palliative exenterations have been and remain a controversial area within the exenteration literature. From a clinical view point, while there are studies that suggest improved symptom control and survival, others have not. From a quality of life viewpoint, Quyn et al. reviewed the quality of life of 39 patients who underwent pelvic exenteration with a palliative intent [26]. Survival of patients who underwent palliative exenteration was significantly better compared to patients who underwent palliative surgery alone (e.g. formation of colostomy), but quality of life trajectories showed a significant drop after surgery and this was followed by a continued gradual decline, with no sustained improvement in subsequent quality of life on follow-up. Furthermore, although there was no in-hospital mortality, major morbidity occurred in 34% of patients. In view of this, palliative exenteration remains controversial and should only be offered selectively on a case by case basis.

Predictors of Postoperative Quality of Life

There are some reports in the literature that aimed to investigate if patient demographics and/or clinical characteristics predict a better or worse postoperative quality of life outcome. However, due to the small number of patients included in these reports, only a limited number of predictors could be investigated. Most of the evidence comes from studies investigating potential predictors on patients undergoing pelvic exenteration for gynecological malignancies and rectal malignancies.

Dessole et al. investigated if patient's age and clinical characteristics (i.e. tumor site, clinical setting, extent of exenteration, urinary diversion, colostomy, and number of ostomies) in a population presenting with gynecological malignancies undergoing pelvic exenteration predicts quality of life at a median time point of 36 months post operation [9]. Patients presenting with a higher number of ostomies, an incontinent bladder, and a definitive colostomy were all independent predictors of poor postoperative quality of life. Other reports demonstrated that older patients (> 60 years) were significantly associated with poorer quality of life, physical scores, and social functioning. Vaginal reconstruction was associated with an increased quality of life score [13].

Three reports investigated predictors of postoperative quality of life in patients undergoing pelvic exenteration due to rectal malignancies. Choy et al. investigated if preoperative quality of life, age, gender, bony resection, margin status, extent of exenteration, and American Society of Anesthesiologists (ASA) scores predicted quality of life scores 12 months after pelvic exenteration in 93 patients [17]. A higher preoperative quality of life score was associated with better postoperative quality of life, whereas female gender and having a bony resection as part of pelvic exenteration were significant predictors of poor quality of life at 12 months. Austin et al. reported that male patients had significantly better mental health scores on the SF-36 survey [16].

Pellino et al. investigated if age, gender, multimodal therapy, complications, and margin status were predictors of poor quality of life scores [22]. The multivariate analysis indicated that patients that had an R2 margin status were three times more likely to have worst quality of life scores postoperative when compared to patients that presented with an R0/R1 margin status. Earlier, Austin et al. had also suggested that margin status was a predictor of quality of life, reporting that patients with an R0 resection margin presented better physical component scores on the SF-36 survey [16].

To date, only a limited number of studies have investigated if patients' demographics and clinical characteristics were predictors of postoperative quality of life. However, most of the significant predictors found to influence postoperative quality of life were non-modifiable, such as gender and bony resection. Therefore we should perhaps focus on factors that are modifiable, such as resection margin and baseline quality of life scores. At this point in time, interventions investigating strategies to improve preoperative quality of life and precision of resection margin (R0) as a means to improve postoperative quality of life are warranted.

Patient-Reported Outcome Measures Following Pelvic Exenteration

Pain is a common complaint in the perioperative period among patients undergoing pelvic exenteration, although this has been very poorly investigated [5, 20]. There are only a few studies assessing pain symptoms in patients undergoing pelvic exenteration. Young et al. investigated the course of pain symptom in patients presenting with mixed malignancies over the period of 12 months [2]. Patients presented with a moderate level of pain at the preoperative assessment and not much change occurred during the first month postoperatively. After the first month postoperatively, pain decreased significantly to approximately 50% of the preoperative value by 12 months. However, in another report involving patients undergoing pelvic exenteration due to gynecological malignancies, pain did not change from preoperative to 3, 6, and 12 months postoperative, with patients reporting a constant lower level of pain [14]. In another study by You et al. looking at patients with recurrent rectal cancers, moderate to high pain scores were found in long-term survivors even in the absence of further disease recurrence. Importantly, patients found to have moderate or more pain were also found to have worse long-term survival compared to patients reporting less severe pain at presentation [4].

A recent study by Lim et al. [5] addressed pain in exenteration patients specifically and also looked at perioperative pain management issues in this cohort of patients. In this retrospective study of 99 patients undergoing pelvic exenteration, a third of patients were found to have significant pain prior to surgery. Patients on preoperative opiates also had more challenging pain management postoperatively, with higher pain scores, longer lengths of stays, higher postoperative opiate consumption, and higher requirements for pain specialist review. The need for opiate-sparing regimes would seem preferable in these patients. In combination, what these studies suggest is the need for better pain management and this has implications for cancer survivorship.

Patients undergoing pelvic exenteration present a clinically important level of distress at the preoperative assessment. Psychological support during the preoperative period and early in the postoperative period should be implemented as part of a pelvic exenteration multidisciplinary team. Young et al. investigated the level of distress throughout 12 months using the distress thermometer [2]. Although preoperative distress levels were high, they decreased slightly over the 12 months study period.

Future Directions

Research involving quality of life following pelvic exenteration is in its infancy, due to not only the small number of prospective studies published to date, but also underpowered studies with small sample sizes. Despite the overall survival rate for patients undergoing pelvic exenteration having increased since the 1990s, studies aiming to collect long-term quality of life outcomes struggle to follow a reasonable number of patients, due to patients lost to follow-up, withdrawn consent, and death. Steffens et al. report on one of the largest prospective cohort studies investigating long-term follow-up including quality of life outcomes [28]. Of the 287 patients that consented to the study preoperatively, only 33% were successfully followed at five years postoperatively, due to 114 deaths, 57 missing data or withdrawn consent, and 88 patients that did not reach the five-year time-point. Therefore it may take some time for us to have some in-depth long-term results. Furthermore, this study only presented data from survivors and methods of data imputation should be considered in future investigations.

Most studies conducted thus far use a generic quality of life instrument. Therefore it is also clear that a more specific measure of quality of life is needed for patients presenting with locally advanced or recurrent cancer confined to the pelvis, including gynecological, rectal, and urological neoplasms. Recently, a specific quality of life questionnaire for patients presenting with locally advanced recurrent rectal cancer was proposed, and it is currently being piloted in the UK and Australia [6]. This instrument will be available in the coming years. It is urged that other research centers start developing other quality of life measures that are specific to their population of interest. However, it is also suggested that a validated and reliable generic quality of life instrument is used in pelvic exenteration research, such as the SF-36 and the EQ-5D instruments. This not only will provide reliable quality of life information of the studied population but also would allow for meaningful comparisons with other patient groups, such as patients undergoing pelvic exenteration due to gynecological, rectal, or urological malignancies or other types of cancer surgery.

In addition, researchers are urged to investigate potential modifiable factors that would influence short- and long-term quality of life outcomes, such as pain, nutrition, and physical fitness management, as well as prospective psych-oncological intervention where future target interventions may result in better quality of life.

Summary Box

- At present there is no validated quality of life instrument specific for patients undergoing pelvic exenteration.
- Most studies reporting quality of life in patients undergoing pelvic exenteration have utilized existing validated instruments by combining them. Despite this, the assessment remains ad hoc. This also contributes to the burden of the questionnaire.
- Patients undergoing pelvic exenteration due to gynecological, rectal, and other malignances present a decline of their quality of life and functional outcomes during the first three months postoperatively, with most patients recovering to their preoperative quality of life and functional levels by six months postoperatively.
- Higher number of ostomies, incontinent bladder, definitive colostomy, older age, female gender, bony resection, and R2 margin status were all predictors of poor postoperative quality of life.
- Pain is a major consideration in patients with advanced cancers of the pelvis. Studies suggest that at least one-third of patients have severe preoperative pain and that this in turn exacerbates postoperative pain management.

References

1 Miner, T.J., Jaques, D.P., Paty, P.B. et al. (2003). Symptom control in patients with locally recurrent rectal cancer. *Ann. Surg. Oncol* 10 (1): 72–79.
2 Young, J.M., Badgery-Parker, T., Masya, L.M. et al. (2014). Quality of life and other patient-reported outcomes following exenteration for pelvic malignancy. *Br. J. Surg* 101 (3): 277–287.
3 Fourney, D.R., Rhines, L.D., Hentschel, S.J. et al. (2005). En bloc resection of primary sacral tumors: classification of surgical approaches and outcome. *J. Neurosurg. Spine* 3 (2): 111–122.
4 You, Y.N., Habiba, H., Chang, G.J. et al. (2011). Prognostic value of quality of life and pain in patients with locally recurrent rectal cancer. *Annals of Surgical Oncology* 18 (4): 989–996.
5 Lim, J.S., Koh, C.E., Liu, H. et al. (2018). The price we pay for radical curative pelvic exenterations: prevalence and management of pain. *Dis. Colon Rectum* 61 (3): 314–319.
6 Harji, D.P., Koh, C., Solomon, M. et al. (2015). Development of a conceptual framework of health-related quality of life in locally recurrent rectal cancer. *Colorectal Dis* 17 (11): 954–964.
7 Armbruster, S.D., Sun, C.C., Westin, S.N. et al. (2018;149(3):484–90). Prospective assessment of patient-reported outcomes in gynecologic cancer patients before and after pelvic exenteration. *Gynecolog. Oncol.*

8 Berretta, R., Marchesi, F., Volpi, L. et al. (2016). Posterior pelvic exenteration and retrograde total hysterectomy in patients with locally advanced ovarian cancer: clinical and functional outcome. *Taiwan. J. Obstet. Gynecol* 55 (3): 346–350.

9 Dessole, M., Petrillo, M., Lucidi, A. et al. (2018). Quality of life in women after pelvic exenteration for gynecological malignancies: a multicentric study. *Int. J. Gynecol. Cancer* 28 (2): 267–273.

10 Forner, D.M. and Lampe, B. (2011). Ileal conduit and continent ileocecal pouch for patients undergoing pelvic exenteration: comparison of complications and quality of life. *Int. J. Gynecol. Cancer* 21 (2): 403–408.

11 Hawighorst-Knapstein, S., Fusshoeller, C., Franz, C. et al. (2004). The impact of treatment for genital cancer on quality of life and body image – results of a prospective longitudinal 10-year study. *Gynecol. Oncol* 94 (2): 398–403.

12 Hawighorst-Knapstein, S., Schonefussrs, G., Hoffmann, S.O., and Knapstein, P.G. (1997). Pelvic exenteration: effects of surgery on quality of life and body image – a prospective longitudinal study. *Gynecol. Oncol* 66 (3): 495–500.

13 Martinez, A., Filleron, T., Rouanet, P. et al. (2018). Prospective assessment of first-year quality of life after pelvic exenteration for gynecologic malignancy: a French multicentric study. *Ann. Surg. Oncol* 25 (2): 535–541.

14 Rezk, Y.A., Hurley, K.E., Carter, J. et al. (2013). A prospective study of quality of life in patients undergoing pelvic exenteration: interim results. *Gynecol. Oncol* 128 (2): 191–197.

15 Ngô, C., Abboud, C., Meria, P. et al. (2013). Long term outcome and quality of life after pelvic exenteration for recurrent endometrial and cervical cancers. *Open J. Obstet. Gynecol.* 3 (5A1): 19–27.

16 Austin, K.K., Young, J.M., and Solomon, M.J. (2010). Quality of life of survivors after pelvic exenteration for rectal cancer. *Dis. Colon Rectum* 53 (8): 1121–1126.

17 Choy, I., Young, J.M., Badgery-Parker, T. et al. (2017). Baseline quality of life predicts pelvic exenteration outcome. *ANZ J. Surg* 87 (11): 935–939.

18 Quyn, A.J., Austin, K.K., Young, J.M. et al. (2016). Outcomes of pelvic exenteration for locally advanced primary rectal cancer: overall survival and quality of life. *Eur. J. Surg. Oncol.* 42 (6): 823–828.

19 Beaton, J., Carey, S., Solomon, M.J. et al. (2014). Preoperative body mass index, 30-day postoperative morbidity, length of stay and quality of life in patients undergoing pelvic exenteration surgery for recurrent and locally-advanced rectal cancer. *Ann. Coloproctol* 30 (2): 83–87.

20 Esnaola, N.F., Cantor, S.B., Johnson, M.L. et al. (2002). Pain and quality of life after treatment in patients with locally recurrent rectal cancer. *J. Clin. Oncol* 20 (21): 4361–4367.

21 Guren, M.G., Wiig, J.N., Dueland, S. et al. (2001). Quality of life in patients with urinary diversion after operation for locally advanced rectal cancer. *Eur. J. Surg. Oncol* 27 (7): 645–651.

22 Pellino, G., Sciaudone, G., Candilio, G., and Selvaggi, F. (2015). Effect of surgery on health-related quality of life of patients with locally recurrent rectal cancer. *Dis. Colon Rectum* 58 (8): 753–761.

23 Radwan, R.W., Codd, R.J., Wright, M. et al. (2015). Quality-of-life outcomes following pelvic exenteration for primary rectal cancer. *Br. J. Surg* 102 (12): 1574–1580.

24 Rausa, E., Kelly, M.E., Bonavina, L. et al. (2017). A systematic review examining quality of life following pelvic exenteration for locally advanced and recurrent rectal cancer. *Colorectal Dis.* 19 (5): 430–436.

25 Levy, M., Lipska, L., Visokai, V., and Simsa, J. (2016). Quality of life after extensive pelvic surgery. *Rozh. Chir* 95 (9): 358–462.

26 Quyn, A.J., Solomon, M.J., Lee, P.M. et al. (2016). Palliative pelvic exenteration: clinical outcomes and quality of life. *Dis. Colon Rectum* 59 (11): 1005–1010.

27 Roos, E.J., de Graeff, A., van Eijkeren, M.A. et al. (2004). Quality of life after pelvic exenteration. *Gynecol. Oncol* 93 (3): 610–614.
28 Steffens, D., Solomon, M.J., Young, J.M. et al. (2018). Cohort study of long-term survival and quality of life following pelvic exenteration. *BJS Open* 2 (5): 328–335.
29 Vera, M.I. (1981). Quality of life following pelvic exenteration. *Gynecol. Oncol.* 12: 355–366.

21

Adjuvant Therapy options after Pelvic Exenteration for Advanced Rectal Cancer

Ka On Lam[1], Jeremy Yip[2], and Wai Lun Law[2]

[1] Department of Clinical Oncology, Faculty of Medicine, University of Hong Kong, Hong Kong
[2] Department of Surgery, Faculty of Medicine, University of Hong Kong, Hong Kong

Background

Exenteration is an ultra-major surgery that involves radical en-bloc resection of all pelvic organs including the rectum, sigmoid colon, distal ureter, urinary bladder, internal reproductive organs, regional lymph nodes, and pelvic peritoneum. In order to achieve negative margin (R0 resection), soft tissues, neurovascular bundles, and even bony structures in the proximity may need to be resected. In the setting of recurrent disease, achieving an R0 resection can be technically challenging due to prior distorted anatomy and fibrosis from prior interventions. As a result, R0 resection was only about 50–60% even in highly specialized centers [1] and therefore adjuvant therapy represents a rational approach to eradicate potential microscopic residual disease.

This chapter aims to review the most up-to-date available evidence for adjuvant therapy following pelvic exenteration for colorectal cancer.

Adjuvant Therapy

In the modern era, approximately 6–10% of patients with rectal cancer have locally advanced disease without metastasis at the time of diagnosis. The number of patients is relatively small to support multiple adequately powered phase III randomized controlled studies. Thus, the evidence for adjuvant therapy after pelvic exenteration has largely been generated from retrospective analysis of single-center cohorts until recently. In the report by Kusters et al., the role of adjuvant chemotherapy after exenteration was studied retrospectively in 95 patients with T4 rectal cancer [2]. All patients received neoadjuvant chemotherapy ± radiotherapy followed by radical surgery. A high R0 resection rate of 87% was reported with favorable long-term outcomes: five-year local recurrence rate of 17%, distant metastasis rate of 16%, and overall survival (OS) rate of 62%. Postoperative chemotherapy was given to 33% of patients and omission of adjuvant chemotherapy was the only factor associated with death on multivariable analysis. The five-year OS were 80% vs. 53% (p = 0.016) in patients who were and were not given adjuvant therapy respectively. Although the number of patients was small and details of chemotherapy missing, the results did support the consideration of adjuvant chemotherapy post exenteration.

Bhangu et al. compared the outcomes of 100 patients following exenteration for locally advanced rectal cancer (LARC) and locally

Surgical Management of Advanced Pelvic Cancer, First Edition.
Edited by Michael E. Kelly and Desmond C. Winter.
© 2022 John Wiley & Sons Ltd. Published 2022 by John Wiley & Sons Ltd.

recurrent rectal cancer (LRRC) [3]. Rates of R0 resection were significantly higher in cases of LARC than in LRRC (91% vs. 62%; p = 0.001). Patients with LRRC may have higher risk of distant relapse after exenteration despite R0 resection as the disease-free survival (DFS), but not the local relapse-free survival, was numerically higher in patients with LARC than LRRC (76% vs. 57%; p = 0.212). Similarly, Nielsen et al. reported higher R0 rate and improved five-year survival in LARC than LRRC [4]. Besides the chronicity of disease presentation, lymph node involvement was associated with significantly decreased OS (p = 0.03) and relapse-free survival (p = 0.01) in a Japanese series of 93 patients from 1975 to 2005 [5]. Therefore it has been proposed that chemotherapy treatment in the pre- and postoperative setting of pelvic exenteration should be considered for patients with lymph node involvement. Currently, the main limitation regarding the assessment of outcomes following pelvic exenteration is the relative paucity of prospective data, in particular the lack of evidence regarding adjuvant therapy.

However, in current practice, adjuvant chemotherapy is recommended in a stage-directed manner by major international guidelines irrespective of whether neoadjuvant therapy has been given [6, 7]. Indeed, only a few studies and meta-analyses suggest a benefit of adjuvant 5-FU (fluorouracil)-based chemotherapy in terms of DFS and OS after surgery alone for rectal cancer, with a magnitude of benefit that is relatively smaller than that of colon cancer [8]. The QUASAR trial demonstrated a 3.6% absolute improvement in OS at five years with adjuvant chemotherapy and recommended adjuvant chemotherapy for all patients with stage II rectal cancer after surgery [9]. However, these results may not be directly applicable to those contemporary patients who undergo total mesorectal excision (TME) with or without neoadjuvant therapy. Moreover, following neoadjuvant radiotherapy with or without chemotherapy, the benefit of 5-FU alone postoperatively has not been demonstrated [10–14].

The I-CNR-RT study enrolled 655 patients with clinically T3–4N ± disease to observation alone or adjuvant 5-FU/LV (leucovorin) after neoadjuvant chemoradiotherapy and surgery, but it failed to show any benefit with adjuvant therapy in the overall population and in the subgroup analysis [10]. The PROCTOR-SCRIPT study by the Dutch Colorectal Cancer Group was another negative study that compared observation vs. adjuvant 5FU or capecitabine [11]. Although the EORTC 22921 study suggested a potential benefit of adjuvant 5FU in patients who could be downstaged to ypT0–2 after initial neoadjuvant chemoradiotherapy, the benefit was not confirmed after a median follow-up of 10.4 years [12]. Nevertheless, in the absence of any concluding data from a large prospective study, any downstaging resulting from neoadjuvant chemoradiotherapy should be regarded as prognostic of outcomes rather than being predictive of the benefit from adjuvant therapy.

Oxaliplatin improves the DFS and OS in stage III colon cancer, but its role in patients with rectal cancer after neoadjuvant chemoradiotherapy is not clearly defined. Attempts have then been made to evaluate the benefit of adding oxaliplatin to adjuvant 5-FU-based chemotherapy in rectal cancer. The CHRONICLE study which compared observation vs. XELOX was closed prematurely due to slow accrual [13]. Although numerical improvement was observed, the study was underpowered for demonstrating any significant DFS or OS in the 113 randomized patients. A meta-analysis of individual patient data from the I-CNR-RT, PROCTOR-SCRIPT, CHRONICLE, and EORTC 22921 studies concluded that adjuvant fluoropyrimidine-based therapy did not improve OS, DFS, or distant recurrence [14]. However, patients with upper rectal tumor at 10–15 cm from the anal verge may benefit in terms of DFS and distant recurrence. While the jury is still out on the role of adjuvant oxaliplatin, the phase II ADORE study compared patients who received neoadjuvant chemoradiotherapy to adjuvant 5FU/LV or FOLFOX. After a median follow-up of

38 months, three-year DFS was 71.6% in the FOLFOX group compared with 62.9% in the 5FU/LV group (HR 0.657, 95% CI 0.434–0.994, p = 0.047), suggesting the benefit for combination therapy in this setting. The result can be regarded as hypothesis-generating and further confirmatory phase III studies are eagerly awaited.

In short, definitive evidence for adjuvant therapy in resected rectal cancer, especially for those who have received prior neoadjuvant chemoradiotherapy, is lacking and the use of adjuvant chemotherapy is generally an extrapolation of evidence from that of resected colon cancer. With regard to patients who have undergone exenteration, the evidence is even less robust as the number of patients with T4 disease or exenteration performed was small in the landmark studies (Table 21.1). In addition, the potential benefit of adjuvant chemotherapy in those patients who can be downstaged with neoadjuvant chemoradiotherapy is apparently irrelevant for those who are still judged to require exenteration. Compliance is another challenging issue since as many as a quarter of patients in these landmark studies never started adjuvant treatment despite being randomized. For patients after exenteration the compliance will likely be lower as a result of prolonged recovery from the major surgery. Nevertheless, the benefit of combination chemotherapy was statistically significant and clinically relevant in

Table 21.1 Landmark studies of adjuvant chemotherapy in rectal cancer after neoadjuvant chemoradiotherapy.

	I-CNR-RT[10] (n = 655)	PROCTOR-SCRIPT[11] (n = 470)	EORTC[12] 22921 (n = 1101)	CHRONICLE[13] (n = 113)	ADORE[15] (n = 321)
Phase	III	III	III	III	II
Year of enrolment	1992–2001	2000–2013	1993–2003	2004–2008	2008–2012
Treatment	Observation vs. 5FU/LV	Observation vs. 5FU/LV or capecitabine	Preoperative RT +/− chemo followed by observation vs. postoperative 5FU/LV	Observation vs. XELOX	5FU/LV vs. FOLFOX
T4 disease	13.9%	81.9%[1]	10.0%	6.8%	4% with 5FU/LV and 2% with FOLFOX
Exenteration	0%	0%	NR	NR	0%
Study endpoints	OS	OS	OS	DFS	DFS
Benefit of adjuvant chemotherapy	NS	NS	NS	NS	71.6 vs. 62.9%[2]
Compliance to adjuvant chemotherapy	28% never started; 58.4% received three to six cycles	4.6% never started; 73.6% completed all cycles	26.9% never started; 42.9% completed without delay (95–105% planned dose)	7% never started; 48.1% completed all cycles	95% with 5FU/LV and 97% with FOLFOX completed all cycles

5FU/LV, 5-Fluorouracil/leucovorin; RT, radiotherapy; Chemo, chemotherapy; NR, not reported; OS, overall survival; DFS, disease-free survival; NS, non-significant.
[1] Stage III disease.
[2] Statistically significant.

the ADORE study, which reported excellent compliance of 95–97% in both study arms. Given the high risk of disease recurrence and less favorable prognosis of patients undergoing exenteration, it is reasonable to pursue adjuvant chemotherapy with a combination regimen in those who are fit and willing to comply to treatment for the maximal benefit.

Novel Agents

Antibodies against vascular endothelial growth factor (VEGF) and epithelial growth factor receptor (EGFR) are the standard of care for metastatic colorectal cancer in addition to the conventional chemotherapy backbone [6, 7]. Various multicenter phase III randomized studies have been performed to compare adjuvant chemotherapy with or without targeted therapy, but results have been disappointing. The NSABP C-08 study failed to show the benefit of adjuvant bevacizumab in the 2672 randomized patients with colon cancer, but suggested a time-dependent effect of bevacizumab in addition to oxaliplatin-based chemotherapy [16]. There was a strong effect of bevacizumab on DFS before, but not beyond, the 15-month landmark (HR 0.61, 95% CI 0.48–0.78, $p < 0.001$). Similarly, DFS was not improved in the subsequent AVANT study with the addition of bevacizumab in 3451 randomized patients [17]. Furthermore, the data suggested a potential detrimental effect on OS. More recently, the QUASAR II study echoed the results of the NSABP C-08 and the AVANT study in terms of both DFS and OS [18]. The findings that higher expression of free CD31 correlated with superior five-year DFS was intriguing, but its application remains elusive. With regard to anti-EGFR monoclonal antibodies in the adjuvant setting, both the NCCTG N-0147 [19] and PETACC-08 [20] studies failed to demonstrate improvement in DFS with cetuximab even in KRAS wild-type patients. A meta-analysis by Kim et al. concluded that the addition of targeted agents (both anti-VEGF and anti-EGFR) to standard adjuvant chemotherapy resulted in no improvement of DFS but an increased risk of severe adverse events and treatment-related death [21]. Although most of the above studies recruited colon cancer only and may not be directly applicable to rectal cancer with exenteration, most centers include targeted agents in the adjuvant setting following pelvic exenteration when patients are recruited to clinical trials.

Recognizing how tumor cells evade immune clearance by the host ("immune escape") has been increasingly researched [22]. Programmed-death-1 (PD-1) is a 55-kD type I transmembrane protein primarily expressed on activated T-cells, B-cells, myeloid cells, and antigen-presenting cells [23]. Binding of PD-1 to its ligands, PD-L1 and PD-L2, has been shown to downregulate T-cell activation in both murine and human systems, leading to suppression of immune surveillance and cancer development [24-27]. Pembrolizumab and nivolumab are examples of monoclonal antibody against the PD-1 molecule, while atezolizumab, durvalumab, and avelumab are anti-PD-L1 monoclonal antibodies. Currently, nivolumab and pembrolizumab are indicated for microsatellite instability high or mismatch repair protein-deficient refractory tumors which account for about 5% of metastatic colorectal cancer [6, 28]. Initial clinical studies for nivolumab and pembrolizumab have shown an objective response rate of ~ 30% and durable disease control in heavily pretreated microsatellite instability high or mismatch repair protein-deficient metastatic colorectal cancer [29, 30]. Preclinical studies have shown that radiotherapy can sensitize tumor cells to immune checkpoint inhibitors by recruiting antitumor T-cells into the tumor [31]. Ongoing studies are evaluating the role of pembrolizumab (NCT02921256), atezolizumab (NCT03127007), and avelumab (NCT03854799) in concurrent with neoadjuvant chemoradiotherapy, and nivolumab (NCT02948348) and avelumab (NCT03299660) as sequential therapy to neoadjuvant chemoradiotherapy (Table 21.2).

Table 21.2 Ongoing clinical trials of immune checkpoint inhibitors in locoregionally advanced rectal cancer.

http://clinicaltrials.gov identifier	ICB	Phase	Timing with CRT	Include cT4 disease	Primary objectives
NCT02948348	Nivolumab	Ib/II	Sequential	Yes	pCR rate
NCT03127007	Atezolizumab	Ib/II	Concurrent	Yes	pCR rate and AE rate
NCT02921256	Pembrolizumab and Veliparib	II	Concurrent	Yes	Change in NAR score
NCT03854799	Avelumab	II	Concurrent	Yes	pCR rate
NCT03299660	Avelumab	II	Sequential	Yes	Pathological RR

ICB, Immune checkpoint inhibitor; CRT, chemoradiotherapy; pCR, pathologic complete response; AE, adverse event; NAR score, neoadjuvant rectal score; RR, response rate.

The results of these studies are eagerly awaited and further effort is mandated to fully unleash the power of our own immune system.

Radiotherapy

Pelvic radiotherapy with or without concurrent chemotherapy is an essential component for successful management of rectal cancer. Pelvic radiotherapy is given with 3D conformal technique or intensity-modulated radiotherapy with maneuver to reduce the volume given to the small bowel in the pelvis. Figure 21.1 shows the typical 3D conformal radiotherapy plan with the patient lying prone on a belly board for neoadjuvant treatment of rectal cancer. In the past decades, the pendulum of giving radiotherapy has swung from postoperative to preoperative. The first individual patient data meta-analysis of adjuvant radiotherapy for primary rectal cancer included 8507 patients from 22 randomized trials which showed lower risk of local recurrence ($p = 0.00001$) and death from rectal cancer ($p = 0.0003$) with neoadjuvant radiotherapy than surgery alone despite similar rates of apparently curative resection [32]. On the other hand, adjuvant radiotherapy improved local control but did not reduce the risk of death from rectal cancer significantly. Since the publication of the German CAO/ARO/AIO-94 study [33], neoadjuvant treatment has been the preferred option for those patients in whom chemoradiotherapy is deemed necessary. Indeed, neoadjuvant radiotherapy for all-comers is superior to adjuvant therapy for patients who are selected as a result of positive circumferential resection margin [34]. Results from meta-analysis involving 3363 patients in 16 studies reported that pathological complete response following neoadjuvant chemoradiotherapy is a good prognostic maker with less local recurrence (OR 0.25, $p = 0.002$), fewer distant metastasis (OR 0.23, $p < 0.001$), and improved survival (OR 3.28, $p = 0.001$) [35].

In general, radiotherapy with or without chemotherapy should be given in the neoadjuvant manner for primary LARC, but this is discussed elsewhere (see Chapter 4). The role of radiotherapy in the setting of LRRC is more controversial [36–39].

The outcomes of patients with R1/2 resection are almost as poor as patients with metastatic disease, but there is debate as to the benefit of intraoperative radiotherapy (IORT) when margins are close and service/expertise is available. IORT is the delivery of irradiation at the time of operation. This is performed with different techniques including intraoperative electron beam and high-dose-rate brachytherapy. IORT allows high dose of radiation to be delivered to the site at risk and at the same time avoid surrounding dose-limiting critical

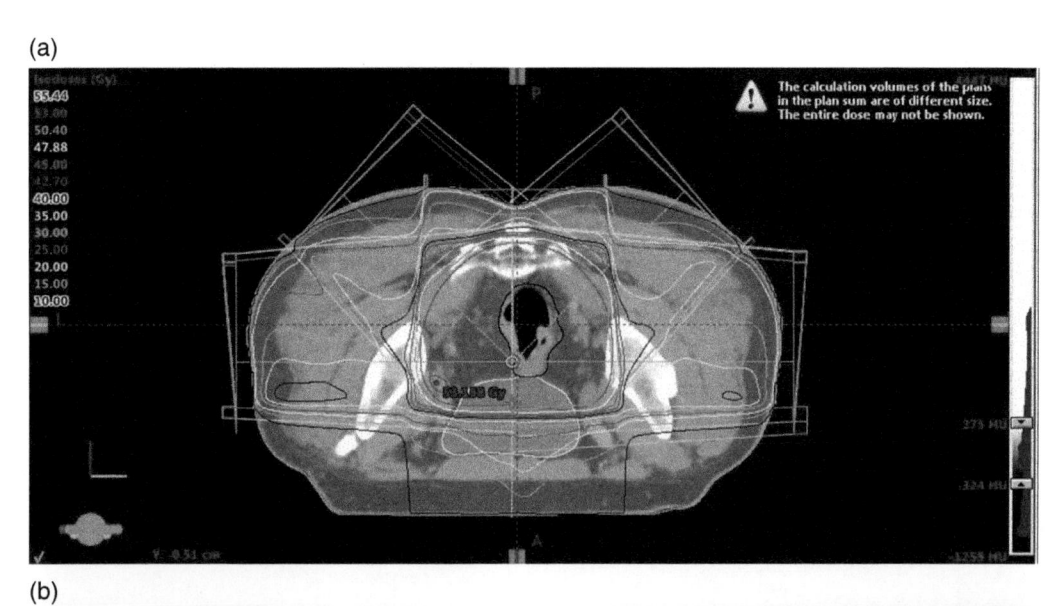

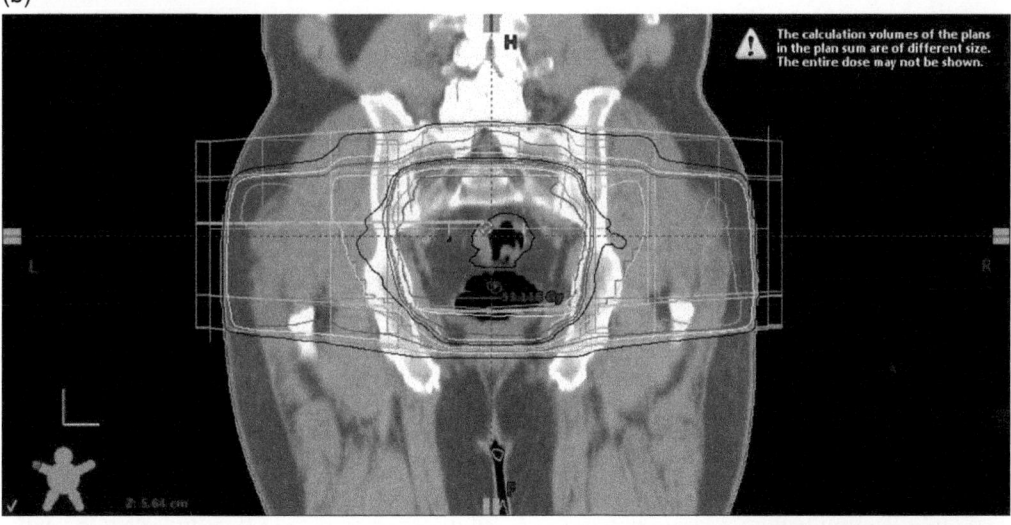

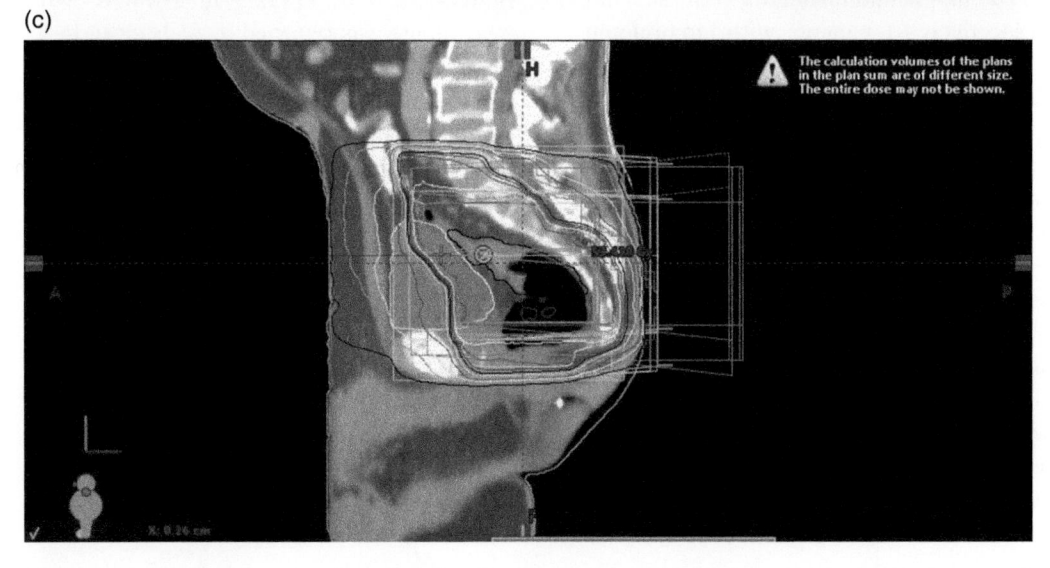

Figure 21.1 Three-dimensional conformal radiotherapy plan with belly board with target volumes and isodose lines. (a) Axial; (b) coronal; (c) sagittal; (d) 3D beam arrangement.

(d)

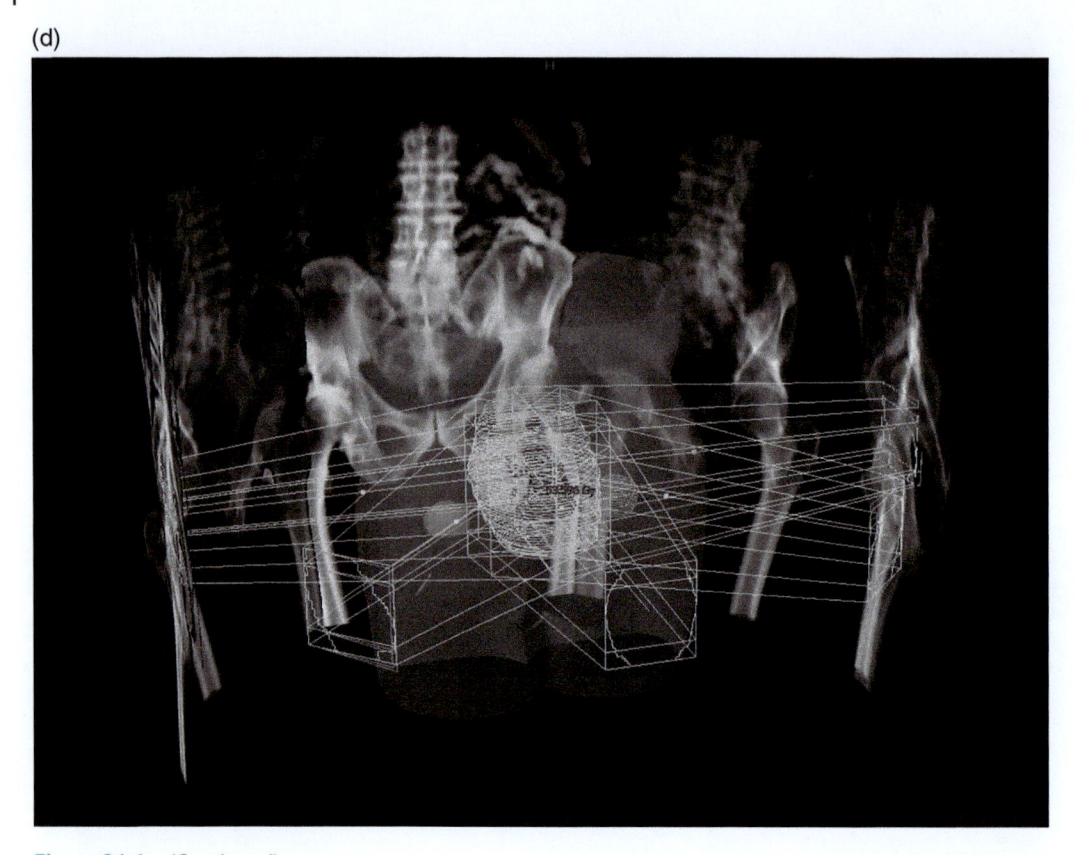

Figure 21.1 (Continued)

structures. These advantages potentially translate into improved local tumor control and reduced complication. Alberda et al. analyzed retrospectively 91 patients with circumferential resection margin ≤ 2 mm in which those with macroscopically involved margins were not included [40]. The clinical benefit of IORT was restricted to those with microscopically involved circumferential resection margin but not in those with close margin. The procedure was also safe without significant increase in complication rate. In another retrospective series, Hyngstrom et al. reported excellent outcomes with IORT for both LARC and LRRC [41]. IORT was delivered with high-dose-rate brachytherapy at a median of 12.5 Gy. The five-year local control was 94 and 56% for LARC and LRRC respectively. A small prospective study of IORT was performed at the Peter MacCallum Cancer Centre which demonstrated a 2.5-year local control of 68% and grade 3/4 toxicities of 37% [42]. Similarly, IORT with orthovoltage was reported by Daly et al. in 55 patients with 61 recurrent sites who achieved a respectable two-year local control rate of 69% [43]. Due to the dosimetric advantages of IORT, it has also been evaluated as modality for re-irradiation. Pezner et al. reviewed 15 patients with pelvic recurrence within the previously irradiated regions [44]. Half of the patients had undergone exenteration and IORT dose was 15–20 Gy. The three-year local control rate was just 25% for the overall population but reached 42% for patients with less extensive recurrent disease (non-fixed transmural recurrence, isolated pelvic node metastasis, and rectal recurrence following local excision). Proton therapy is another area of active research, but studies in

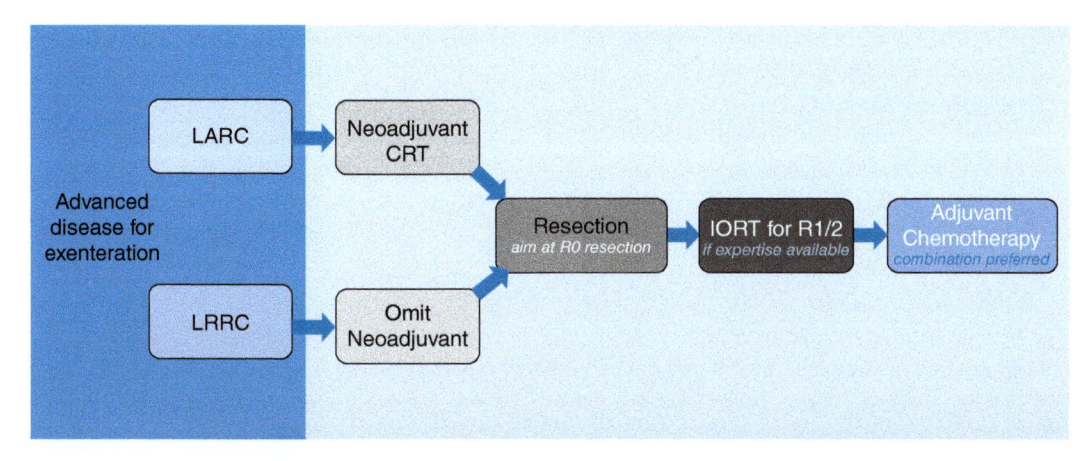

Figure 21.2 Treatment algorithm for LARC and LRRC with regard to exenteration. CRT, Chemoradiotherapy; IORT, intraoperative radiotherapy.

rectal cancer are mostly on feasibility and dosimetry at present [45–47].

Future Directions

Adjuvant management of rectal cancers that require exenteration is a great clinical challenge and controversies exist in various aspects due to the paucity of high-quality data. When deciding on the adjuvant therapy for exenteration, the classification of LARC and LRRC is essential as it provides useful guidance for when and what additional treatment should be given. Figure 21.2 is the proposed treatment algorithm.

Summary Box
• The role of adjuvant therapy following pelvic exenteration is heterogenous.   • There is a lack of high-quality prospective trial data regarding its benefit to patient survival.   • There is a considerable move towards upfront neoadjuvant therapy and selective adjuvant therapy use.   • IORT and proton therapy may be helpful in the setting of R1/2 resection, but both expertise and facilities are not widely available.

References

1 Yang, T.X., Morris, D.L., and Chua, T.C. (2013). Pelvic exenteration for rectal cancer: a systematic review. *Dis. Colon Rectum* 56 (4): 519–531.

2 Kusters, M., Austin, K.K.S., Solomon, M.J. et al. (2015). Survival after pelvic exenteration for T4 rectal cancer. *Br. J. Surg.* 102 (1): 125–131.

3 Bhangu, A., Ali, S.M., Brown, G. et al. (2014). Indications and outcome of pelvic exenteration for locally advanced primary and recurrent rectal cancer. *Ann. Surg.* 259 (2): 315–322.

4 Nielsen, M.B., Rasmussen, P.C., Lindegaard, J.C., and Laurberg, S. (2012). A 10-year experience of total pelvic exenteration for primary advanced and locally recurrent rectal

cancer based on a prospective database. *Colorectal Dis.* 14 (9): 1076–1083.

5 Ishiguro, S., Akasu, T., Fujita, S. et al. (2009). Pelvic exenteration for clinical T4 rectal cancer: oncologic outcome in 93 patients at a single institution over a 30-year period. *Surgery* 145 (2): 189–195.

6 National Comprehensive Cancer Network (2019). NCCN Guidelines on Rectal Cancer. Version 1. https://www.nccn.org/professionals/physician_gls.

7 Glynne-Jones, R., Wyrwicz, L., Tiret, E. et al. (2017). Rectal cancer: ESMO clinical practice guidelines for diagnosis, treatment and follow-up. *Ann. Oncol.* 28 (suppl 4): iv22–iv40.

8 Petersen, S.H., Harling, H., Kirkeby, L.T. et al. (2012). Postoperative adjuvant chemotherapy in rectal cancer operated for cure. *Cochrane Database Syst. Rev.* 3: CD004078.

9 Gray, R., Barnwell, J., McConkey, C. et al. (2007). Adjuvant chemotherapy versus observation in patients with colorectal cancer: a randomised study. *Lancet* 370 (9604): 2020–2029.

10 Sainato, A., Cernusco Luna Nunzia, V., Valentini, V. et al. (2014). No benefit of adjuvant fluorouracil leucovorin chemotherapy after neoadjuvant chemoradiotherapy in locally advanced cancer of the rectum (LARC): long term results of a randomized trial (I-CNR-RT). *Radiother. Oncol.* 113 (2): 223–229.

11 Breugom, A.J., van Gijn, W., Muller, E.W. et al. (2015). Adjuvant chemotherapy for rectal cancer patients treated with preoperative (chemo)radiotherapy and total mesorectal excision: a Dutch Colorectal Cancer Group (DCCG) randomized phase III trial. *Ann. Oncol.* 26 (4): 696–701.

12 Bosset, J.F., Calais, G., Mineur, L. et al. (2014). Fluorouracil-based adjuvant chemotherapy after preoperative chemoradiotherapy in rectal cancer: long-term results of the EORTC 22921 randomised study. *Lancet Oncol.* 15 (2): 184–190.

13 Glynne-Jones, R., Counsell, N., Quirke, P. et al. (2014). CHRONICLE: results of a randomised phase III trial in locally advanced rectal cancer after neoadjuvant chemoradiation randomising postoperative adjuvant capecitabine plus oxaliplatin (XELOX) versus control. *Ann. Oncol.* 25 (7): 1356–1362.

14 Breugom, A.J., Swets, M., Bosset, J.F. et al. (2015). Adjuvant chemotherapy after preoperative (chemo)radiotherapy and surgery for patients with rectal cancer: a systematic review and meta-analysis of individual patient data. *Lancet Oncol.* 16 (2): 200–207.

15 Hong, Y.S., Nam, B.H., Kim, K.P. et al. (2014). Oxaliplatin, fluorouracil, and leucovorin versus fluorouracil and leucovorin as adjuvant chemotherapy for locally advanced rectal cancer after preoperative chemoradiotherapy (ADORE): an open-label, multicentre, phase 2, randomised controlled trial. *Lancet Oncol.* 15 (11): 1245–1253.

16 Allegra, C.J., Yothers, G., O'Connell, M.J. et al. (2011). Phase III trial assessing bevacizumab in stages II and III carcinoma of the colon: results of NSABP protocol C-08. *J. Clin. Oncol.* 29 (1): 11–16.

17 de Gramont, A., Van Cutsem, E., Schmoll, H.J. et al. (2012). Bevacizumab plus oxaliplatin-based chemotherapy as adjuvant treatment for colon cancer (AVANT): a phase 3 randomised controlled trial. *Lancet Oncol.* 13 (12): 1225–1233.

18 Kerr, R.S., Love, S., Segelov, E. et al. (2016). Adjuvant capecitabine plus bevacizumab versus capecitabine alone in patients with colorectal cancer (QUASAR 2): an open-label, randomised phase 3 trial. *Lancet Oncol.* 17 (11): 1543–1557.

19 Alberts, S.R., Sargent, D.J., Nair, S. et al. (2012). Effect of oxaliplatin, fluorouracil, and leucovorin with or without cetuximab on survival among patients with resected stage III colon cancer a randomized trial. *JAMA* 307 (13): 1383–1393.

20 Taieb, J., Tabernero, J., Mini, E. et al. (2014). Oxaliplatin, fluorouracil, and leucovorin with or without cetuximab in patients with resected stage III colon cancer (PETACC-8): an open-label, randomised phase 3 trial. *Lancet Oncol.* 15 (8): 862–873.

21 Kim, B.J., Jeong, J.H., Kim, J.H. et al. (2017). The role of targeted agents in the adjuvant treatment of colon cancer: a meta-analysis of randomized phase III studies and review. *Oncotarget* 8 (19): 31112–31118.

22 Swann, J.B. and Smyth, M.J. (2007). Immune surveillance of tumors. *J. Clin. Invest.* 117 (5): 1137–1146.

23 Keir, M.E., Butte, M.J., Freeman, G.J., and Sharpe, A.H. (2008). PD-1 and its ligands in tolerance and immunity. *Annu. Rev. Immunol.* 26: 677–704.

24 Freeman, G.J., Long, A.J., Iwai, Y. et al. (2000). Engagement of the PD-1 immunoinhibitory receptor by a novel B7 family member leads to negative regulation of lymphocyte activation. *J. Exp. Med.* 192 (7): 1027–1034.

25 Latchman, Y., Wood, C.R., Chernova, T. et al. (2001). PD-L2 is a second ligand for PD-I and inhibits T cell activation. *Nat. Immunol.* 2 (3): 261–268.

26 Carter, L.L., Fouser, L.A., Jussif, J. et al. (2002). PD-1:PD-L inhibitory pathway affects both CD4(+)and CD8(+) T cells and is overcome by IL-2. *Eur. J. Immunol.* 32 (3): 634–643.

27 Barber, D.L., Wherry, E.J., Masopust, D. et al. (2006). Restoring function in exhausted CD8 T cells during chronic viral infection. *Nature* 439 (7077): 682–687.

28 Le, D.T., Uram, J.N., Wang, H. et al. (2015). PD-1 blockade in tumors with mismatch-repair deficiency. *N. Engl. J. Med.* 372 (26): 2509–2520.

29 Overman, M.J., McDermott, R., Leach, J.L. et al. (2017). Nivolumab in patients with metastatic DNA mismatch repair-deficient or microsatellite instability-high colorectal cancer (CheckMate 142): an open-label, multicentre, phase 2 study. *Lancet Oncol.* 18 (9): 1182–1191.

30 Le, D.T., Kavan, P., Kim, T.W. et al. (2018). KEYNOTE-164: Pembrolizumab for patients with advanced microsatellite instability high (MSI-H) colorectal cancer. *J. Clin. Oncol.* 36 (15): 3514.

31 Demaria, S., Coleman, C.N., and Formenti, S.C. (2016). Radiotherapy: changing the game in immunotherapy. *Trends Cancer.* 2 (6): 286–294.

32 Colorectal Cancer Collaborative Group (2001). Adjuvant radiotherapy for rectal cancer: a systematic overview of 8,507 patients from 22 randomised trials. *Lancet* 358 (9290): 1291–1304.

33 Sauer, R., Becker, H., Hohenberger, W. et al. (2004). Preoperative versus postoperative chemoradiotherapy for rectal cancer. *N. Engl. J. Med.* 351 (17): 1731–1740.

34 Sebag-Montefiore, D., Stephens, R.J., Steele, R. et al. (2009). Preoperative radiotherapy versus selective postoperative chemoradiotherapy in patients with rectal cancer (MRC CR07 and NCIC-CTG C016): a multicentre, randomised trial. *Lancet* 373 (9666): 811–820.

35 Martin, S.T., Heneghan, H.M., and Winter, D.C. (2012). Systematic review and meta-analysis of outcomes following pathological complete response to neoadjuvant chemoradiotherapy for rectal cancer. *Br. J. Surg.* 99 (7): 918–928.

36 PelvEx Collaborative (2018). Factors affecting outcomes following pelvic exenteration for locally recurrent rectal cancer. *Br. J. Surg.* 105 (6): 650–757.

37 Rombouts, A.J., Koh, C.E., Young, J.M. et al. (2015). Does radiotherapy of the primary rectal cancer affect prognosis after pelvic exenteration for recurrent rectal cancer? *Dis. Colon Rectum* 58 (1): 65–73.

38 Valentini, V., Morganti, A.G., Gambacorta, M.A. et al. (2006). Preoperative hyperfractionated chemoradiation for locally recurrent rectal cancer in patients previously irradiated to the pelvis: a multicentric phase II study. *Int. J. Radiat. Oncol. Biol. Phys.* 64 (4): 1129–1139.

39 Jensen, G., Tao, R., Eng, C. et al. (2018). Treatment of primary rectal adenocarcinoma after prior pelvic radiation: the role of hyperfractionated accelerated reirradiation. *Adv. Radiat. Oncol.* 3 (4): 595–600.

40 Alberda, W.J., Verhoef, C., Nuyttens, J.J. et al. (2014). Intraoperative radiation therapy reduces local recurrence rates in patients with microscopically involved circumferential resection margins after resection of locally advanced rectal cancer. *Int. J. Radiat. Oncol. Biol. Phys.* 88 (5): 1032–1040.

41 Hyngstrom, J.R., Tzeng, C.W., Beddar, S. et al. (2014). Intraoperative radiation therapy for locally advanced primary and recurrent colorectal cancer: ten-year institutional experience. *J. Surg. Oncol.* 109 (7): 652–658.

42 Tan, J., Heriot, A.G., Mackay, J. et al. (2013). Prospective single-arm study of intraoperative radiotherapy for locally advanced or recurrent rectal cancer. *J. Med. Imaging Radiat. Oncol.* 57 (5): 617–625.

43 Daly, M.E., Kapp, D.S., Maxim, P.G. et al. (2012). Orthovoltage intraoperative radiotherapy for locally advanced and recurrent colorectal cancer. *Dis. Colon Rectum* 55 (6): 695–702.

44 Pezner, R.D., Chu, D.Z., and Ellenhorn, J.D. (2002). Intraoperative radiation therapy for patients with recurrent rectal and sigmoid colon cancer in previously irradiated fields. *Radiother. Oncol.* 64 (1): 47–52.

45 Dionisi, F., Batra, S., Kirk, M. et al. (2013). Pencil beam scanning proton therapy in the treatment of rectal cancer. *Int. J. Radiat. Oncol. Biol. Phys.* 87 (2): S341–S342.

46 Berman, A.T., Both, S., Sharkoski, T. et al. (2014). Proton reirradiation of recurrent rectal cancer: dosimetric comparison, toxicities, and preliminary outcomes. *Int. J. Part Ther.* 1 (1): 2–13.

47 Ogi, Y., Yamaguchi, T., Kinugasa, Y. et al. (2018). Effect and safety of proton beam therapy for locally recurrent rectal cancer. *J. Clin. Oncol.* 36 (4): 743.

22

Adjuvant Therapy Options after Pelvic Exenteration for Gynecological Malignancy

Nisha Jagasia

Department of Gynecological Oncology, Mater Adults Hospital, Brisbane, Australia

Background

Pelvic exenteration is offered in only selective cases of gynecological malignancy, usually in the setting of centrally recurrent pelvic disease post pelvic radiation. In most instances the surgery is performed with curative intent and the aim to achieve complete gross resection with negative surgical margins. In a large series of 75 patients undergoing pelvic exenteration for gynecological cancers (cervical [1], vaginal [2], and uterine [3] cancers) Berek et al. [4] reported survival for patients with cervical and vaginal cancer as 73% at one year and 57% at three years. Survival for patients with uterine cancer was 86% at one year and 62% at three years. Survival for patients who underwent exenteration with negative margins was 81% at one year and 64% at three years, while those with positive margins had a poor survival of 25% at one year and 0% at three years [4]. Similarly, a series from the Memorial Sloan-Kettering Cancer Center showed that no patients with positive margins at extended pelvic resection were alive at five years [5]. This underscores the importance of careful patient selection and limiting potentially morbid exenteration to those patients who will derive survival benefit as a result of complete resection.

Despite careful patient selection and advances in surgical techniques, recurrence occurs in 35–50% of cases [5, 6] and the five-year survival post pelvic exenteration for various indications ranges from 20 to 73% [5, 7–10]. These figures suggest that a significant proportion of patients may benefit from adjuvant therapy after pelvic exenteration to reduce the risk of recurrence or treat recurrent disease.

In a US series, the authors assessed the utilization of adjuvant chemotherapy in 42 patients undergoing pelvic exenteration for gynecological malignancy. In this series all patients had a complete gross (R0) resection. However, 26% were referred for adjuvant chemotherapy because of adverse or high-risk pathological features. The study demonstrated that adjuvant systemic therapy was feasible in patients post pelvic exenteration; 88% of those undergoing chemotherapy completing at least four cycles and the median interval from pelvic exenteration to initiation of chemotherapy was 71 days. Three out of the eight patients who had systemic therapy post exenteration recurred – all recurring in the pelvis. The three-year progression-free survival (PFS) and overall survival (OS) were 58 and 54% respectively [3]. Despite chemotherapy, recurrence after pelvic exenteration remains a significant

---

Surgical Management of Advanced Pelvic Cancer, First Edition.
Edited by Michael E. Kelly and Desmond C. Winter.
© 2022 John Wiley & Sons Ltd. Published 2022 by John Wiley & Sons Ltd.

therapeutic challenge because chemotherapy may be less effective in previously irradiated tissue. In many patients, targeted therapies may be explored either as stand-alone treatments or in combination with chemotherapy.

This chapter explores the role of adjuvant chemotherapy and options for targeted therapies for patients who recur post pelvic exenteration for gynecological malignancies or in whom therapy may be utilized because of a high risk of recurrence.

Cervical Cancer

Patients with early-stage cervical cancer are treated with radical surgery and/or chemoradiotherapy depending on disease volume, tumor characteristics, and/or patient risk characteristics. Adjuvant radiotherapy is delivered to those with risk factors for recurrence including positive resection margins, parametrial involvement, or node-positive disease [11]. Adjuvant radiation is also prescribed to those who meet intermediate-risk clinicopathological criteria based on presence of lymphovascular invasion (LVI), tumor size, and extent of cervical stromal invasion (Gynecologic Oncology Group (GOG) score/Sedlis' criteria). The risk of recurrence and death in the presence of these factors is up to 30% after surgery alone [12, 13]. Adjuvant radiotherapy reduces the risk of progression by 40% [11]. Locally advanced disease, node-positive disease, and bulky tumors are treated with primary chemoradiotherapy (weekly tissue sensitizing cisplatin and pelvic radiation delivered with external beam and brachytherapy). Surgery in these patients is unlikely to be curative. The role of hysterectomy after primary chemoradiotherapy is not well defined, with a lack of evidence showing that this improves survival.

Patients with high-risk disease such as those treated with adjuvant radiation after surgery or primary chemoradiotherapy undergo close surveillance after treatment; the main goal of this is to aid early detection of pelvic recurrence that may be amenable to salvage with pelvic exenteration. Patients with partial response to primary chemoradiotherapy and those with evidence of recurrence on follow-up of cervical cancer may be candidates for pelvic exenteration. Criteria used to help identify ideal patients are those with a central pelvic recurrence without sidewall fixation or associated hydronephrosis. In addition, those with a long disease-free interval and recurrences of less than 3 cm in diameter are also favorable. Patients who develop para-aortic nodal or distant metastatic disease are not suitable for exenteration surgery.

Five-year survival post pelvic exenteration for recurrent cervical cancer in selected patients ranges from 30 to 40% [14, 15]. In more contemporary series, five-year OS rates of up to 50% are reported [2]. Given that these patients have all had high-dose pelvic radiation prior to exenteration, further adjuvant pelvic radiation is not appropriate. While intraoperative radiotherapy (IORT) requires further investigation, there may be a role in patients having surgery for locally recurrent cervical cancer. Barney et al. [16] assessed 73 patients with locally recurrent cervical cancer that received IORT following pelvic exenteration or sidewall resection and showed a three-year cancer-specific survival (CSS) and OS of 31 and 25% respectively. In another series of 36 patients with recurrent disease treated with IORT, the 10-year in-field control rate was 46% [17].

As outlined above, systemic chemotherapy may be utilized post exenteration for recurrent cervical cancer if negative margins are not achieved; however, this would be deemed a failure to achieve curative intent. Systemic chemotherapy is also offered to those patients who have previously been treated with radiation and are not candidates for surgical resection. Patients who develop recurrent or metastatic disease following pelvic exenteration are managed depending on location and extent of metastatic disease.

For patients with isolated or limited metastatic disease in a radiation naïve region (isolated para-aortic node, solitary lung nodule), treatment can be focally directed to the site of disease with radiation therapy, and in selected cases patients could be considered for surgical (oligometastatic) resection [18]. Otherwise, the mainstay of treatment for metastatic disease remains platinum-based combination chemotherapy with anti-angiogenic vascular endothelial growth factor (VEGF-A) inhibitor (bevacizumab). Meta-analysis of five randomized trials assessing 1114 participants revealed significantly lower response rates in the group that received cisplatin alone compared to the group that received combination chemotherapy (relative risk [RR] = 0.60, 95% CI 0.44–0.81) [19]. Women who have received prior chemotherapy also have a lower response rate compared to chemotherapy naïve patients. The GOG 240 trial [20] randomized women with metastatic, persistent, or recurrent cervical cancer to chemotherapy with or without bevacizumab and observed a significant improvement in overall response rate (ORR), PFS (HR 0.68), and OS (HR 0.77) with the addition of bevacizumab to chemotherapy. However, the addition of bevacizumab was associated with a higher rate of complications. The same trial compared two chemotherapy combinations and noted that cisplatin and paclitaxel was superior to topotecan and paclitaxel. Carboplatin is a reasonable substitute for cisplatin, particularly for patients with medical comorbidities (e.g. pre-existing renal failure) and those patients previously treated with cisplatin-based chemoradiation [21]. Currently, there is no standard second-line systemic therapy for advanced cervical cancer. Patients should be considered for clinical trials whenever feasible, including the use of novel targeted agents and immunotherapy like pembrolizumab (a programed cell death ligand 1 (PD L1) inhibitor). Alternatively, several biological agents are currently in development, aiming at inhibiting angiogenesis, targeting epidermal growth factor receptor (EGFR), cell cycle, histone deacetylases, cyclooxygenase-2 (COX-2), or mammalian target of rapamycin (mTOR) [22].

Vaginal Cancer

The treatment paradigm for vaginal cancers is similar to that of cervical cancers. At diagnosis, patients with small stage I tumors may be treated with surgical excision; however, larger tumors (stage II–IV) are treated with primary chemoradiotherapy. Central recurrence following chemoradiotherapy can be considered for pelvic exenteration on a case-by-case basis. Adjuvant therapy follows protocols as per recurrent/metastatic cervical cancer.

Vulval Cancer

Vulval cancer often stays confined to the pelvis until advanced stages. Less than 10% of vulval cancers are stage III–IV at diagnosis, in developed countries [23]. Whether patients are managed with upfront surgery ± adjuvant therapy or have primary non-surgical treatment depends on the stage of the disease and patient-related factors. In patients with involvement of the urethra or anus, fixed inguinofemoral nodes, or pelvic lymphadenopathy, or the medically frail, chemoradiotherapy is the preferred approach. Primary chemoradiotherapy achieves complete remission in one-third of cases, and in those women who respond partially, survival is improved if the residual disease can be surgically excised. Primary pelvic exenteration may be considered in rare cases of vulval cancer presenting with extensive involvement of the rectum or bladder, in women presenting with locally advanced vulval cancers where radiation therapy is contraindicated, or in selected cases of localized recurrence following radiotherapy.

Unfortunately, there are few studies directly comparing chemoradiotherapy to pelvic exenteration surgery in advanced or recurrent vulval cancer. Forner and Lampe [24] presented a retrospective review of 27 cases of stage III or stage IV vulval cancer undergoing exenteration, of which 9 resections were for primary disease and 18 for recurrent disease. In their cohort the five-year survival rate for primary and recurrent disease after exenteration was 67 and 59% respectively. Another study on pelvic exenteration for recurrent vulval cancer found that almost 70% of patients had further recurrence and all were in the pelvis [25]. This underscores the importance of nodal assessment prior to attempted exenteration for recurrent vulval cancers.

In those patients who undergo primary surgery, adjuvant chemoradiotherapy is indicated for those with close (< 8 mm) or positive margins, particularly if re-excision of margins is not feasible. Lymph-node-positive patients benefit from chemoradiotherapy in terms of PFS but not OS when compared to those who just receive adjuvant chemotherapy [26]. Chemoradiotherapy in the adjuvant setting consists of weekly cisplatin 40 mg/m^2 concurrently with radiation. Patients with stage IVB disease at presentation or those with recurrent disease involving other adjacent pelvic organs are offered systemic therapy with carboplatin and paclitaxel (evidence largely extrapolated from metastatic cervical cancer). For patients who progress after first-line chemotherapy, treatment options also mirror those for women with metastatic cervical cancer.

Endometrial Cancer

A National Cancer Database series [27] examined the outcomes of 652 women with uterine malignancy undergoing pelvic exenteration and found that women with positive lymph nodes or presence of distant disease at time of diagnosis had poorer outcomes post exenteration compared with women without these features. The authors suggest that women with positive lymph nodes should be counseled before undergoing exenteration as it is unlikely to increase their long-term survival. Recurrent endometrial cancer is relatively uncommon and rarely presents with isolated pelvis disease. In the small group that have central pelvic recurrence post primary surgery or post radiotherapy, a pelvic exenteration could be considered.

The endometrial cancer population is generally older and more comorbid compared to patients being considered for pelvic exenteration for cervical cancer and this must be considered when counseling patients. Even in expert centers, the morbidity of such procedures is high, reported at 30–80%, and OS poor, at 14–45%. [28–30]. In a series of 44 patients with recurrent endometrial cancer undergoing pelvic exenteration, 80% had major postoperative complication and only 20% achieved long-term disease control (more than five years) [31]. In a carefully selected cohort with contemporary preoperative imaging, Schmidt et al. [30] achieved a five-year survival rate of 61%. Similarly, Chiantera et al. [32] reported a complete resection rate of 86% and OS of 60%.

In the setting of positive margins post exenteration, radiotherapy may be indicated in patients who have previously not been exposed to pelvic radiation. Re-irradiation of a previously irradiated field is possible, especially with the utilization of specialized tailored radiotherapy techniques such as intensity-modulated radiation therapy (IMRT). Some units have assessed the role of IORT in combination with extended surgical resection for recurrent endometrial cancer [33]; however, this multimodality aggressive surgical approach requires further investigation. In patients with high risk features such as pelvic recurrences (vs. isolated vaginal recurrence), incomplete resection, LVI, high tumor grade, and in those in whom pelvic radiation has already been utilized, systemic adjuvant therapy is warranted. The choice between chemotherapy and endocrine therapy is determined by patient performance status, previous adjuvant treatment, and the histologic and molecular features of the tumor.

Unfortunately, the efficacy of systemic and endocrine therapies in recurrent endometrial cancer is limited. Single-agent chemotherapy with cisplatin, paclitaxel, or doxorubicin has shown overall response rates in the order of 20–30%, with few patients achieving complete response [34–36]. Response rates with multi-agent chemotherapy range from 10 to 45% but are associated with significant toxicity and PFS of approximately six months [37–42]. GOG 209 [43] compared cisplatin-based triplet chemotherapy regimens with carboplatin plus paclitaxel and found the doublet therapy to be non-inferior to the more toxic triplet. The three-drug regimen paclitaxel/doxorubicin/cisplatin has shown benefit over cisplatin and paclitaxel and is an alternative but is less preferred due to increased toxicity [44]. Endocrine treatment with progestogen with or without tamoxifen similarly shows response rates of 15–30%, with higher response rates in hormone receptor positive low-grade tumors [45, 46]. In the majority of cases, endocrine therapy achieves partial remission or stable disease, but some patients may remain progression-free for extended periods of time [47]. Endocrine therapy is an alternative to first- or second-line chemotherapy, or it may be used as a later-line option for those who have progressed on chemotherapy. Aromatase inhibitors such as letrozole and anastrozole have limited activity in endometrial cancer, with response rates < 10% [48, 49]. In patients with uterine serous papillary carcinoma (USPC) and human epidermal growth factor receptor 2 (HER2) overexpression (approximately 30% of USPC) the addition of trastuzumab is suggested. A randomized phase II study of chemotherapy with or without trastuzumab in the advanced stage or recurrent HER2 overexpressed USPC noted that the addition of trastuzumab conferred a statistically significant 4.5-month PFS advantage with no difference in toxicity between the two arms [50]. Bevacizumab also has activity in recurrent or metastatic endometrial cancer. When combined with carboplatin and paclitaxel it showed higher ORR and improved median PFS and OS compared to platinum-based chemotherapy alone [51, 52].

In patients who progress on chemotherapy, mismatch repair gene (MMR) status should be evaluated using the primary tumor or tissue obtained at the time of metastatic disease, as this may direct patients toward immunotherapy with immune checkpoint inhibitor pembrolizumab. Immune checkpoint inhibitors have shown efficacy in many advanced solid tumors, particularly among MMR-deficient (dMMR) or cancers with microsatellite instability (MSI) [1, 53]. Phase II studies of pembrolizumab in dMMR non-colorectal metastatic carcinomas have shown response rates of 57–71% and median PFS of up to 26 months [54, 55]. Additionally, the combination of pembrolizumab and VEGF inhibitor levatinib has been tested on 94 patients with metastatic endometrial carcinoma with some favorable results [56]. However, 3% of patients experience fatal adverse reactions.

Ovarian Cancer

Several modified pelvic exenterative resections have been reported for both primary and recurrent epithelial ovarian cancer (EOC). For example, rectosigmoid colectomy is not uncommonly performed in advanced ovarian cancer to achieve optimal cytoreduction. Less commonly, partial bladder or ureteric resection may be required. Adjuvant therapy in EOC is a vast topic and outside the scope of this chapter. Suffice to say that platinum-based chemotherapy combinations form the cornerstone of adjuvant therapy in EOC. Maintenance with poly ADP ribose polymerase (PARP) inhibitors is recommended in those individuals with high-grade serous pathology who respond to frontline platinum chemotherapy, with the most benefit to PFS seen in those with germline mutations in BRCA1 or BRCA2 and those with homologous DNA repair-deficient tumors [57–59]. Bevacizumab has been shown to improve PFS but not OS in a subset of women with advanced EOC (women without a known mutation in BRCA1 or BRCA2 who have a high risk of recurrence (e.g. those with pleural effusions or ascites or those with >1 cm of residual disease post maximal effort cytoreduction)) [60].

Summary Box

- Survival and presumptive cure are possible in approximately one-half of women undergoing exenteration as salvage therapy for pelvic cancers.
- Patients need to be carefully selected so that complete resection with negative margins is achieved and reconstruction is tailored to allow patients good functional outcomes and improved quality of life.
- Despite careful selection, a subset of patients will require adjuvant therapy post exenteration for positive margins or recurrent disease.
- Platinum-based chemotherapy regimens remain the mainstay of treatment for recurrent and metastatic gynecological carcinoma.
- Targeted therapies may offer a therapeutic benefit particularly in the presence of targetable mutations, and eligible patients should continue to be enrolled in clinical trials of these agents.

References

1 Piulats, J.M. and Matias-Guiu, X. (2016). Immunotherapy in endometrial cancer: in the nick of time. *Clin. Cancer Res.* 22 (23): 5623.

2 Li, L., Ma, S.Q., Tan, X.J. et al. (2018). Pelvic exenteration for recurrent and persistent cervical cancer. *Chin. Med. J. (Engl.)* 131 (13): 1541–1548.

3 Andikyan, V., Khoury-Collado, F., Sandadi, S. et al. (2013). Feasibility of adjuvant chemotherapy after pelvic exenteration for gynaecological malignancies. *Int. J. Gynecol. Cancer* 23: 923–928.

4 Berek, J.S., Howe, C., Lagasse, L.D., and Hacker, N.F. (2005). Pelvic exenteration for recurrent gynaecological malignancy: survival and morbidity analysis of the 45-year experience at UCLA. *Gynecol. Oncol.* 99: 153–159.

5 Andikyan, V., Khoury-Collado, F., Sonoda, Y. et al. (2012). Extended pelvic resections for recurrent or persistent uterine and cervical malignancies: an update on out of the box surgery. *Gynecol. Oncol.* 125: 404–408.

6 Kaur, M., Joniau, S., and D'Hoore, A. (2014). Vergote I indications, techniques and outcomes for pelvic exenteration in gynecological malignancy. *Curr. Opin. Oncol.* 26: 514–520.

7 Caceres, A., Mourton, S.M., Bochner, B.H. et al. (2008). Extended pelvic resections for recurrent uterine and cervical cancer: out-of-the-box surgery. *Int. J. Gynecol. Cancer* 18: 1139–1144.

8 Morris, M., Alvarez, R.D., Kinney, W.K., and Wilson, T.O. (1996). Treatment of recurrent adenocarcinoma of the endometrium with pelvic exenteration. *Gynecol. Oncol.* 60: 288–291.

9 Goldberg, G., Sukumvanich, P., Einstein, M.H. et al. (2006). Total pelvic exenteration: the Albert Einstein College of Medicine/Montefiore Medical Center Experience (1987 to 2003). *Gynecol. Oncol.* 101: 261–268.

10 Hoeckel, M. (2003). Laterally extended endopelvic resection. Novel surgical treatment of locally recurrent cervical carcinoma involving the pelvic side wall. *Gynecol. Oncol.* 91: 369–377.

11 Rogers, L., Siu, S.S., Luesley, D. et al. (2012). Radiotherapy and chemoradiation after surgery for early cervical cancer. *Cochrane Database Syst. Rev.* 5 (5): CD007583.

12 Sedlis, A., Bundy, B.N., Rotman, M.Z. et al. (1999). A randomized trial of pelvic radiation therapy versus no further therapy in selected patients with stage IB carcinoma of the cervix after radical hysterectomy and pelvic lymphadenectomy: a Gynecologic Oncology Group study. *Gynecol. Oncol.* 73 (2): 177.

13 Rotman, M., Sedlis, A., Piedmonte, M.R. et al. (2006). A phase III randomized trial of postoperative pelvic irradiation in stage IB cervical carcinoma with poor prognostic features: follow-up of a Gynecologic Oncology Group study. *Int. J. Radiat. Oncol. Biol. Phys.* 65 (1): 169.

14 Rutledge, S., Carey, M.S., Prichard, H. et al. (1994). Conservative surgery for recurrent or persistent carcinoma of the cervix following irradiation: is exenteration always necessary? *Gynecol. Oncol.* 52 (3): 353.

15 Maneo, A., Landoni, F., Cormio, G. et al. (1999). Radical hysterectomy for recurrent or persistent cervical cancer following radiation therapy. *Int. J. Gynecol. Cancer* 9 (4): 295.

16 Barney, B.M., Petersen, I.A., Dowdy, S.C. et al. (2013). Intraoperative electron beam radiotherapy (IOERT) in the management of locally advanced or recurrent cervical cancer. *Radiat. Oncol.* 8: 80.

17 Martínez-Monge, R., Jurado, M., Aristu, J.J. et al. (2001). Intraoperative electron beam radiotherapy during radical surgery for locally advanced and recurrent cervical cancer. *Gynecol. Oncol.* 82 (3): 538.

18 Lim, M.C., Lee, H.S., Seo, S.S. et al. (2010). Pathologic diagnosis and resection of suspicious thoracic metastases in patients with cervical cancer through thoracotomy or video-assisted thoracic surgery. *Gynecol. Oncol.* 116 (3): 478.

19 Alberts, D.S., Kronmal, R., Baker, L.H. et al. (1987). Phase II randomized trial of cisplatin chemotherapy regimens in the treatment of recurrent or metastatic squamous cell cancer of the cervix: a Southwest Oncology Group study. *J. Clin. Oncol.* 5 (11): 1791–1795.

20 Tewari, K.S., Sill, M.W., Penson, R.T. et al. (2017). Bevacizumab for advanced cervical cancer: final overall survival and adverse event analysis of a randomised, controlled, open-label, phase 3 trial (Gynecologic Oncology Group 240). *Lancet* 390 (10103): 1654.

21 Kitagawa, R., Katsumata, N., Shibata, T. et al. (2015). Paclitaxel plus carboplatin versus paclitaxel plus cisplatin in metastatic or recurrent cervical cancer: the open-label randomized phase III trial JCOG0505. *J. Clin. Oncol.* 33 (19): 2129.

22 Zagouri, F., Sergentanis, T.N., Chrysikos, D. et al. (2012). Molecularly targeted therapies in cervical cancer. A systematic review. *Gynecol. Oncol.* 126 (2): 291–303. Comprehensive review of currently available targeted therapies in cervical cancer.

23 Beller, U., Quinn, M.A., Benedet, J.L. et al. (2006). Carcinoma of the vulva. FIGO 6th Annual Report on the Results of Treatment in Gynecological Cancer. *Int. J. Gynaecol. Obstet.* 95: S7–S27.

24 Forner, M. and Lampe, B. (2012). Exenteration in the treatment of stage III/IV vulvar cancer. *Gynecol. Oncol.* 124: 87–91.

25 Miller, B., Morris, M., Levenback, C. et al. (1995). Pelvic exenteration for primary and recurrent vulvar cancer. *Gynecol. Oncol.* 58: 202–205.

26 Gill, B.S., Bernard, M.E., Lin, J.F. et al. (2015). Impact of adjuvant chemotherapy with radiation for node-positive vulvar cancer: a National Cancer Database (NCDB) analysis. *Gynecol. Oncol.* 137 (3): 365–372.

27 Seagle, B.L., Dayno, M., Strohl, A.E. et al. (2016). Survival after pelvic exenteration for uterine malignancy: a National Cancer Database study. *Gynecol. Oncol.* 143 (3): 472–478.

28 Barber, H.R.K. and Brunschwig, A. (1968). Treatment and results of recurrent cancer of the corpus uteri in patients receiving

anterior and total pelvic exenteration 1947–1963. *Cancer* 22: 949–955.

29 Morris, M., Alvarez, R.D., Kinney, W.K., and Wilson, T.O. (1996). Treatment of recurrent adenocarcinoma of the endometrium with pelvic exenteration. *Gynecol. Oncol.* 60 (2): 288–291.

30 Schmidt, A., Imesch, P., Fink, D., and Egger, H. (2016). Pelvic exenterations for advanced and recurrent endometrial cancer: clinical outcomes of 40 patients. *Int. J. Gynecol. Cancer* 26 (4): 716–720.

31 Barakat, R.R., Goldman, N.A., Patel, D.A. et al. (1999). Pelvic exenteration for recurrent endometrial cancer. *Gynecol. Oncol.* 75 (1): 99–102.

32 Chiantera, P.V., Rossi, M., De Iaco, P. et al. (2014). Pelvic exenteration for recurrent endometrial adenocarcinoma: a retrospective multi-institutional study about 21 patients. *Int. J. Gynecol. Cancer* 24 (5): 880–884.

33 Dowdy, S.C., Mariani, A., Cliby, W.A. et al. (2006). Radical pelvic resection and intraoperative radiation therapy for recurrent endometrial cancer: technique and analysis of outcomes. *Gynecol. Oncol.* 101 (2): 280–286.

34 Thigpen, J.T., Blessing, J.A., Homesley, H. et al. (1989). Phase II trial of cisplatin as first-line chemotherapy in patients with advanced or recurrent endometrial carcinoma: a Gynecologic Oncology Group study. *Gynecol. Oncol.* 33: 68–70.

35 Thigpen, T., Blessing, J., Homesley, H. et al. (1993). Phase III trial of doxorubicin +/− cisplatin in advanced or recurrent endometrial carcinoma: a Gynecologic Oncology Group (GOG) study. *Proc. Am. Soc. Clin. Oncol.* 12: 261.

36 Ball, H.G. (1996). A phase II trial of paclitaxel in patients with advanced or recurrent adenocarcinoma of the endometrium: a Gynecologic Oncology Group study. *Gynecol. Oncol.* 622: 278–281.

37 Burke, T.W., Stringer, C.A., Morris, M. et al. (1991). Prospective treatment of advanced or recurrent endometrial carcinoma with cisplatin, doxorubicin, and cyclophosphamide. *Gynecol. Oncol.* 40: 264–267.

38 Gallion, H.H., Brunetto, V.L., Cibull, M. et al. (2003). Randomized phase III trial of standard timed doxorubicin plus cisplatin versus circadian timed doxorubicin plus cisplatin in stage III and IV or recurrent endometrial carcinoma: a Gynecologic Oncology Group study. *J. Clin. Oncol.* 21: 3808–3813.

39 Muggia, F.M., Blessing, J.A., Sorosky, J., and Reid, G.C. (2002). Phase II trial of the pegylated liposomal doxorubicin in previously treated metastatic endometrial cancer: a Gynecologic Oncology Group study. *J. Clin. Oncol.* 20: 2360–2364.

40 Pierga, J.Y., Dieras, V., Beuzeboc, P. et al. (1997). Phase II trial of doxorubicin, 5-fluorouracil, etoposide, and cisplatin in advanced or recurrent endometrial carcinoma. *Gynecol. Oncol.* 66: 246–249.

41 Scudder, S.A., Liu, P.Y., Wilczynski, S.P. et al. (2005). Paclitaxel and carboplatin with amifostine in advanced, recurrent, or refractory endometrial adenocarcinoma: a phase II study of the Southwest Oncology Group. *Gynecol. Oncol.* 96: 610–615.

42 Thigpen, J.T., Blessing, J.A., DiSaia, P.J. et al. (1994). A randomized comparison of doxorubicin alone versus doxorubicin plus cyclophosphamide in the management of advanced or recurrent endometrial carcinoma: a Gynecologic Oncology Group study. *J. Clin. Oncol.* 12: 1408–1414.

43 Miller, D., Filiaci, V., Fleming, G. et al. (2012). Late-breaking abstract 1: randomized phase III noninferiority trial of first line chemotherapy for metastatic or recurrent endometrial carcinoma: a Gynecologic Oncology Group study. *Gynecol Oncol.* 125S: 771.

44 Fleming, G.F., Brunetto, V.L., Cella, D. et al. (2004). Phase III trial of doxorubicin plus cisplatin with or without paclitaxel plus filgrastim in advanced endometrial carcinoma: a Gynecologic Oncology Group study. *J. Clin. Oncol.* 22 (11): 2159.

45 Moore, T.D., Phillips, P.H., Nerenstone, S.R., and Cheson, B.D. (1991). Systemic treatment of advanced and recurrent carcinoma: current status and future directions. *J. Clin. Oncol.* 9: 1071–1088.

46 Decruze, S.B. and Green, J.A. (2007). Hormone therapy in advanced and recurrent endometrial cancer: a systematic review. *Int. J. Gynecol. Cancer* 17 (5): 964.

47 Markman, M. (2005). Hormonal therapy of endometrial cancer. *Eur. J. Cancer* 41 (5): 673.

48 Rose, P.G., Brunetto, V.L., VanLe, L. et al. (2000). A phase II trial of anastrozole in advanced recurrent or persistent endometrial carcinoma: a Gynecologic Oncology Group study. *Gynecol. Oncol.* 78 (2): 212.

49 Ma, B.B., Oza, A., Eisenhauer, E. et al. (2004). The activity of letrozole in patients with advanced or recurrent endometrial cancer and correlation with biological markers – a study of the National Cancer Institute of Canada Clinical Trials Group. *Int. J. Gynecol. Cancer* 14 (4): 650.

50 Fader, A.N., Roque, D.M., Siegel, E. et al. (2018). Randomized phase II trial of carboplatin-paclitaxel versus carboplatin-paclitaxel-trastuzumab in uterine serous carcinomas that overexpress human epidermal growth factor receptor 2/neu. *J. Clin. Oncol.* 36 (20): 2044.

51 Aghajanian, C.A., Filaci, V.L., Dizon, D.S. et al. (2015). A randomized phase II study of paclitaxel/carboplatin/bevacizumab, paclitaxel/carboplatin/temsirolimus and ixabepilone/carboplatin/bevacizumab as initial therapy for measurable stage III or IVA, stage IVB or recurrent endometrial cancer, GOG-86P. *J. Clin. Oncol.* 33S: 5500.

52 Lorusso, D., Ferrandina, G., Colombo, N. et al. (2015). Randomized phase II trial of carboplatin-paclitaxel (CP) compared to carboplatin-paclitaxel-bevacizumab (CP-B) in advanced (stage III–IV) or recurrent endometrial cancer: the MITO END-2 trial. *J. Clin. Oncol.* 33S: 5502.

53 Howitt, B.E., Shukla, S.A., Sholl, L.M. et al. (2015). Association of polymerase e-mutated and microsatellite-instable endometrial cancers with neoantigen load, number of tumor-infiltrating lymphocytes, and expression of PD-1 and PD-L1. *JAMA Oncol.* 1 (9): 1319.

54 Le, D.T., Uram, J.N., Wang, H. et al. (2015). PD-1 blockade in tumors with mismatch-repair deficiency. *N. Engl. J. Med.* 372 (26): 2509.

55 Ott, P.A., Bang, Y.J., Berton-Rigaud, D. et al. (2017). Safety and antitumor activity of pembrolizumab in advanced programmed death ligand 1-positive endometrial cancer: results from the KEYNOTE-028 study. *J. Clin. Oncol.* 35 (22): 2535.

56 Lenvatinib capsules, for oral use. United States Prescribing Information. US National Library of Medicine. https://www.accessdata.fda.gov/drugsatfda_docs/label/2019/206947s011lbl.pdf (accessed September 17, 2019).

57 Ray-Coquard, I., Pautier, P., Pignata, S. et al. (2019). Olaparib plus bevacizumab as first-line maintenance in ovarian cancer. *N. Engl. J. Med.* 381 (25): 2416.

58 González-Martín, A., Pothuri, B., Vergote, I. et al. (2019). Niraparib in patients with newly diagnosed advanced ovarian cancer. *N. Engl. J. Med.* 381 (25): 2391.

59 Coleman, R.L., Fleming, G.F., Brady, M.F. et al. (2019). Veliparib with first-line chemotherapy and as maintenance therapy in ovarian cancer. *N. Engl. J. Med.* 381 (25): 2403.

60 Oza, A.M., Cook, A.D., Pfisterer, J. et al. (2015 Aug). Standard chemotherapy with or without bevacizumab for women with newly diagnosed ovarian cancer (ICON7): overall survival results of a phase 3 randomised trial. *Lancet Oncol* 16 (8): 928–936.

23

Adjuvant Therapy Options for Urological Neoplasms

Gregory J. Nason[1], Clare O'Connell[2], and Paul K. Hegarty[3]

[1] Division of Uro-Oncology, University of Toronto, Ontario, Canada
[2] Department of Urology, Tallaght University Hospital, Dublin 24, Ireland
[3] Department of Urology, Mater Hospital, Cork, Ireland

Background

Common urological cancers of the pelvis include bladder and prostate cancer, as well as rarer diseases such as penile cancer. Both are in the top 10 most common cancers worldwide and represent disease spectra with huge variation. A significant proportion of the urology referral workload worldwide is taken up by diagnostic pathways for investigation of these two cancers. Development of rapid-access prostate cancer diagnostic pathways and hematuria clinics aim to improve detection at earlier-stage disease. Despite this, a significant proportion of prostate and bladder cancers present with locally advanced or metastatic disease and requiring multimodal therapy. This chapter focuses on adjuvant therapies used after radical surgical resection of prostate and bladder cancer, and provides an introduction to systemic therapies used in these diseases.

Prostate Cancer

Radiation Therapy

As well as its use upfront for curative intent, radiation therapy is used as part of multimodal treatment strategies after prostatectomy. Adjuvant radiation therapy (ART) can be considered in men who have high-risk pathological features in their prostatectomy specimen (high Gleason score, presence of extracapsular extension, seminal vesicle involvement, or positive margins) [1]. Also, radiation therapy is used in the "salvage" setting (salvage radiotherapy (SRT)) for biochemical recurrence (detectable prostate-specific antigen (PSA) after a period of observation following prostatectomy) – 20% of men under radical prostatectomy will experience disease recurrence and the percentage is higher for those with adverse pathological features [2]. The debate continues as to the optimal treatment strategy in the adjuvant setting for men with locally advanced prostate cancer after prostatectomy. Proponents of ART argue that waiting for biochemical recurrence to occur before offering radiation may miss the treatment window to cure disease and prevent development of distant metastasis. Proponents of waiting to offer radiation at the time of subsequent biochemical recurrence argue that some men with locally advanced disease will be cured by surgery alone, thus sparing them the side effects of radiation, and of hormone deprivation therapy that is usually given concurrently.

Surgical Management of Advanced Pelvic Cancer, First Edition.
Edited by Michael E. Kelly and Desmond C. Winter.
© 2022 John Wiley & Sons Ltd. Published 2022 by John Wiley & Sons Ltd.

Three randomized controlled trials have compared adjuvant radiation for locally aggressive prostate cancer to observation and found ART to increase biochemical recurrence-free survival and disease-specific survival [3–5]. However, these studies did not directly compare ART to observation with early salvage radiation therapy (esRT) when biochemical recurrence is detected. A more recent study compared long-term metastasis-free survival (MFS) and overall survival (OS) in 510 patients with locally advanced (≥ T3) prostate cancer with undetectable PSA after radical prostatectomy who underwent ART vs. initial observation with esRT when biochemical recurrence occurred. Of 267 who underwent initial observation, 141 experienced biochemical recurrence and received esRT. There was no significant difference in MFS or OS eight years after radical prostatectomy between the two groups, suggesting that there is no disadvantage to waiting until biochemical recurrence is detected to use adjuvant radiation [6]. On the basis of this study, it would spare a signification proportion of men from the side effects of radiation.

Brachytherapy

Brachytherapy utilizes radioactive seeds permanently implanted in the prostate bed and is a widely accepted option as monotherapy for carefully selected patients with prostate-confined disease [7]. Brachytherapy has also been described in the adjuvant setting, for the salvage of recurrent disease after radiation treatment in several phase II trials and case series [8]. The main concern with using brachytherapy after external beam radiation is the excess of genitourinary toxicity from using two radiation modalities in sequence [9–12]. Salvage brachytherapy remains an investigative approach for the time being.

Hormonal Therapy: Gonadotropin-Releasing Hormone (GnRH) Analogs

The role of hormone therapy in combination with radiation for prostate cancer has been proven to be superior to radiation alone for prostate cancer, as demonstrated by several phase III randomized control trials [13–17]. Androgen deprivation therapy (ADT) is given in the form of luteinizing hormone releasing hormone (LHRH) analogs, leading to gonadal suppression and chemical castration. Duration of hormonal therapy depends on disease features, with six months ADT recommended for intermediate risk and three years recommended for high-risk disease [1]. LHRH analogs are a hugely important development in the management of high-risk and metastatic prostate cancer, where previously men underwent bilateral orchidectomy to achieve suppression of testosterone [18]. LHRH agonists lead to a decrease in serum testosterone by binding to GnRH receptors in the pituitary gland, leading to an initial stimulus of luteinizing hormone (LH) and follicle-stimulating hormone (FSH), followed by sustained downregulation, while LHRH antagonists block the release of LH and FSH by reversible competitive binding to GnRH receptors [19]. However, the effects of GnRH blockade are transient, and most patients progress to castration-resistant prostate cancer (CRPC) within 18–30 months [20].

Abiraterone Acetate

Abiraterone acetate inhibits the enzyme CYP17A1 and is used in addition to GnRH analogs in metastatic castration-resistant prostate cancer (mCRPC) and metastatic castration-sensitive high-risk prostate cancer (mCSPC). CYP17A1 catalyzes the conversion of pregnenolone and progesterone to their 17α-hydroxy derivatives, and subsequently converts these proteins to dehydroepiandrosterone (DHEA) and androstenedione, precursors of testosterone [21].

In mCRPC, abiraterone in combination with prednisone improves OS from 30.3 months with placebo to 34.7 months [22]. It is also now being investigated and used in mCSPC. A seminal study published in the *New England Journal of Medicine* examined the use of abiraterone with prednisone in men starting hormonal therapy for the first time, with locally advanced or metastatic disease. The addition of abiraterone and prednisone to standard ADT significantly improved OS in patients with and without metastatic disease [23].

Enzalutamide

Enzalutamide is a second-generation androgen receptor (AR) antagonist, with additional antisignaling activity as well as antagonist activity compared to first-generation drugs such as bicalutamide [24]. The PREVAIL study was a randomized double-blind placebo controlled trial which compared enzalutamide to placebo for men with progressive metastatic prostate cancer despite treatment with ADT. The treatment arm saw significant increases in both overall and progression-free survival and delayed time to initiation of chemotherapy [25]. Enzalutamide has also been compared head-to-head against a first-generation AR antagonist, bicalutamide, and was found to increase progression-free survival from 5.8 to 15.7 months [26].

Chemotherapy

Docetaxel is a taxane chemotherapeutic agent used in the treatment of high-risk prostate cancer. Docetaxel prevents microtubule disassembly between metaphase and anaphase, leading to microtubule accumulation inside the cell causing apoptosis [27]. Compared with mitoxantrone, the SWOG 99-16 trial revealed that docetaxel chemotherapy improves median OS by two months for mCRPC [28]. Another study from the STAMPEDE trial compared use of docetaxel to abiraterone with prednisone in combination with standard of care (ADT ± radiation therapy) and found no significant difference in OS between the two groups [29].

Second-line Treatment for Metastatic Prostate Cancer

As abiraterone and docetaxel have equivalent oncologic outcomes and completely different mechanisms of action, these drugs can be used in sequence if resistance develops. Median OS for patients with mCRPC who progressed on docetaxel was 15.8 months when treated with abiraterone and compared to placebo [30]. Enzalutamide has also been shown to improve OS when used in patients who have progressive prostate cancer on chemotherapy, with a five-month OS benefit when compared to placebo [31].

Cabazitaxel is a novel taxane chemotherapy which has been found to have benefit in patients with mCRPC who have progressed on docetaxel [32]. In the first-line setting it has not been shown to be superior to docetaxel, and continues to be reserved for second-line therapy [33].

Radium-223 is an alpha particle emitter which selectively targets bone metastases. In conjunction with standard of care, in comparison to placebo, six injections of radium-223 at a dose of 50 kBq per kilogram of body weight at four-weekly intervals increased OS from 11.2 to 14 months [34]. The addition of radium-223 to abiraterone for mCRPC did not, however, improve skeletal event-free survival and there was an increased rate of pathological fractures seen in this study with the use of radium-223 [35].

Bladder Cancer

The recommended approach for patients with muscle invasive bladder cancer (MIBC) is neoadjuvant cisplatin-based chemotherapy [36–38]. Two large randomized control trials have demonstrated a survival advantage with the use of neoadjuvant chemotherapy (NAC). Grossman et al. demonstrated a 31-month survival advantage with the use of NAC and a 23% increase in pT0 rates at radical cystectomy (RC) [39]. The long-term results of the BA06 30894 trial and international phase 3 trial of 976 patients with an eight-year follow-up showed a 16% decrease in risk of death following NAC [40]. Despite this guideline recommendation, many patients do not receive it [41–43].

Chemotherapy

Although the evidence is contentious, the adjuvant use of a cisplatin-based regimen is generally advocated in healthy individuals who did not receive NAC. It is unlikely a definitive randomized trial will ever fully accrue to address the role of adjuvant treatment for advanced bladder cancer. Numerous historical randomized clinical trials have explored the efficacy of adjuvant chemotherapy (AC) in locally advanced bladder cancer. These trials demonstrated feasibility but used suboptimal chemotherapy regimens and were underpowered [44–47]. More recent trials evaluated contemporary chemotherapy regimens in the adjuvant setting in patients with locally advanced bladder cancer. Unfortunately, these trials closed early because of poor accrual [48, 49]. Although an updated meta-analysis of nine randomized controlled trials recently demonstrated an OS benefit with the use of immediate postoperative cisplatin-based chemotherapy [50], the latest randomized comparison of AC versus deferred chemotherapy at the time of relapse failed to confirm these results [51].

An observational study of the National Cancer Database (NCDB) compared the effectiveness of AC versus observation following RC for patients with T3/4 disease and/or pathological nodal disease [52]. A total of 5653 patients were analyzed; 23% received AC following RC. The median time to initiation of AC was 52 days. Chemotherapy-treated patients were younger and had adverse pathological findings such as node-positive disease and positive surgical margins. Stratified analyses adjusted for propensity score demonstrated an improvement in OS with AC (HR 0.70, 95% CI 0.64–0.76). The association between AC and improved OS was consistent in subset analyses and across performance status. In a similar multi-institutional prospective observational study across 18 units in Europe, 224 patients with T3/4 disease and/or nodal disease were compared – 37% underwent AC within three months of RC while the rest were observed [53]. The rate of three-year OS in patients who received AC vs. observation was 62.1 vs. 40.9% respectively (HR 0.47, 95% CI 0.25–0.86, $p = 0.014$).

Interestingly, Seisen et al. assessed the use of AC in patients who had already received NAC and RC [54]. The median follow-up was 45.7 months and median OS was significantly longer for NAC and RC followed by AC (29.9 months) vs. observation (24.2 months).

Immunotherapy

Prior to the emergence of programed death-1 (PD-1)/PD L1 checkpoint inhibitors, systemic chemotherapy with cisplatin-based regimens was the standard of care, with a median survival of around one year [55]. For patients with cisplatin-refractory disease, the median survival was only six to nine months [56]. Furthermore, up to 30–50% of patients with bladder cancer are ineligible to receive cisplatin due to comorbidities, limiting treatment options [57]. With the approval of several PD-1/PD L1 inhibitors, several combinations of chemotherapeutics and immunotherapeutic agents have been investigated in bladder cancer. In the metastatic setting, atezolizomab, pembrolizumab, nivolumab, durvalumab, and avelumab have all been approved for cisplatin ineligible or refractory patients [58–63]. There are currently three registered randomized controlled trials assessing the role of anti-PD-1/PD L1 agents with placebo or observation in patients with MIBC and locally advanced bladder cancer [64–66]. These are likely to change practice in the adjuvant setting in the coming years.

Radiotherapy

Traditionally, radiotherapy has been used in patients with MIBC who are unfit for cystectomy or for palliative symptom control. The National Comprehensive Cancer Network (NCCN) guidelines recommend considering

AR after RC in patients with ≥ pathological T3, positive lymph nodes, or high-grade bladder cancer [38], whereas the European Association of Urology guidelines do not feel there is sufficient evidence to support this [36]. One randomized controlled trial demonstrated a beneficial effect of AR in patients with locally advanced bladder cancer resulting in a significant improvement of recurrence-free survival (RFS) (49% for AR vs. 25% for RC only) [67].

Conclusion

Patients with advanced pelvic urological malignancies often require a multimodal approach both for oncological and functional outcomes as well as for symptom relief. There is a need for a multidisciplinary approach to tailor an individualized care plan for each patient.

Summary Box

- A multimodal approach is often utilized for adjuvant therapy for urological malignancies.
- A combination of adjuvant radiation treatment, chemotherapy, and hormonal axis targets are used for prostate cancer.
- Neoadjuvant chemotherapy is preferred in bladder cancer.
- Immunotherapy has emerged as a viable adjuvant option in advanced bladder cancer.

References

1 Heidenreich, A., Bastian, P.J., Bellmunt, J. et al. (2014). EAU guidelines on prostate cancer. Part 1: screening, diagnosis, and local treatment with curative intent – update 2013. *Eur. Urol.* 65 (1): 124–137.

2 Lobo, J.M., Stukenborg, G.J., Trifiletti, D.M. et al. (2016). Reconsidering adjuvant versus salvage radiation therapy for prostate cancer in the genomics era. *J. Comp. Eff. Res.* 5 (4): 375–382.

3 Bolla, M., van, Poppel, H., Tombal, B. et al. (2012). Postoperative radiotherapy after radical prostatectomy for high-risk prostate cancer: long-term results of a randomised controlled trial (EORTC trial 22911). *Lancet* 380 (9858): 2018–2027.
Seminal paper highlighting the benefit of adjuvant radiation treatment following radical prostatectomy with 10-year follow-up.

4 Wiegel, T., Bartkowiak, D., Bottke, D. et al. (2014). Adjuvant radiotherapy versus wait-and-see after radical prostatectomy: 10-year follow-up of the ARO 96-02/AUO AP 09/95 trial. *Eur. Urol.* 66 (2): 243–250.

5 Thompson, I.M., Tangen, C.M., Paradelo, J. et al. (2009). Adjuvant radiotherapy for pathological T3N0M0 prostate cancer significantly reduces risk of metastases and improves survival: long-term follow-up of a randomized clinical trial. *J. Urol.* 181 (3): 956–962.

6 Fossati, N., Karnes, R.J., Boorjian, S.A. et al. (2017). Long-term impact of adjuvant versus early salvage radiation therapy in pT3N0 prostate cancer patients treated with radical prostatectomy: results from a multi-institutional series. *Eur. Urol.* 71 (6): 886–893.

7 Ash, D., Flynn, A., Battermann, J. et al. (2000). ESTRO/EAU/EORTC recommendations on permanent seed implantation for localized prostate cancer. *Radiother. Oncol.* 57 (3): 315–321.

8 Baumann, B.C., Baumann, J.C., Christodouleas, J.P., and Soffen, E. (2017). Salvage of locally recurrent prostate cancer after external beam radiation using reduced-dose brachytherapy with neoadjuvant plus adjuvant androgen deprivation. *Brachytherapy* 16 (2): 291–298.

9 Peters, M., Moman, M.R., van der Poel, H.G. et al. (2013). Patterns of outcome and toxicity after salvage prostatectomy, salvage cryosurgery and salvage brachytherapy for prostate cancer recurrences after radiation therapy: a multi-center experience and literature review. *World J. Urol.* 31 (2): 403–409.

10 Yamada, Y., Kollmeier, M.A., Pei, X. et al. (2014). A phase II study of salvage high-dose-rate brachytherapy for the treatment of locally recurrent prostate cancer after definitive external beam radiotherapy. *Brachytherapy* 13 (2): 111–116.

11 Chen, C.P., Weinberg, V., Shinohara, K. et al. (2013). Salvage HDR brachytherapy for recurrent prostate cancer after previous definitive radiation therapy: 5-year outcomes. *Int. J. Radiat. Oncol. Biol. Phys.* 86 (2): 324–329.

12 Nguyen, P.L., Chen, M.H., D'Amico, A.V. et al. (2007). Magnetic resonance image-guided salvage brachytherapy after radiation in select men who initially presented with favorable-risk prostate cancer: a prospective phase 2 study. *Cancer* 110 (7): 1485–1492.

13 Denham, J.W., Joseph, D., Lamb, D.S. et al. (2019). Short-term androgen suppression and radiotherapy versus intermediate-term androgen suppression and radiotherapy, with or without zoledronic acid, in men with locally advanced prostate cancer (TROG 03.04 RADAR): 10-year results from a randomised, phase 3, factorial trial. *Lancet Oncol.* 20 (2): 267–281.

14 Pilepich, M.V., Winter, K., Lawton, C.A. et al. (2005). Androgen suppression adjuvant to definitive radiotherapy in prostate carcinoma – long-term results of phase III RTOG 85-31. *Int. J. Radiat. Oncol. Biol. Phys.* 61 (5): 1285–1290.

15 Roach, M., Bae, K., Speight, J. et al. (2008). Short-term neoadjuvant androgen deprivation therapy and external-beam radiotherapy for locally advanced prostate cancer: long-term results of RTOG 8610. *J. Clin. Oncol.* 26 (4): 585–591.

16 D'Amico, A.V., Chen, M.H., Renshaw, A.A. et al. (2008). Androgen suppression and radiation vs radiation alone for prostate cancer: a randomized trial. *JAMA* 299 (3): 289–295.

17 Bolla, M., de, Reijke, T.M., Van, Tienhoven, G. et al. (2009). Duration of androgen suppression in the treatment of prostate cancer. *N. Engl. J. Med.* 360 (24): 2516–2527.

18 Damber, J.E. (2005). Endocrine therapy for prostate cancer. *Acta Oncol.* 44 (6): 605–609.

19 Crona, D.J. and Whang, Y.E. (2017). Androgen receptor-dependent and -independent mechanisms involved in prostate cancer therapy resistance. *Cancers (Basel)* 9 (6):67.

20 Oudard, S. (2013). Progress in emerging therapies for advanced prostate cancer. *Cancer Treat. Rev.* 39 (3): 275–289.

21 Attard, G., Belldegrun, A.S., and De Bono, J.S. (2005). Selective blockade of androgenic steroid synthesis by novel lyase inhibitors as a therapeutic strategy for treating metastatic prostate cancer. *BJU Int.* 96 (9): 1241–1246.

22 Ryan, C.J., Smith, M.R., Fizazi, K. et al. (2015). Abiraterone acetate plus prednisone versus placebo plus prednisone in chemotherapy-naive men with metastatic castration-resistant prostate cancer (COU-AA-302): final overall survival analysis of a randomised, double-blind, placebo-controlled phase 3 study. *Lancet Oncol* 16 (2): 152–160.

23 James, N.D., de, Bono, J.S., Spears, M.R. et al. (2017). Abiraterone for prostate cancer not previously treated with hormone therapy. *N. Engl. J. Med* 377 (4): 338–351.

24 Antonarakis, E.S. (2013). Enzalutamide: the emperor of all anti-androgens. *Transl. Androl. Urol.* 2 (2): 119–120.

25 Beer, T.M., Armstrong, A.J., Rathkopf, D.E. et al. (2014). Enzalutamide in metastatic prostate cancer before chemotherapy. *N. Engl. J. Med.* 371 (5): 424–433.

26 Shore, N.D., Chowdhury, S., Villers, A. et al. (2016). Efficacy and safety of enzalutamide versus bicalutamide for patients with metastatic prostate cancer (TERRAIN): a randomised, double-blind, phase 2 study. *Lancet Oncol.* 17 (2): 153–163.

27 Herbst, R.S. and Khuri, F.R. (2003). Mode of action of docetaxel – a basis for combination with novel anticancer agents. *Cancer Treat. Rev.* 29 (5): 407–415.

28 Petrylak, D.P., Tangen, C.M., Hussain, M.H. et al. (2004). Docetaxel and estramustine compared with mitoxantrone and prednisone for advanced refractory prostate cancer. *N. Engl. J. Med.* 351 (15): 1513–1520.

29 Sydes, M.R., Spears, M.R., Mason, M.D. et al. (2018). Adding abiraterone or docetaxel to long-term hormone therapy for prostate cancer: directly randomised data from the STAMPEDE multi-arm, multi-stage platform protocol. *Ann. Oncol* 29 (5): 1235–1248.

30 Fizazi, K., Scher, H.I., Molina, A. et al. (2012). Abiraterone acetate for treatment of metastatic castration-resistant prostate cancer: final overall survival analysis of the COU-AA-301 randomised, double-blind, placebo-controlled phase 3 study. *Lancet Oncol.* 13 (10): 983–992.

31 Scher, H.I., Fizazi, K., Saad, F. et al. (2012). Increased survival with enzalutamide in prostate cancer after chemotherapy. *N. Engl. J. Med.* 367 (13): 1187–1197.

32 De Bono, J.S., Oudard, S., Ozguroglu, M. et al. (2010). Prednisone plus cabazitaxel or mitoxantrone for metastatic castration-resistant prostate cancer progressing after docetaxel treatment: a randomised open-label trial. *Lancet* 376 (9747): 1147–1154.

33 Sartor, A.O., Oudard, S., Sengelov, L. et al. (2017). Cabazitaxel vs docetaxel in chemotherapy-naive (CN) patients with metastatic castration-resistant prostate cancer (mCRPC): a three-arm phase III study (FIRSTANA). *J. Clin. Oncol.* 35 (28): 3189–3197.

34 Parker, C., Nilsson, S., Heinrich, D. et al. (2013). Alpha emitter radium-223 and survival in metastatic prostate cancer. *N. Engl. J. Med.* 369 (3): 213–223.

35 Smith, M., Parker, C., Saad, F. et al. (2019). Addition of radium-223 to abiraterone acetate and prednisone or prednisolone in patients with castration-resistant prostate cancer and bone metastases (ERA 223): a randomised, double-blind, placebo-controlled, phase 3 trial. *Lancet Oncol* 20 (3): 408–419.

36 Alfred Witjes, J., Lebret, T., Compérat, E.M. et al. (2017). Updated 2016 EAU guidelines on muscle-invasive and metastatic bladder cancer. *Eur. Urol.* 71 (3): 462–475.

37 Chang, S.S., Bochner, B.H., Chou, R. et al. (2017). Treatment of non-metastatic muscle-invasive bladder cancer: AUA/ASCO/ASTRO/SUO guideline. *J. Urol.* 198 (3): 552–559.

38 Spiess, P.E., Agarwal, N., Bangs, R. et al. (2017). Bladder cancer, version 5.2017, NCCN Clinical Practice Guidelines in Oncology. *J. Natl. Compr. Cancer Netw* 15 (10): 1240–1267.

39 Grossman, H.B., Natale, R.B., Tangen, C.M. et al. (2003). Neoadjuvant chemotherapy plus cystectomy compared with cystectomy alone for locally advanced bladder cancer. *N. Engl. J. Med.* 349 (9): 859–866.
NAC improves survival following RC.

40 Griffiths, G., Hall, R., Sylvester, R. et al. (2011). International phase III trial assessing neoadjuvant cisplatin, methotrexate, and vinblastine chemotherapy for muscle-invasive bladder cancer: long-term results of the BA06 30894 trial. *J. Clin. Oncol* 29 (16): –2171, 7.

41 Booth, C.M., Siemens, D.R., Peng, Y. et al. (2014). Delivery of perioperative chemotherapy for bladder cancer in routine clinical practice. *Ann. Oncol.* 25 (9): 1783–1788.

42 Reardon, Z.D., Patel, S.G., Zaid, H.B. et al. (2015). Trends in the use of perioperative chemotherapy for localized and locally advanced muscle-invasive bladder cancer: a sign of changing tides. *Eur. Urol.* 67 (1): 165–170.

43 Krabbe, L.M., Westerman, M.E., Margulis, V. et al. (2015). Changing trends in utilization of neoadjuvant chemotherapy in muscle-invasive bladder cancer. *Can. J. Urol.* 22 (4): 7865–7875.

44 Freiha, F., Reese, J., and Torti, F.M. (1996). A randomized trial of radical cystectomy versus radical cystectomy plus cisplatin, vinblastine and methotrexate chemotherapy for muscle invasive bladder cancer. *J. Urol.* 155 (2): 495–499. discussion 499–500.

45 Studer, U.E., Bacchi, M., Biedermann, C. et al. (1994). Adjuvant cisplatin chemotherapy following cystectomy for bladder cancer: results of a prospective randomized trial. *J. Urol.* 152 (1): 81–84.

46 Stöckle, M., Meyenburg, W., Wellek, S. et al. (1992). Advanced bladder cancer (stages pT3b, pT4a, pN1 and pN2): improved survival after radical cystectomy and 3 adjuvant cycles of chemotherapy. Results of a controlled prospective study. *J. Urol.* 148 (2 Pt 1): 302–306; discussion 306–7.

47 Skinner, D.G., Daniels, J.R., Russell, C.A. et al. (1991). The role of adjuvant chemotherapy following cystectomy for invasive bladder cancer: a prospective comparative trial. *J. Urol.* 145 (3): 459–464; discussion 464–7.

48 Cognetti, F., Ruggeri, E.M., Felici, A. et al. (2012). Adjuvant chemotherapy with cisplatin and gemcitabine versus chemotherapy at relapse in patients with muscle-invasive bladder cancer submitted to radical cystectomy: an Italian, multicenter, randomized phase III trial. *Ann. Oncol.* 23 (3): 695–700.

49 Sternberg, C.N., Skoneczna, I., Kerst, J.M. et al. (2015). Immediate versus deferred chemotherapy after radical cystectomy in patients with pT3-pT4 or N+ M0 urothelial carcinoma of the bladder (EORTC 30994): an intergroup, open-label, randomised phase 3 trial. *Lancet Oncol* 16 (1): 76–86. Supports timing of AC.

50 Leow, J.J., Martin-Doyle, W., Rajagopal, P.S. et al. (2014). Adjuvant chemotherapy for invasive bladder cancer: a 2013 updated systematic review and meta-analysis of randomized trials. *Eur. Urol.* 66 (1): 42–54.

51 Sternberg, C.N., de Mulder, P.H., Schornagel, J.H. et al. (2001). Randomized phase III trial of high-dose-intensity methotrexate, vinblastine, doxorubicin, and cisplatin (MVAC) chemotherapy and recombinant human granulocyte colony-stimulating factor versus classic MVAC in advanced urothelial tract tumors: European Organization for Research and Treatment of Cancer protocol no. 30924. *J. Clin. Oncol* 19 (10): 2638–2646.

52 Galsky, M.D., Stensland, K.D., Moshier, E. et al. (2016). Effectiveness of adjuvant chemotherapy for locally advanced bladder cancer. *J. Clin. Oncol.* 34 (8): 825–832.

53 Vetterlein, M.W., Seisen, T., May, M. et al. (2018). Effectiveness of adjuvant chemotherapy after radical cystectomy for locally advanced and/or pelvic lymph node-positive muscle-invasive urothelial carcinoma of the bladder: a propensity score-weighted competing risks analysis. *Eur. Urol. Focus* 4 (2): 252–259.

54 Seisen, T., Jamzadeh, A., Leow, J.J. et al. (2018). Adjuvant chemotherapy vs observation for patients with adverse pathologic features at radical cystectomy previously treated with neoadjuvant chemotherapy. *JAMA Oncol* 4 (2): 225–229.

55 von der Maase, H., Hansen, S.W., Roberts, J.T. et al. (2000). Gemcitabine and cisplatin versus methotrexate, vinblastine, doxorubicin, and cisplatin in advanced or metastatic bladder cancer: results of a large, randomized, multinational, multicenter, phase III study. *J. Clin. Oncol.* 18 (17): 3068–3077.

56 McCaffrey, J.A., Hilton, S., Mazumdar, M. et al. (1997). Phase II trial of docetaxel in patients with advanced or metastatic transitional-cell carcinoma. *J. Clin. Oncol.* 15 (5): 1853–1857.

57 Galsky, M.D., Hahn, N.M., Rosenberg, J. et al. (2011). Treatment of patients with metastatic urothelial cancer "unfit" for cisplatin-based chemotherapy. *J. Clin. Oncol.* 29 (17): 2432–2438.

58 Rosenberg, J.E., Hoffman-Censits, J., Powles, T. et al. (2016). Atezolizumab in patients with locally advanced and metastatic

urothelial carcinoma who have progressed following treatment with platinum-based chemotherapy: a single-arm, multicentre, phase 2 trial. *Lancet* 387 (10031): 1909–1920.

59 Balar, A.V., Galsky, M.D., Rosenberg, J.E. et al. (2017). Atezolizumab as first-line treatment in cisplatin-ineligible patients with locally advanced and metastatic urothelial carcinoma: a single-arm, multicentre, phase 2 trial. *Lancet* 389 (10064): 67–76.

60 Bellmunt, J., de Wit, R., Vaughn, D.J. et al. (2017). Pembrolizumab as second-line therapy for advanced urothelial carcinoma. *N. Engl. J. Med.* 376 (11): 1015–1026.

61 Sharma, P., Callahan, M.K., Bono, P. et al. (2016). Nivolumab monotherapy in recurrent metastatic urothelial carcinoma (CheckMate 032): a multi-centre, open-label, two-stage, multi-arm, phase 1/2 trial. *Lancet* 17 (11): 1590–1598.

62 Powles, T., O'Donnell, P.H., Massard, C. et al. (2017). Efficacy and safety of durvalumab in locally advanced or metastatic urothelial carcinoma: updated results from a phase 1/2 open-label study. *JAMA Oncol.* 3 (9): e172411.

63 Apolo, A.B., Infante, J.R., Balmanoukian, A. et al. (2017). Avelumab, an anti-programmed death-ligand 1 antibody, in patients with refractory metastatic urothelial carcinoma: results from a multicenter, phase IB study. *J. Clin. Oncol.* 35 (19): 2117–2124.

64 ClincalTrials.gov. Testing MK-3475 (pembrolizumab) after surgery for localized muscle-invasive bladder cancer and locally advanced urothelial cancer (AMBASSADOR). https://clinicaltrials.gov/ct2/show/NCT03244384 (accessed December 16, 2019).

65 ClincalTrials.gov. An investigational immuno-therapy study of nivolumab, compared to placebo, in patients with bladder or upper urinary tract cancer, following surgery to remove the cancer (CheckMate 274). https://clinicaltrials.gov/ct2/show/NCT02632409 (accessed December 16, 2019).

66 ClincalTrials.gov. A study of atezolizumab versus observation as adjuvant therapy in participants with high-risk muscle-invasive urothelial carcinoma (UC) after surgical resection (IMvigor010). https://clinicaltrials.gov/ct2/show/NCT02450331 (accessed December 16, 2019).

67 Zaghloul, M.S., Awwad, H.K., Akoush, H.H. et al. (1992). Postoperative radiotherapy of carcinoma in bilharzial bladder: improved disease free survival through improving local control. *Int. J. Radiat. Oncol. Biol. Phys.* 23 (3): 511–517.

24

The Role of Re-irradiation for Locally Recurrent Rectal Cancer

Johannes H.W. de Wilt[1] and Jacobus W.A. Burger[2]

[1] *Department of Surgery, Radboud University Hospital, Nijmegen, The Netherlands*
[2] *Department of Surgery, Catharina Hospital Eindhoven, The Netherlands*

Background

Treatment of colorectal cancer has improved significantly due to advances in chemo- and/or radiotherapy and better surgical management [1–4]. Local recurrence in the modern era of rectal surgery occurs in approximately 4–11% of patients [2, 5, 6]. The role of (chemo)radiation therapy to further reduce recurrence rates in primary treatment of rectal cancer patients is well established [5, 6]. On the other hand, when locally recurrent disease becomes apparent, optimal treatment becomes more difficult [7]. Previously irradiated patients with a recurrence present often with simultaneous metastatic disease and their median survival is reduced [8]. van den Brink et al. observed that previously irradiated patients in the Dutch total mesorectal excision (TME) trial died within three years after being diagnosed with a recurrence [9]. Others have demonstrated that locally recurrent rectal cancer (LRRC) patients who previously received radiotherapy for primary rectal cancer had worse oncological outcomes than those who had not received radiotherapy [7].

Traditionally, there has been a hesitance toward re-irradiation due to concerns regarding toxicity [10–12]. Nevertheless, re-irradiation has been reported to be safe [13], and several early studies observed promising results, with acceptable long-term outcomes [14, 15].

Despite this, the treatment of LRRC in previously irradiated patients poses difficulties and the risks and benefits of re-irradiation do require further assessment [16]. This chapter outlines the current evidence regarding re-irradiation of LRRC.

Treatment of Locally Recurrent Rectal Cancer

Curative resection of LRRC is the most important factor for survival [12]. Surgical salvage of LRRC is challenging because of previous rectal surgery, fibrosis, and obliteration of surgical planes [17]. This may influence the ability to achieve complete surgical margins (R0 resection), which is the single most important predictor of long-term survival in patients with LRRC [18, 19]. Re-irradiation may potentially increase the rate of R0 resections and as such could provide better results. To optimize treatment, the tumor should receive a high total dose, while sparing the surrounding normal tissue and avoiding toxicity. Re-irradiation is therefore challenging because the surrounding tissues have already received doses near the

Surgical Management of Advanced Pelvic Cancer, First Edition.
Edited by Michael E. Kelly and Desmond C. Winter.
© 2022 John Wiley & Sons Ltd. Published 2022 by John Wiley & Sons Ltd.

Table 24.1 Patient and previous radiotherapy characteristics.

Author, year	Center, country	Number of re-irradiated patients	Age (years)	Median previous radiotherapy dose (Gy)	Time from previous treatment (months)
Tao et al., 2017 [20]	MD Anderson Cancer Center, USA	102	58 (range 35–77)	50.4 (range 25–63)	30 (range 5–789)
Susko et al., 2016 [21]	Duke Cancer Center, USA	33	63 (IQR 58–70)	Not mentioned	39 (range 25–50)
Alberda et al., 2014 [22]	Erasmus MC Cancer Institute, Netherlands	28	63 (range 55–70)	50 (range 25–50)	20 (range 12–30)
Bosman et al., 2014 [23]	Catherina Hospital, Netherlands	135	63 (range 30–84)	50 (range 25–50)	34 (range 7–198)
Ng et al., 2013 [24]	Peter MacCallum Cancer Centre, Australia	56	69 (range 26–88)	50.4 (range 21–64)	30 (range 8–176)
Sun et al., 2012 [25]	Shandong University, China	72	59 (range 29–78)	< 50	25 (range 13–77)
Koom et al., 2012 [26]	Yonsei University College of Medicine, South Korea	22	50 (range 33–64)	54 (range 45–59.4)	26 (range 5–72)

IQR, Interquartile range.

organ-specific tolerance dose during the primary treatment [12].

Data from published studies since 2012 demonstrate that re-irradiation is performed only in a few expert centers worldwide (Table 24.1). Average age of treated patients is between 50 and 69 years, which means that this group represents a relatively young group of colorectal cancer patients [20–26]. The majority of patients were previously treated with chemoradiation up to a radiation dose of 54 Gy. However, in the studies by Alberda et al. [27] and Bosman et al. [23] many patients were treated with short-course radiotherapy for the primary tumor. The interval between treatment of the primary rectal cancer and re-irradiation was 26–39 months.

Among all studies, re-irradiation dosages varied between 27 and 50 Gy (Table 24.2). Several techniques were used, with most centers using one dose of external beam radiation therapy (EBRT) per day [22, 23, 28–30]. Alternatively, hyperfractioning of EBRT twice daily is considered [15, 20]. The number of fractions varied substantially between the different protocols in each center [15].

Morbidity After Re-irradiation

Toxicity as a result of re-irradiation has been reported in several studies in the literature [12]. Generally, toxicity is modest, with grade 3 or higher acute toxicity reported in 2–4% [14, 24], nausea/vomiting in 4% [31], skin damage in 5–8% [14, 24], and acute diarrhea in 10–20% of patients [14, 15, 24–26]. Tao et al. [20] reported a three-year actuarial grade 3–4 toxicity of 34% of all patients that had re-irradiation. Patients who underwent surgery had a significantly higher rate of grade 3–4 toxicity of 54% versus 16% in the non-surgery group. This was comparable with results in the large cohort study by Bosman et al. who reported 39.7% grade 3–5 complications in their group of surgically treated patients. Overall, toxicity following

Table 24.2 Re-irradiation details and outcome.

Author, year	Re-irradiated dose (Gy)	Number of fractions	Concurrent chemotherapy	Surgical resection	Median survival in surgery group (months)
Tao et al., 2017 [20]	39 (range 30–45)	26	91%	45% (67% R0)	47
Susko et al., 2016 [21]	30 (range 18–36)	Not mentioned	—	42% (71% R0)	32 (range 13–48)
Alberda et al., 2014 [22]	27–30	19–28	100% (from 2006)	100% (46% R0)	32 (range 4–86)
Bosman et al., 2014 [23]	30–30.6	19–28	87%	100% (56% R0)	±38[1]
Ng et al., 2013 [24]	39.6 (range 20–39.6)	10–22	80%	21% (75% R0)	39
Sun et al., 2012 [25]	36	30	100%	25% (89% R0)	32 (all patients)
Koom et al., 2012 [26]	50 (range 28–66)	Not mentioned	73%	23%	21 (all patients)

[1] Based on Kaplan–Meier survival curves.

re-irradiation is well tolerated but is increased in those undergoing surgery. The PelvEx Collaborative also observed that neoadjuvant therapy in LRRC patients was associated with higher rates of readmission, complications, and radiological reinterventions [19].

Primary Outcome after Re-irradiation for LRRC

There is considerable heterogeneity across the available literature, with not all studies presenting data on patients' management with curative intent. A substantial number of patients are treated with palliative intention and the number of patients undergoing a surgical procedure varied between 21 and 100% (Table 24.2). A wide variety of surgical techniques were reported, such as low anterior resection, abdomino-perineal resection, and pelvic exenterations with or without sacrectomy. In some studies [22, 23], surgical resection was combined with intraoperative radiotherapy (IORT) at a single dose varying from 10 to 17.5 Gy. The number of complete surgical resections (R0) ranged between 46 and 89% across the various studies. Adjuvant chemotherapy was not routinely administered in all patients, and the type of chemotherapy schedule and length were not specified.

Local control (LC) was reported in both palliative and curatively treated patients and therefore it is difficult to tease out specific results. However, the largest study to date from Bosman and colleagues examined patients who were all treated with surgery following re-irradiation. They report a five-year local recurrence-free survival of 51% [23]. Median survival of all surgically treated patients ranged between 32 and 47 months (Table 24.2).

Survival of patients is variable but consistently better when patients have R0 resections [12, 23–29]. A wide variety of surgical techniques and approaches have been described, with more radical resections including bony and vascular resection needed to ensure complete oncological resection [7, 32]. Though complete resection is the goal of treatment [18], the adjunct of re-irradiation has benefit in select cases, with tolerable risks of toxicity and low specific procedure-related complications [8, 14, 15, 23, 26, 29, 31, 33, 34]. Re-irradiation is an inseparable part of multimodality treatment containing IORT, which is considered the standard of care in some countries. Perioperative mortality, after re-irradiation and extensive resections, is generally low in experienced centers. However, perioperative morbidity is not reported uniformly and might be underestimated due to the retrospective nature of most studies. Although surgery for LRRC has a high rate of morbidity, this seems to be increased by re-irradiation. On the other hand, since re-irradiation is associated with a relatively high number of more complete resections, this might positively affect long-term prognosis [14, 15, 23, 28, 35].

In the treatment of locally advanced (primary) rectal cancer, there is strong evidence that preoperative timing of (chemo)radiotherapy is more effective than postoperative [8, 36]. Preoperative tumor volume reduction which can be caused by preoperative radiotherapy increased the likelihood of complete resections [28].

In most studies, concomitant chemotherapy was used in combination with re-irradiation instead of radiotherapy only. In primary rectal cancer patients, chemoradiation resulted in better LC than radiotherapy alone, without a positive effect on overall survival [37–40]. A study by Yu et al. demonstrated that responses for LRRC were significantly lower compared to primary rectal cancer, which justifies future investigations into improving or intensifying chemotherapy and radiotherapy for LRRC patients [34].

The addition of systemic chemotherapy to the neoadjuvant treatment of LRRC is rapidly gaining popularity. This development followed promising results in the treatment of locally advanced primary rectal cancer, where the combination of neoadjuvant chemotherapy and chemoradiotherapy was reported to increase the rate of R0 resection rates [41–44]. The role of systemic chemotherapy in the neoadjuvant treatment of LRRC is even less clear. A recent study from van Zoggel et al. [45] demonstrates high pathological complete response (pCR) rates in patients with LRRC after a new sequential neoadjuvant regimen consisting of induction chemotherapy followed by chemoradiation therapy. The reported pCR rate of 17% is comparable to results in patients treated with chemoradiotherapy for locally advanced primary rectal cancer [46]. The use of intensified neoadjuvant treatment regimens generates a new hypotheses with regard to the treatment of LRRC and requires further validation in future study designs. The multicenter randomized controlled PelvEx II trial will start accrual in September 2020, with 365 patients with LRRC after partial mesorectal excision (PME)/TME surgery receiving either neoadjuvant chemoradiotherapy alone or induction chemotherapy and chemoradiotherapy prior to surgery. This study will start in seven expert centers centers in the Netherlands. International partners from across The PelvEx Collaborative will join the study in 2021.

Summary Box

- LRRC in previously irradiated patients is a heterogeneous disease and complete surgical resection should be the primary goal of treatment.
- Preoperative tumor volume reduction by re-irradiation appears to be safe and seems to be of additional value to obtaining R0 resections.
- Evidence to support routine re-irradiation is lacking. Further research and trials are needed to establish the value of re-irradiation in recurrent rectal cancer.
- Patients should be treated in dedicated centers that prospectively collect information and collaborate with other international units.

References

1 Ferlay, J., Steliarova-Foucher, E., Lortet-Tieulent, J. et al. (2013). Cancer incidence and mortality patterns in Europe: estimates for 40 countries in 2012. *Eur. J. Cancer* 49 (6): 1374–1403.

2 den Dulk, M., Krijnen, P., Marijnen, C.A. et al. (2008). Improved overall survival for patients with rectal cancer since 1990: the effects of TME surgery and pre-operative radiotherapy. *Eur. J. Cancer* 44 (12): 1710–1716.

3 MacFarlane, J.K., Ryall, R.D., and Heald, R.J. (1993). Mesorectal excision for rectal cancer. *Lancet* 341 (8843): 457–460.

4 Brouwer, N.P.M., Bos, A., Lemmens, V. et al. (2018). An overview of 25 years of incidence, treatment and outcome of colorectal cancer patients. *Int. J. Cancer* 143 (11): 2758–2766.

5 van Gijn, W., Marijnen, C.A., Nagtegaal, I.D. et al. (2011). Preoperative radiotherapy combined with total mesorectal excision for resectable rectal cancer: 12-year follow-up of the multicentre, randomised controlled TME trial. *Lancet Oncol* 12 (6): 575–582.

6 Sebag-Montefiore, D., Stephens, R.J., Steele, R. et al. (2009). Preoperative radiotherapy versus selective postoperative chemoradiotherapy in patients with rectal cancer (MRC CR07 and NCIC-CTG C016): a multicentre, randomised trial. *Lancet* 373 (9666): 811–820.

7 Rombouts, A.J., Koh, C.E., Young, J.M. et al. (2015). Does radiotherapy of the primary rectal cancer affect prognosis after pelvic exenteration for recurrent rectal cancer? *Dis. Colon Rectum* 58 (1): 65–73.

8 Glimelius, B., Gronberg, H., Jarhult, J. et al. (2003). A systematic overview of radiation therapy effects in rectal cancer. *Acta Oncol* 42 (5–6): 476–492.

9 van den Brink, M., Stiggelbout, A.M., van den Hout, W.B. et al. (2004). Clinical nature and prognosis of locally recurrent rectal cancer after total mesorectal excision with or without preoperative radiotherapy. *J. Clin. Oncol* 22 (19): 3958–3964.

10 Owens, R. and Muirhead, R. (2018). External beam re-irradiation in rectal cancer. *Clin. Oncol* 30 (2): 116–123.

11 Glimelius, B. (2003). Recurrent rectal cancer. The pre-irradiated primary tumour: can more radiotherapy be given? *Colorectal Dis* 5 (5): 501–503.

12 Guren, M.G., Undseth, C., Rekstad, B.L. et al. (2014). Reirradiation of locally recurrent rectal cancer: a systematic review. *Radiother. Oncol* 113 (2): 151–157.

13 van der Meij, W., Rombouts, A.J., Rutten, H. et al. (2016). Treatment of locally recurrent rectal carcinoma in previously (chemo) irradiated patients: a review. *Dis. Colon Rectum* 59 (2): 148–156.

14 Mohiuddin, M., Marks, G., and Marks, J. (2002). Long-term results of reirradiation for patients with recurrent rectal carcinoma. *Cancer* 95 (5): 1144–1150.

15 Valentini, V., Morganti, A.G., Gambacorta, M.A. et al. (2006). Preoperative hyperfractionated chemoradiation for locally recurrent rectal cancer in patients previously irradiated to the pelvis: a multicentric phase II study. *Int. J. Radiat. Oncol. Biol. Phys* 64 (4): 1129–1139.

16 Beyond, T.C. (2013). Consensus statement on the multidisciplinary management of patients with recurrent and primary rectal cancer beyond total mesorectal excision planes. *Br. J. Surg* 100 (8): E1–E33.

17 de Wilt, J.H., Vermaas, M., Ferenschild, F.T., and Verhoef, C. (2007). Management of locally advanced primary and recurrent rectal cancer. *Clinics Colon Rectal Surg* 20 (3): 255–263.

18 Bhangu, A., Ali, S.M., Darzi, A. et al. (2012). Meta-analysis of survival based on resection margin status following surgery for recurrent rectal cancer. *Colorectal Dis* 14 (12): 1457–1466.

19 PelvEx Collaborative (2018). Factors affecting outcomes following pelvic

exenteration for locally recurrent rectal cancer. *Br. J. Surg* 105 (6): 650–657.
20 Tao, R., Tsai, C.J., Jensen, G. et al. (2017). Hyperfractionated accelerated reirradiation for rectal cancer: an analysis of outcomes and toxicity. *Radiother. Oncol* 122 (1): 146–151.
21 Susko, M., Lee, J., Salama, J. et al. (2016). The use of re-irradiation in locally recurrent, non-metastatic rectal cancer. *Ann. Surg. Oncol* 23 (11): 3609–3615.
22 Alberda, W.J., Verhoef, C., Nuyttens, J.J. et al. (2014). Outcome in patients with resectable locally recurrent rectal cancer after total mesorectal excision with and without previous neoadjuvant radiotherapy for the primary rectal tumor. *Ann. Surg. Oncol* 21 (2): 520–526.
23 Bosman, S.J., Holman, F.A., Nieuwenhuijzen, G.A. et al. (2014). Feasibility of reirradiation in the treatment of locally recurrent rectal cancer. *Br. J. Surg* 101 (10): 1280–1289.
24 Ng, M.K., Leong, T., Heriot, A.G., and Ngan, S.Y. (2013). Once-daily reirradiation for rectal cancer in patients who have received previous pelvic radiotherapy. *J. Med. Imaging Radiat. Oncol* 57 (4): 512–518.
25 Sun, D.S., Zhang, J.D., Li, L. et al. (2012). Accelerated hyperfractionation field-involved re-irradiation combined with concurrent capecitabine chemotherapy for locally recurrent and irresectable rectal cancer. *Br. J. Radiol* 85 (1011): 259–264.
26 Koom, W.S., Choi, Y., Shim, S.J. et al. (2012). Reirradiation to the pelvis for recurrent rectal cancer. *J. Surg. Oncol* 105 (7): 637–642.
27 Alberda, W.J., Verhoef, C., Nuyttens, J.J. et al. (2014). Intraoperative radiation therapy reduces local recurrence rates in patients with microscopically involved circumferential resection margins after resection of locally advanced rectal cancer. *Int. J. Radiat. Oncol. Biol. Phys* 88 (5): 1032–1040.
28 Dresen, R.C., Gosens, M.J., Martijn, H. et al. (2008). Radical resection after IORT-containing multimodality treatment is the most important determinant for outcome in patients treated for locally recurrent rectal cancer. *Ann. Surg. Oncol* 15 (7): 1937–1947.
29 Kim, T.H., Kim, D.Y., Jung, K.H. et al. (2010). The role of omental flap transposition in patients with locoregional recurrent rectal cancer treated with reirradiation. *J. Surg. Oncol* 102 (7): 789–795.
30 Park, J.K., Kim, Y.W., Hur, H. et al. (2009). Prognostic factors affecting oncologic outcomes in patients with locally recurrent rectal cancer: impact of patterns of pelvic recurrence on curative resection. *Langenbecks Arch. Surg* 394 (1): 71–77.
31 Das, P., Delclos, M.E., Skibber, J.M. et al. (2010). Hyperfractionated accelerated radiotherapy for rectal cancer in patients with prior pelvic irradiation. *Int. J. Radiat. Oncol. Biol. Phys* 77 (1): 60–65.
32 Bhangu, A., Ali, S.M., Brown, G. et al. (2014). Indications and outcome of pelvic exenteration for locally advanced primary and recurrent rectal cancer. *Ann. Surg.* 259 (2): 315–322.
33 Mohiuddin, M., Marks, G.M., Lingareddy, V., and Marks, J. (1997). Curative surgical resection following reirradiation for recurrent rectal cancer. *Int. J. Radiat. Oncol. Biol. Phys* 39 (3): 643–649.
34 Yu, S.K., Bhangu, A., Tait, D.M. et al. (2014). Chemoradiotherapy response in recurrent rectal cancer. *Cancer Med* 3 (1): 111–117.
35 Asoglu, O., Karanlik, H., Muslumanoglu, M. et al. (2007). Prognostic and predictive factors after surgical treatment for locally recurrent rectal cancer: a single institute experience. *Eur. J. Surg. Oncol* 33 (10): 1199–1206.
36 Sauer, R., Becker, H., Hohenberger, W. et al. (2004). Preoperative versus postoperative chemoradiotherapy for rectal cancer. *New Engl. J. Med* 351 (17): 1731–1740.
37 Bonnetain, F., Bosset, J.F., Gerard, J.P. et al. (2012). What is the clinical benefit of

preoperative chemoradiotherapy with 5FU/leucovorin for T3–4 rectal cancer in a pooled analysis of EORTC 22921 and FFCD 9203 trials: surrogacy in question? *Eur. J. Cancer* 48 (12): 1781–1790.

38 Bosset, J.F., Collette, L., Calais, G. et al. (2006). Chemotherapy with preoperative radiotherapy in rectal cancer. *New Engl. J. Med* 355 (11): 1114–1123.

39 Braendengen, M., Tveit, K.M., Berglund, A. et al. (2008). Randomized phase III study comparing preoperative radiotherapy with chemoradiotherapy in nonresectable rectal cancer. *J. Clin. Oncol* 26 (22): 3687–3694.

40 Gerard, J.P., Conroy, T., Bonnetain, F. et al. (2006). Preoperative radiotherapy with or without concurrent fluorouracil and leucovorin in T3–4 rectal cancers: results of FFCD 9203. *J. Clin. Oncol* 24 (28): 4620–4625.

41 Chau, I., Brown, G., Cunningham, D. et al. (2006). Neoadjuvant capecitabine and oxaliplatin followed by synchronous chemoradiation and total mesorectal excision in magnetic resonance imaging-defined poor-risk rectal cancer. *J. Clin. Oncol* 24 (4): 668–674.

42 Chua, Y.J., Barbachano, Y., Cunningham, D. et al. (2010). Neoadjuvant capecitabine and oxaliplatin before chemoradiotherapy and total mesorectal excision in MRI-defined poor-risk rectal cancer: a phase 2 trial. *Lancet Oncol* 11 (3): 241–248.

43 Cercek, A., Goodman, K.A., Hajj, C. et al. (2014). Neoadjuvant chemotherapy first, followed by chemoradiation and then surgery, in the management of locally advanced rectal cancer. *J. Natl Compr. Canc. Netw* 12 (4): 513–519.

44 Cercek, A., Roxburgh, C.S.D., Strombom, P. et al. (2018). Adoption of total neoadjuvant therapy for locally advanced rectal cancer. *JAMA Oncol* 4 (6): e180071.

45 van, Zoggel, D., Bosman, S.J., Kusters, M. et al. (2018). Preliminary results of a cohort study of induction chemotherapy-based treatment for locally recurrent rectal cancer. *Br. J. Surg* 105 (4): 447–452.

46 Maas, M., Nelemans, P.J., Valentini, V. et al. (2010). Long-term outcome in patients with a pathological complete response after chemoradiation for rectal cancer: a pooled analysis of individual patient data. *Lancet Oncol* 11 (9): 835–844.

25

Palliative Pelvic Exenteration

Hidde M. Kroon[1,2] and Tarik Sammour[1,2]

[1] *Colorectal Unit, Department of Surgery, Royal Adelaide Hospital, Adelaide, Australia*
[2] *Faculty of Health and Medical Science, School of Medicine, University of Adelaide, Adelaide, Australia*

Background

Locally advanced or recurrent pelvic malignancy can result in debilitating symptoms, causing a significant impact on the quality of life (QoL) of affected patients [1–3]. Symptoms often include intractable pain, bleeding, pelvic sepsis, obstruction, and fistula formation. Pelvic exenterative surgery (PES) with curative intent, defined as the radical en-bloc resection of multiple endopelvic and exopelvic structures with clear margins (R0 resection), followed by reconstruction or diversion of visceral functions, can relieve symptoms and improve QoL, and is potentially lifesaving.

Pelvic exenteration, however, is major surgery with long operating times (5–14 hours), significant blood loss, and high perioperative morbidity and mortality rates (40–90% and 0–24% respectively), despite gradual improvements in surgical technique and perioperative practice [4]. Therefore indications for curative exenteration are carefully assessed and the procedure is normally reserved for selected patients without extrapelvic disease and who are considered to be in good general health.

Patients in whom an R0 resection is unlikely to be achieved or those with distant metastatic disease are typically not considered candidates for pelvic exenteration. These patients may, however, benefit from palliative treatments such as chemotherapy and radiotherapy or palliative procedures such as formation of a colostomy or urinary diversion for symptom relief. In some centers, palliative exenteration is considered for symptom relief in highly selective patients. However, this topic remains controversial. Some argue that there is no indication for palliative exenteration as the high procedural morbidity is not suitable in palliative patients with a limited overall survival (OS). To date, there are limited data on the role of palliative exenteration in patients with severe symptoms due to advanced pelvic malignancies [3, 5–8].

Historical Perspective

Pelvic exenteration was first reported by Brunschwig in 1948 and was actually proposed as a palliative procedure for locally advanced or locally recurrent malignancies [9]. It was indicated for patients without distant metastases, but with locally advanced tumors causing disabling symptoms such as pain, bleeding, pelvic sepsis, and fistulae, in whom other treatment options were exhausted. Initially, results were quite discouraging, with perioperative mortality rates of 23–33% and

Surgical Management of Advanced Pelvic Cancer, First Edition.
Edited by Michael E. Kelly and Desmond C. Winter.
© 2022 John Wiley & Sons Ltd. Published 2022 by John Wiley & Sons Ltd.

quite significant morbidity. However, the potential benefits were clearly expressed by Brunschwig himself: "Because of the advanced stage of disease, it is not to be anticipated that many patients will survive for prolonged periods. On the other hand, of those surviving, not one has expressed the feeling that they would have preferred to have remained as they were and not to have had the operation." [9]

In the following years, exenteration was increasingly performed and the technique was further refined. Importantly, a consensus was formed regarding relative and absolute contraindications based on incurability: distant and peritoneal metastases and invasion into major nerves, common iliac vessels, and/or pelvic bones precluding R0 resection [10–14]. The indications for pelvic exenteration have continued to gradually expand higher and wider with increased experience, the advent of better imaging, and multimodality strategies involving coordinated specialties. Due to this, exenteration is now a well-established curative-intent option with acceptable morbidity and mortality in locally advanced primary or recurrent colorectal, urological, gynecological, and soft tissue malignancies [15–17]. With this broader indication for curative pelvic exenteration developing over time, the indication for palliative exenteration has become less well defined. The first report on palliative exenteration that would equate to current standards stems back to 1976, when Deckers et al. argued that pelvic exenteration as intentional palliation can be of benefit to selected patients [13]. However, there is still no real international consensus with regards to the definition and the indication for palliative exenteration [5, 7, 18–21].

Definition

The World Health Organization emphasizes that palliative care neither hastens nor postpones death, but provides relief from distressing symptoms [22]. In view of this, surgery can have a palliative role if the benefits in terms of symptoms relief outweigh the potential disadvantages in terms of postoperative morbidity [23, 24]. A recent systematic review for malignant bowel obstruction, however, showed that palliative surgery does come at a high cost, in particular with regards to prolonged convalescence relative to the patient's remaining survival time [25]. This probably also holds true for palliative exenteration, and it is clear that surgeons should present realistic expectations of palliative surgery in this setting.

The definition of what constitutes palliative pelvic exenteration remains ill-defined, with considerable heterogeneity to date [2, 3, 5–8, 19, 26]. Quyn et al., for instance, defined an exenteration as palliative if there is known presence of extrapelvic disease and/or if clear margins cannot be achieved [3]. Schmidt et al. defined palliative exenteration as the presence of distant metastasis, positive peritoneal lavage, or perforation into the pouch of Douglas, as well as in cases when complete tumor removal was not possible [26]. Finlayson et al. offered three definitions of palliative exenteration and differentiated between patients operated on specifically for symptom control, those operated on as part of salvage therapy, and patients operated on with curative intent in whom surgical findings indicated incurable disease [2], while Magrina et al. defined palliative exenteration as tumor extension to the lateral pelvic wall, or positive pelvic/para-aortic lymph nodes [19], and Stanhope et al. used a similar criterion with the addition of bony involvement or distant metastases [27]. Additionally, it should be noted that some articles mention the word palliative when the procedure was actually performed with curative intent but was unsuccessful [28–30].

Summarizing the above information, we propose the following definition of palliative exenteration: a pelvic exenteration performed with the aim of symptom relief in patients with known distant metastases, peritoneal disease, retroperitoneal or para-aortic lymph node metastases, and/or pelvic disease where an R0 resection with curative intent is expected not to be possible.

Indications

There is varying indication for palliative exenteration across the literature (Table 25.1). At one of the spectrum, many surgeons still consider it to be contraindicated in all patients, as the morbidity of the surgery is likely to always outweigh any potential QoL benefits [2, 5, 6, 31–34]. This is compounded by the fact that it is quite difficult to select patients and consent them successfully in this setting, as the stakes are quite high and not always predictable. As a result, some stress the use of less maximally invasive palliative treatments to alleviate symptoms such as a diverting colostomy, endoscopic stent placement, suprapubic catheter, or palliative radiotherapy and/or chemotherapy, in addition to palliative pain and symptom management [3, 14, 24, 32, 35–37].

Some physicians do not completely out-rule palliative exenteration, but consider it an absolute last resort to alleviate symptoms [1, 2, 38, 39]. There are advocates that call for the selecting of patients with severe symptoms who are physically and emotionally able to tolerate the surgery and may benefit from it even in the setting of extensive local and/or distal disease [8, 13, 40]. However, most offering selective palliative exenteration do not in patients with a life expectancy of less than six months (in view of the recovery time following the surgery), or in those with severe comorbidities (such as cardiac, pulmonary, renal, dementia, or cachexia due to distant metastases), or those with extensive local tumor progression who

Table 25.1 Reported indications for PPES.

Origin of tumor	Main indication	Extent of tumor
Colorectal	Pain	Locally irradical tumor progression
Colon	Bleeding	Nodal metastases
Rectal	Hematuria	Pelvic/lateral
Anal	Rectal	Inguinal
Gynecological	Vaginal	Para-aortic
Vulval	Obstruction	Peritoneal metastases
Vaginal	Urine	Distant metastases
Cervical	Bowel	
Uterine/endometrial	Incontinence	
Ovarian	Urine	
Urological	Fecal	
Urethra	Fistula	
Prostate	Recto-vesical	
Bladder	Recto-prostatic	
Melanoma	Recto-vaginal	
Sarcoma	Vesico-vaginal	
	Ulcerative/fungating tumor	
	Pelvic sepsis	
	Fever	
	Malodorous	

require high sacral resections or have lower limb lymphedema, and patients who will unlikely benefit from the procedure with regards to symptom relief [41, 42].

> *In summary, the ideal candidate for a palliative pelvic exenteration would be a fit patient, with limited and chemo-responsive distant disease, who has pelvic symptoms that are thought treatable with exenteration, and who cannot be equally palliated with a less-invasive option.*

Selecting eligible patients for palliative exenteration is a difficult and clouded process [13]. Therefore it is advisable that patients are discussed in a specialized multidisciplinary team (MDT) meeting. Quyn et al. reported that advances in preoperative imaging and the introduction of an exenteration MDT meeting improved assessments of disease and operative planning. This resulted in a reduction in the percentage of patients undergoing palliative exenteration from 11 to 8% [3].

When a patient is found surgically and medically eligible for a palliative exenteration after MDT consensus, the treating clinician must inform the patient and their relatives thoroughly and discuss the procedure in detail, providing them with a realistic assessment regarding its efficacy in terms of palliation and potential adverse outcomes. It is also important to clearly discuss limits on subsequent care, and an open, frank, shared decision-making process should be actively encouraged.

Outcomes

One of the difficulties of analyzing the results from palliative exenteration series is the considerable heterogeneity that exists in terms of tumor location, the definition of palliative exenteration, and the indications used [3, 7, 14, 19, 27]. Furthermore, studies are mostly retrospective and do not have a uniform definition for outcome reporting [3, 8, 27, 40].

Nevertheless, an overview of the results is given in Table 25.2.

Morbidity and Mortality

Despite advances in surgical techniques and better perioperative care, one of the main concerns with palliative exenteration is the associated high rates of morbidity and mortality [3, 8, 49, 56]. Some would go as far as to suggest that the significant mortality and morbidity associated with pelvic exenteration preclude its use as a palliative procedure [57]. Overall, the median (range) in-hospital morbidity rate is 53% (13–100%) [3, 8, 19, 27, 39, 40, 43, 46, 48, 49, 52]. Most reported major surgical complications relate to flap failure and urosepsis/urine leak. In-hospital mortality directly related to palliative exenteration is 10% (0–67%) [3, 5, 7–9, 11, 13, 18, 19, 26, 27, 39, 40, 43, 45, 46, 48, 49, 52, 54].

Quyn et al. reported results after 39 palliative exenterations for a variety of malignancies for symptom control. Though there were no in-hospital deaths, one-third of patients experienced a major morbidity [3]. They concluded that in view of comorbidities, palliative exenteration can be performed in an expert center, since their complication rates approached those having curative resections.

Symptom Relief

To date, 12 studies have been published on symptom relief following palliative exenteration. Seventy-six percent of patients experienced some reduction in reported symptoms (50–100%) [6–9, 13, 40, 43, 58–62]. Six studies observed a median duration of symptom relief of 14 months (8–18 months) [7, 13, 43, 58, 61, 62]. However, these results must be interpreted with caution as there was no mention of which symptoms were being palliated in the majority of these studies. As shown in Table 25.2, many studies did not mention symptom relief at all. Quyn et al., for instance, reported mainly on QoL after palliative exenteration mainly

Table 25.2 Historical overview of selected series in the English literature reporting on outcomes of PPES.

Author, year	Number of patients	Cancer types (%)	Disease progression beyond pelvis (%)	Main indication/ reason palliative	Type of exenteration performed (%)	Hospital stay (days)	Hospital morbidity (%)	Hospital mortality (%)	Postoperative QoL	Symptom relief (%)	Median symptom-free survival (months)	Median OS (months)	Conclusion on palliative exenteration
Quyn et al., 2016 [3]	39	Colorectal (79; recurrent 56 and primary 23) Gynecological (8) Bladder (5) Sarcoma (5) Melanoma (4)	Liver mets (12) Nodal mets (21) Peritoneal mets (21) Irradical pelvic resection (48)	Pain Bleeding Fistula Prognosis	Resection of tumor and 2+ adjacent organs/bone/ neurovascular structures, involving 3/5 or more pelvic compartments	18	34 (grade III/IV 21%)	0	Worse than preoperative	—	—	24	Controversial and questionable effect
Pathiraja et al., 2014 [40]	18	Cervical (67) Vulvar (27) Endometrial (6)	Irradical pelvic resection	Pain Malodor Bleeding Fistula	Total (50) Anterior (27) Posterior (22)	24	78 (long term: 39)	0	—	78	—	11	Technically feasible in carefully selected patients
Schmidt et al., 2012 [26]	149	Cervical	Distant mets Peritoneal mets Irradical pelvic resection (R1)	> 5 cm tumor Fistula Recurrences meeting the criteria for primary exenteration	Total (96) Anterior (2) Posterior (2)	—	51[1]	5[1]	—	—	—	14	Previous contraindication should be reconsidered
Guimarães et al., 2011 [8]	13	Cervical (69) Endometrial (15) Leiomyosarcoma (15)	Distant mets Retroperitoneal nodal mets Peritoneal mets Irradical pelvic resection	Fistula Pain Malodor Bleeding	Total	15	38.4	15	Improved	100	—	5	In highly selected patients only: role yet to be established
Fotopoulou et al., 2010 [39]	22	Cervical Vaginal Ovarian[1]	Distant mets/ para-aortic lymph nodes Peritoneal mets	Bleeding Bowel obstruction Fistula	Total Anterior Posterior[1]	29[1]	82	8.5[1]	—	—	—	4	Considerable in highly selected patients to improve QoL

Author	N	Cancer type	Indications	Symptoms	Type of exenteration						Comments
Nishio et al., 2009 [48]	14	Colorectal	Irradical pelvic resection	Postoperative due to irradical	Total	143[1]	—	12[1]	—	14	Total exenteration may have better outcomes when performed with curative intent
Marnitz et al., 2006 [46]	18	Cervical	Preoperative irradical pelvic resection expected	No alternative treatment available	Total (93) Posterior (5) Anterior (2)[5]	37.6[1]	58[1]	5.5[1]	—	8	Should be offered in recurrent disease where radical resection seems unlikely
Vieira et al., 2004 [49]	9	Colorectal	R1 and R2 resections Abdominal or systemic mets	Pain Weight loss Bleeding Change in bowel habits Mucorrhea Fistula Fever Pneumaturia[5]	Colectomy and en-bloc one or more organs/structures	11[1]	77.8	66.7	—	3.1	Could benefit selected patients when cautiously indicated
Kamat et al., 2003 [43]	14	Prostate	None	Pain Dysuria Hematuria Fecal and urinary incontinence	Total	—	50	0	79	14.1	24	Feasible in highly selected patients
Magrina et al., 1997 [19]	30	Cervical Endometrial Vaginal Colorectal Vulval	Nodal mets (pelvic, aorta, sidewall)	Bleeding Malodorous Pain Irresectable nodal mets	Total Anterior Posterior "Extended"	26.6[1]	57[1]	6.7[1]	—	14	Shorter survival after palliative exenteration

(Continued)

Table 25.2 (Continued)

Author, year	Number of patients	Cancer types (%)	Disease progression beyond pelvis (%)	Main indication/reason palliative	Type of exenteration performed (%)	Hospital stay (days)	Hospital morbidity (%)	Hospital mortality (%)	Postoperative QoL	Symptom relief (%)	Median symptom-free survival (months)	Median OS (months)	Conclusion on palliative exenteration
Woodhouse et al., 1995 [7]	10	Colorectal Bladder Vulval/vaginal Cervical Anal	Local nodal mets (pelvic, sidewall) Bone involvement Irradical pelvic resection None	Pain Discharge Hematuria/dysuria	Total (60) Anterior (39)	—	Early: 20 Late: 60	0	Improved in 80%	80	>18	17	In highly selected patients and appropriate multispeciality care, exenteration can be of palliative value
Brophy, et al. 1994 [5]	35	Colorectal Bladder/renal/urethral Cervical/Ovarian	Distant mets Irradical pelvic resection (R1/R2) None	Pain (33) Bleeding (31) Fistula (20) Obstruction (17)	Total (31) Anterior (37) Posterior (31) (Extended in 48%)	—	47	3	Improved in 88%	—	—	20	Aggressive treatment can be considered in selected patients after a multimodality approach
Stanhope et al., 1990 [18]	16	Cervical adenocarcinoma	Nodal mets (para-aortic/pelvic) Irradical pelvic resection	Intraoperatively due to no curative resection possible	Total Anterior Posterior	—	38[1]	4.2[1]	—	—	—	14	Better imaging may improve patient selection
Rutledge and McGuffee, 1987 [45]	44	Cervical Vaginal Endometrial Vulval Urethral Colorectal	Nodal mets	Intraoperatively positive nodes found	Total Anterior Posterior	—	—	6.8	—	—	—	26.3%[2]	Futile in case of irradical resections or distant mets. May be justified in selected patients with regional nodes
Stanhope and Symmonds, 1985 [27]	59	Cervical Vaginal/vulvar Endometrial Colorectal Bladder/urethral Melanoma	Nodal mets (para-aortic/pelvic 66) Peritoneal mets (15) Distant mets (10) Irradical pelvic resection (8)	Fistula Intraoperatively due to no curative resection possible	Total (57) Anterior (41) Posterior (2)	22	—	5.1	—	—	—	19	Reasonable in selected patients by experienced pelvic surgeons if good clearance of cancer can be achieved

Study	N	Tumour type (%)	Exclusion criteria	Complications	Type of exenteration			Mortality (%)	Symptom improvement		5-year survival (%)	Conclusion
Rutledge et al., 1977 [52]	53	Cervical / Colorectal / Bladder / Vulval / Bladder/urethral	Nodal mets (pelvis/inguinal 57) / Irradical pelvic resection (43)	Intraoperative due to nodal mets / Postoperative due to irradical pelvic resection	Total / Anterior / Posterior	—	70[1]	13.5[1]	—	—	6%[2]	Not advisable; palliative benefit doubtful due to short survival
Deckers et al., 1976 [13]	8	Cervical (50) / Bladder (25) / Colorectal (25)	Distant mets / Peritoneal mets / Nodal mets (para-aortic) / Non-cancerous (hydronephrosis, dementia, cardiac)	Fistula / Pain / Bleeding / Infections / Incontinence	Total (63) / Anterior (36)	—	13	0	Improved in all patients	100	15	15 / To be considered in symptomatic patients
Barber and Jones, 1971 [11]	97	Cervical	Nodal mets	Retrospective upon histopathology	—	—	"high"	21.6	"difficult"	—	—	5.1%[2] / Contraindicated
Brunschwig and Barber, 1969 [54]	26	Colon (35) / Vulval (38) / Vaginal (12) / Cervical (15)	Irradical pelvic resections / Bone involvement	Pain or "desperate circumstances" / Retrospective due to survival time	Total (with/without bone) / Posterior (with/without bone) / Anterior	—	"many"	31	—	—	—	14 (colon) / 9.7 (vulval) / 12 (vaginal) / 10 (cervical) / High complication rates and low survival; however, may be considered in selected patients
Brunschwig, 1948 [9]	22	Cervical (68) / Vaginal/vulval (9) / Sarcoma (5) / Uterus (5) / Colon (5) / Unknown (5)	None	Pain / Discomfort / Fistula / Pelvic sepsis	Total	—	—	23	Improved in all patients still alive and out of hospital (50%)	59	—	8 / Justified in selected patients without extra pelvic spread and whose disease cannot be controlled by other measures

mets, Metastases.
Dashes indicate not reported.
[1] Reported for entire palliative and curative exenteration cohort.
[2] Five-year survival (%).

because there was no durable palliation of symptoms [3].

Quality of Life

There have been several studies looking at QoL after curative pelvic exenteration [1, 51]. Patients reported similar levels of emotional functioning and QoL compared to the healthy population shortly after recovery from surgery [1, 50, 51, 63, 64]. Following palliative pelvic exenteration, QoL has been reported in 10 studies [3, 5, 7–9, 11, 13, 53, 60, 65]. The best-quality study was performed by Quyn et al. who had prospective follow-up QoL questionnaires completed by their patients and showed that, unlike in the curative setting, palliative exenteration patients gradually experienced a sustained decline in QoL after surgery until death [3]. They concluded that no dramatic or durable palliation of symptoms, or improved or sustained QoL was observed after palliative exenteration. Therefore many debate that its role remains questionable.

There was only one other prospective study on QoL after palliative exenteration, reporting an 88% improvement in 35 patients. However, this study used a non-validated questionnaire [5]. Additionally, there were eight lower-quality studies that reported on QoL after palliative exenteration, but they did not mention how the QoL assessment was performed, making interpretation difficult. Of these studies, six mentioned an improvement in QoL, while two studies described a decline in postoperative QoL.

Overall Survival

Median OS following palliative pelvic exenteration is 14 months. However, differences in reports to date (3–40 months) reflect differences in tumor biology, extent of disease, and definitions used [3, 5, 7–9, 11, 13, 18, 19, 26, 27, 39, 40, 43, 45, 46, 48, 49, 52, 54].

You et al. demonstrated a reduced QoL in cases of R2 resection with a similar short life expectancy when compared to non-operative patients [53]. Finally, a meta-analysis of survival based on resection margins for rectal cancer showed that patients with R1 resections have a significantly reduced survival compared to R0 resections, while there is no survival benefit compared to less-invasive palliative measures after an R2 resection [66].

Despite the heterogeneity of most palliative pelvic exenteration studies, there are some reports on single tumor types. Twelve studies have been published on colorectal palliative exenteration with a median OS of 10 months (3–14 months) [6, 15, 44, 47–49, 55, 60–62, 67, 68]. Six studies have reported OS after palliative exenteration for cervical cancer with a median of 14 months (5–14 months) [10, 11, 18, 26, 46, 58]. There are two studies that reported on palliative exenteration for prostate carcinoma showing median survival rates of 17 and 24 months respectively [43, 59]. In summary, OS after palliative pelvic exenterative surgery (PPES) is short for all tumor types. However, survival is clearly not the best measure of success in this patient category.

Future Directions

Since the first report on exenterative surgery in 1948, the definition and indications for palliative have changed significantly, likely due to increasing experience, improvements in radiology and adjuvant therapy, and the introduction of new techniques. It is likely that these definitions and indications will continue to evolve in the future with the introduction of more effective systemic and local therapies, such as immunotherapy, precision radiotherapy, and radiological chemo-embolization. The role for minimally invasive surgery remains undefined, but there are increasing reports of the feasibility of this in the literature, with case series on laparoscopic and robot palliative exenteration becoming available [28, 40, 69].

Despite this, there is simply no good evidence regarding the current role of palliative exenteration, which makes it difficult to either recommend or deny surgical management for these patients [2, 3, 14, 40]. Future prospective studies are needed to establish palliative exenteration as a treatment option, using validated instruments of QoL.

Summary Box

- The definition of PPES has evolved since first described in 1948.
- Proposed current definition: PPES is a pelvic exenteration performed with the aim of symptom relief in patients with known distant metastases, peritoneal disease, retroperitoneal or para-aortic lymph node metastases, and/or pelvic disease where an R0 resection with curative intent is expected not to be possible.
- Evidence for PPES is scarce. Only limited, single-center, highly selected cohort studies are available.
- Reported postoperative morbidity and mortality after PPES are higher than those reported after curative PES.
- A palliative pelvic exenteration should only be considered in selected fit patients, with limited and chemo-responsive distant disease, who have pelvic symptoms that are thought treatable with exenteration, and who cannot be equally palliated with a less-invasive option

---

References

1 Harji, D.P., Griffiths, B., Velikova, G. et al. (2016). Systematic review of health-related quality of life in patients undergoing pelvic exenteration. *Eur. J. Surg. Oncol.* 42: 1132–1145.

2 Finlayson, C.A. and Eisenberg, B.L. (1996). Palliative pelvic exenteration: patient selection and results. *Oncology (Williston Park)* 10: 479–484.
   Study that defined the role of PPES best.

3 Quyn, A.J., Solomon, M.J., Lee, P.M. et al. (2016). Palliative pelvic exenteration: clinical outcomes and quality of life. *Dis. Colon Rectum* 59: 1005–1010.
   Good quality cohort study on outcomes following palliative exenteration. Includes prospective data with QoL with validated questionnaires.

4 Brown, K.G., Solomon, M.J., and Koh, C.E. (2017). Pelvic exenteration surgery: the evolution of radical surgical techniques for advanced and recurrent pelvic malignancy. *Dis. Colon Rectum* 60: 745–754.

5 Brophy, P.F., Hoffman, J.P., and Eisenberg, B.L. (1994). The role of palliative pelvic exenteration. *Am. J. Surg.* 167: 386–390.

6 Yeung, R.S., Moffat, F.L., and Falk, R.E. (1993). Pelvic exenteration for recurrent and extensive primary colorectal adenocarcinoma. *Cancer* 72: 1853–1858.

7 Woodhouse, C.R., Plail, R.O., Schlesinger, P.E. et al. (1995). Exenteration as palliation for patients with advanced pelvic malignancy. *Br. J. Urol.* 76: 315–320.

8 Guimarães, G.C., Baiocchi, G., Ferreira, F.O. et al. (2011). Palliative pelvic exenteration for patients with gynecological malignancies. *Arch. Gynecol. Obstet.* 283: 1107–1112.

9 Brunschwig, A. (1948). Complete excision of pelvic viscera for advanced carcinoma; a one-stage abdominoperineal operation with end colostomy and bilateral ureteral implantation into the colon above the colostomy. *Cancer* 1: 177–183.
   First study to report on pelvic exenteration, calling it a palliative procedure, but by today's

standards Brunschwig actually performed curative PES.

10 Creasman, W.T. and Rutledge, F. (1974). Is positive pelvic lymphadenopathy a contraindication to radical surgery in recurrent cervical carcinoma? *Gynecol. Oncol.* 2: 482–485.
11 Barber, H.R. and Jones, W. (1971). Lymphadenectomy in pelvic exenteration for recurrent cervix cancer. *JAMA* 22 (215): 1945–1949.
12 Morley, G.W., Lindenauer, S.M., and Cerny, J.C. (1971). Pelvic exenterative therapy in recurrent pelvic carcinoma. *Am. J. Obstet. Gynecol.* 109: 1175–1186.
13 Deckers, P.J., Olsson, C., Williams, L.A., and Mozden, P.J. (1976). Pelvic exenteration as palliation of malignant disease. *Am. J. Surg.* 131: 509–515.
14 Hope, J.M. and Pothuri, B. (2013). The role of palliative surgery in gynecologic cancer cases. *Oncologist* 18: 73–79.
15 Ike, H., Shimada, H., Yamaguchi, S. et al. (2003). Outcome of total pelvic exenteration for primary rectal cancer. *Dis. Colon Rectum* 46: 474–480.
16 Nielsen, M.B., Rasmussen, P.C., Lindegaard, J.C., and Laurberg, S. (2012). A 10-year experience of total pelvic exenteration for primary advanced and locally recurrent rectal cancer based on a prospective database. *Colorectal Dis.* 14: 1076–1083.
17 Vermaas, M., Ferenschild, F.T., Verhoef, C. et al. (2007). Total pelvic exenteration for primary locally advanced and locally recurrent rectal cancer. *Eur. J. Surg. Oncol.* 33: 452–458.
18 Stanhope, C.R., Webb, J.M., and Podratz, K.C. (1990). Pelvic exenteration for recurrent cervical cancer. *Clin. Obstet. Gynecol.* 33: 897–909.
19 Magrina, J.F., Stanhope, C.R., and Waever, A.L. (1997). Pelvic exenterations: supralevator, infralevator, and with vulvectomy. *Gynecol. Oncol.* 64: 130–135.
20 Crowe, P.J., Temple, W.J., Lopez, M.J., and Ketcham, A.S. (1999). Pelvic exenteration for advanced pelvic malignancy. *Semin. Surg. Oncol.* 17: 152–160.
21 Lambrou, N.C., Pearson, J.M., and Averette, H.E. (2005). Pelvic exenteration of gynecologic malignancy: indications, and technical and reconstructive considerations. *Surg. Oncol. Clin. North Am.* 14: 289–300.
22 WHO. WHO Definition of Palliative Care. http://www.who.int/cancer/palliative/definition/en (accessed June 25, 2020)
23 McCahill, L.E., Krouse, R., Chu, D. et al. (2002). Indications and use of palliative surgery – results of Society of Surgical Oncology survey. *Ann. Surg. Oncol.* 9: 104–112.
24 Dunn, G.P. (2015). Surgery, palliative care, and the American College of Surgeons. *Ann. Palliat. Med.* 4: 5–9.
25 Paul Olson, T.J., Pinkerton, C., Brasel, K.J., and Schwarze, M.L. (2014). Palliative surgery for malignant bowel obstruction from carcinomatosis: a systematic review. *JAMA Surg.* 149: 383–392.
26 Schmidt, A.M., Imesch, P., Fink, D., and Egger, H. (2012). Indications and long-term clinical outcomes in 282 patients with pelvic exenteration for advanced or recurrent cervical cancer. *Gynecol. Oncol.* 125: 604–609. Largest patient cohort reporting on indication and outcomes following PPES.
27 Stanhope, C.R. and Symmonds, R.E. (1985). Palliative exenteration – what, when, and why? *Am. J. Obstet. Gynecol.* 152: 12–16.
28 Boustead, G.B. and Feneley, M.R. (2010). Pelvic exenterative surgery for palliation of malignant disease in the robotic era. *Clin. Oncol. (R. Coll. Radiol.)* 22: 740–746.
29 Touran, T., Frost, D.B., and O'Connell, T.X. (1990). Sacral resection. *Arch. Surg.* 125: 911–913.
30 Boey, J., Wong, J., and Ong, G.B. (1982). Pelvic exenteration for locally advanced colorectal carcinoma. *Ann. Surg.* 195: 513–518.
31 Guo, C.C., Pisters, L.L., and Troncoso, P. (2009). Prostate cancer invading the rectum: a clinical pathological study of 18 cases. *Pathology* 41: 539–543.

32 Barber, H.R. (1969). Relative prognostic significance of preoperative and operative findings in pelvic exenteration. *Surg. Clin. North Am.* 49: 431–447.

33 Rodriguwz-Bigas, M.A. and Petrelli, N.J. (1996). Pelvic exenteration and its modifications. *Am. J. Surg.* 171: 293–298.

34 Bacalbasa, N. and Balescu, I. (2015). Palliative pelvic exenteration for pelvic recurrence invading the sciatic foramen with chronic cutaneous perineal fistula after radical surgery for cervical cancer: a case report. *Anticancer Res.* 35: 4877–4880.

35 Ito, Y., Ohtsu, A., Ishikura, S. et al. (2003). Efficacy of chemoradiotherapy on pain relief in patients with intrapelvic recurrence of rectal cancer. *Jpn J. Clin. Oncol.* 33: 180–185.

36 Larsen, S.G., Wiig, J.N., Tretli, S., and Giercksky, K.E. (2006). Surgery and pre-operative irradiation for locally advanced or recurrent rectal cancer in patients over 75 years of age. *Colorectal Dis.* 8: 177–185.

37 Rhomberg, W., Eiter, H., Hergan, K., and Schneider, B. (1994). Inoperable recurrent rectal cancer: results of a prospective trial with radiation therapy and razoxane. *Int. J. Radiat. Oncol. Biol. Phys.* 30: 419–425.

38 Saunders, N. (1995). Pelvic exenteration: by whom and for whom? *Lancet* 345: 5–6.

39 Fotopoulou, C., Neumann, U., Kraetschell, R. et al. (2010). Longterm clinical outcome of pelvic exenteration in patients with advanced gynaecological malignancies. *J. Surg. Oncol.* 101: 507–512.

40 Pathiraja, P., Sandhu, H., Instone, M. et al. (2014). Should pelvic exenteration for symptomatic relief in gynaecology malignancies be offered? *Arch. Gynecol. Obstet.* 289: 657–662.

41 Fazio, V.W. (2004). Indications and surgical alternatives for palliation of rectal cancer. *J. Gastrointest. Surg.* 8: 262–265.

42 Sasson, A.R. and Sigurdson, E.R. (2000). Management of locally advanced rectal cancer. *Surg. Oncol.* 9: 193–204.

43 Kamat, A.M., Huang, S.F., Bermejo, C.E. et al. (2003). Total pelvic exenteration: effective palliation of perineal pain in patients with locally recurrent prostate cancer. *J. Urol.* 170: 1868–1871.

44 Maetani, S., Onodera, H., Nishikawa, T. et al. (1998). Total pelvic exenteration: effective palliation of perineal pain in patients with locally recurrent prostate cancer. Significance of local recurrence of rectal cancer as a local or disseminated disease. *Br. J. Surg.* 85: 521–525.

45 Rutledge, F.N. and McGuffee, V.B. (1987). Pelvic exenteration: prognostic significance of regional lymph node metastasis. *Gynecol. Oncol.* 26: 374–380.

46 Marnitz, S., Köhler, C., Müller, M. et al. (2006). Indications for primary and secondary exenterations in patients with cervical cancer. *Gynecol. Oncol.* 103: 1023–1030.

47 Wanebo, H.J., Koness, R.J., Turk, P.S. et al. (1992). Composite resection of posterior pelvic malignancy. *Ann. Surg.* 215: 685–693.

48 Nishio, M., Sakakura, C., Nagata, T. et al. (2009). Outcomes of total pelvic exenteration for colorectal cancer. *Hepato-Gastroenterology* 56: 1637–1641.

49 Vieira, R.A., Lopes, A., and Almeida, P.A. (2004). Prognostic factors in locally advanced colon cancer treated by extended resection. *Rev. Hosp. Clin. Fac. Med. Sao Paulo* 59: 361–368.

50 Quyn, A.J., Austin, K.K., Young, J.M. et al. (2016). Outcomes of pelvic exenteration for locally advanced primary rectal cancer: overall survival and quality of life. *Eur. J. Surg. Oncol.* 42: 823–828.

51 Austin, K.K., Young, J.M., and Solomon, M.J. (2010). Quality of life of survivors after pelvic exenteration for rectal cancer. *Dis. Colon Rectum* 53: 1121–1126.

52 Rutledge, F.N., Smith, J.P., Wharton, J.T., and O'Quinn, A.G. (1977). Pelvic exenteration: analysis of 296 patients. *Am. J. Obstet. Gynecol.* 15 (129): 881–892.

53 You, Y.N., Habiba, H., Chang, G.J. et al. (2011). Prognostic value of quality of life and

pain in patients with locally recurrent rectal cancer. *Ann. Surg. Oncol.* 18: 989–996.

54 Brunschwig, A. and Barber, H.R.K. (1969). Pelvic exenteration combined with resection of segments of bony pelvis. *Surgery* 65: 417–420.

55 Shirouzu, K., Isomoto, H., and Kakegawa, T. (1996). Total pelvic exenteration for locally advanced colorectal carcinoma. *Br. J. Surg.* 83: 32–35.

56 Hafner, G.H., Herrera, L., and Petrelli, N.J. (1992). Morbidity and mortality after pelvic exenteration for colorectal adenocarcinoma. *Ann. Surg.* 215: 63–67.

57 Lawhead, R.A. Jr., Clark, D.G., and Smith, D.H. (1989). Pelvic exenteration for recurrent or persisting gynecologic malignancies: a 10-year review of the memorial Sloan-Kettering Cancer Centre experience (1972–1981). *Gynecol. Oncol.* 33: 279–282.

58 Puntambekar, S.P., Agarwal, G.A., Puntambekar, S.S. et al. (2009). Stretching the limits of laparoscopy in gynecological oncology: technical feasibility of doing a laparoscopic total pelvic exenteration for palliation in advanced cervical cancer. *Int. J. Biomed. Sci.* 5: 17–22.

59 Leibovici, D., Pagliaro, L., Rosser, C.J., and Pisters, L.L. (2005). Salvage surgery for bulky local recurrence of prostate cancer following radical prostatectomy. *J. Urol.* 173: 781–783.

60 Temple, W.J. and Ketcham, A.S. (1990). Surgical palliation for recurrent rectal cancers ulcerating in the perineum. *Cancer* 65: 1111–1114.

61 Pearlman, N.W., Stiegmann, G.V., and Donohue, R.E. (1989). Extended resection of fixed rectal cancer. *Cancer* 63: 2438–2441.

62 Wanebo, H.J. and Marcove, R.C. (1981). Abdominal sacral resection of locally recurrent rectal cancer. *Ann. Surg.* 194: 458–471.

63 Roos, E.J., de Graeff, A., van Eijkeren, M.A. et al. (2004). Quality of life after pelvic exenteration. *Gynecol. Oncol.* 93: 610–614.

64 Young, J.M., Badgery-Parker, T., Masya, L.M. et al. (2014). Quality of life and other patient-reported outcomes following exenteration for pelvic malignancy. *Br. J. Surg.* 101: 277–287.

65 McCullough, W.M. and Nahhas, W.A. (1987). Palliative pelvic exenteration – futility revisited. *Gynecol. Oncol.* 27: 97–103.

66 Bhangu, A., Ali, S.M., Darzi, A. et al. (2012). Meta-analysis of survival based on resection margin status following surgery for recurrent rectal cancer. *Colorectal Dis.* 14: 1457–1466.

67 Kakuda, J.T., Lamont, J.P., Chu, D.Z., and Paz, I.B. (2003). The role of pelvic exenteration in the management of recurrent rectal cancer. *Am. J. Surg.* 186: 660–664.

68 Yamada, K., Ishizawa, T., Niwa, K. et al. (2002). Pelvic exenteration and sacral resection for locally advanced primary and recurrent rectal cancer. *Dis. Colon Rectum* 45: 1078–1084.

69 Puntambekar, S., Sharma, V., Jamkar, A.V. et al. (2016). Our experience of laparoscopic anterior exenteration in locally advanced cervical carcinoma. *J. Minim. Invasive Gynecol.* 23: 396–340.

26

Outcomes of Pelvic Exenteration for Locally Advanced and Recurrent Rectal Cancer

Awad M. Jarrar and Scott R. Steele

Department of Colorectal Surgery, Cleveland Clinic, Cleveland, OH, USA

Background

Since the late 1990s, the oncologic outcomes for primary rectal cancer have significantly improved, in part due to refinements in neoadjuvant chemoradiotherapy and revising the surgical approach to rectal cancer resection. The concepts of total mesorectal excision (TME) and circumferential resection margin (CRM) radicalized rectal cancer surgery and translated into an improved local and distal recurrence, along with prolonged overall survival. TME refers to complete removal of the lymph node bearing mesorectum along with its intact enveloping fascia. TME dissection occurs in the areolar plane between the visceral fascia that envelops the rectum and mesorectum and the parietal fascia that envelops the pelvic wall structures. The CRM corresponds to the non-peritonealized surface of the resection specimen created by the dissection of the subperitoneal aspect of the rectum. Reported five-year rates of local recurrence, even without radiotherapy, were as low as 5% [1, 2] and less than 10% for transmural or node-positive rectal cancers [3–5]. This is in contrast to local recurrence rates of 14–40% in series published before the use of TME dissection.

Studies have demonstrated a local recurrence rate of 55% for cases with tumor at the CRM vs. 28% for cases with tumor 1 mm or less from the CRM [6, 7]. Despite these improvements, a 10% rate of local recurrence [3] remains a considerable burden [8]. In the UK, 14 000 new cases of rectal cancer are diagnosed every year, and 40 000 in the USA, of which between 5 and 10% are locally invasive (T4) at presentation [9, 10]. By definition, this cohort has a compromised CRM, adjacent organ involvement, and a worse oncological outcome. Historically, local invasion into other organs/structures was a contraindication to surgery, resulting in a median survival of less than one year and a five-year overall survival of less than 5% [11–13]. However, pelvic exenteration entailing multi-organ resection will increase the five-year survival rate for the locally advanced disease to a range between 22 and 66% [14–17]. It is important to take into account the lack of uniformity in defining locally advanced rectal cancer (LARC) when interpreting related studies. For patients who develop local recurrent rectal cancer (LRRC), the five-year survival ranges from 28 to 35% after curative surgery [18–22]. The complexities behind LARC and LRRC are summed up by tumor-specific factors (e.g. lack of clear delineation between failure of surgical technique vs. aggressive biology in dictating tumor recurrence, lack of an early screening tool to detect recurrence, the eventual therapy resistance emerging in recurrent tumors), patient-specific factors (e.g. poor quality of life after pelvic exenteration, poor overall survival), and surgery-specific factors (e.g. high postoperative morbidity rates, very complex surgery particularly when the anatomy is disrupted because of previous irradiation and surgical resections). Standard TME is rarely sufficient in LARC and LRRC, and therefore techniques to achieve extended multivisceral resections are required (Figures 26.1 and 26.2). Table 26.1 describes the relative and absolute contraindications of LARC and LLRC.

Tumor Biology and its Effect on Oncological Outcomes

The anatomical basis of the TME hypothesis assumes that the rectum and its mesorectum constitute a single self-contained one embryonic entity. Lymph nodes are randomly distributed within the mesorectum, the majority of which are neither all visible nor palpable. The size of the normal mesorectal lymph nodes in approximately 80% of cases is less than 3 mm. Most of these are located posteriorly, and 92% of the posterior lymph nodes lie within the superior half of the upper two-thirds of the rectum [23]. Original models explaining the improved outcome of TME assumed that metastasis spread via the lymph node route. TME allows the removal of the mesorectum

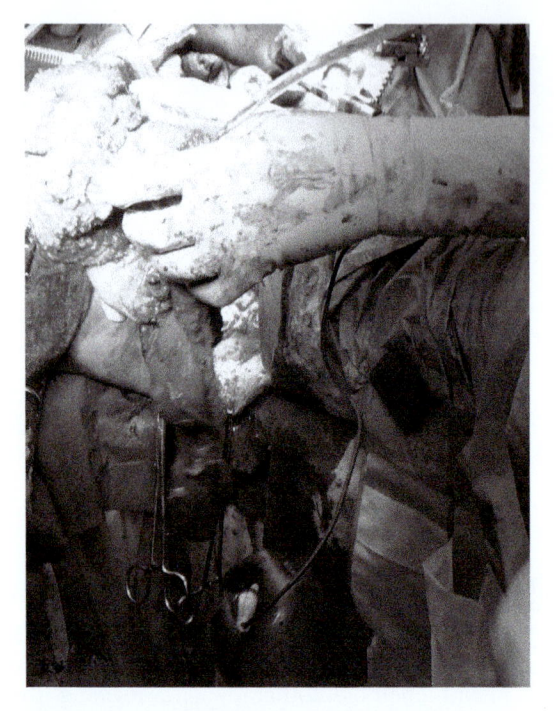

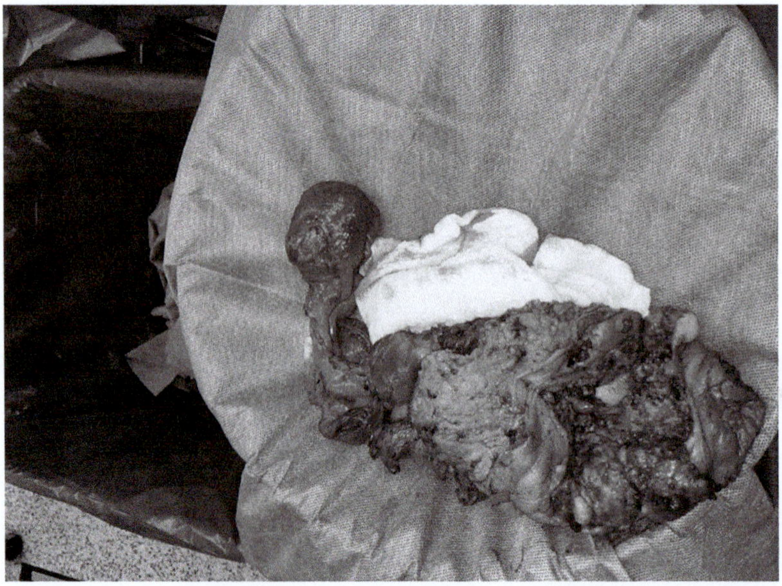

Figure 26.1 Intraoperative locally advanced tumor via multivisceral resection. *Source:* Awad M. Jarrar and Scott R. Steele.

Figure 26.2 Total pelvic exenteration specimen. *Source:* Awad M. Jarrar and Scott R. Steele.

Table 26.1 Contraindications for LARC and LLRC.

Relative contraindication	Absolute contraindication
Metastasis to retroperitoneal/aortic chain nodes	Peritoneal metastasis
Sciatic nerve encasement.	Multiple metastases at other distant sites, such as pulmonary metastases that are not resectable.
High sacral invasion (> S2–S3).	
Lateral bone invasion.	
Iliac vessel involvement.	
The clinical triad of leg edema, ureteral obstruction, and leg pain is almost pathognomonic for disease extending to the pelvic sidewall and, historically, has generally been considered a contraindication to surgery. However, some surgeons have reported on an even more radical resection, the laterally extended endopelvic resection (LEER), which extends the lateral extent of the resection to include structures of the pelvic sidewall, including striated muscle and vessels. Further study is required to evaluate the indications and outcomes of these procedures.	

and any extramural spread contained within its fascia, preventing further vertical lymphatic spread beyond the mesorectum.

Detailing the biological processes that dictate tumor metastasis is beyond the scope of this chapter. However, in brief terms, we will emphasize certain aspects that can lead to improved oncological outcomes after exenteration. Rectal cancer can metastasize via two mechanisms: single-cell dissemination through a process called the epithelial–mesenchymal transition (EMT) where the epithelial cancer cells activate a mesenchymal program that allows them to invade, grow in an anchorage-independent manner, intravasate in the hematogenous circulation, and extravasate in distant organs where cancer metastasis will ensue. Another model of tumor spread is called collective migration, where cancer cells located at the tumor's invasive edge move as spearheads, led by cells showing mesenchymal invasive phenotype, and dragging behind a group of cells with an epithelial phenotype. Collective cell migration is associated with direct invasion into adjacent structures, while hematogenous and lymphatic spread causes distal seeding [24]. The newly emerging clinicopathological term to describe collective migration is tumor budding at the invasive front. In colorectal cancer (CRC), high budding correlated with worse overall survival and distal recurrence [25–28]. Consequently, high budding also correlated with lower five-year disease-free survival (DFS) [25, 29]. Tumor budding was associated with higher T stage [30], lymphatic invasion, venous invasion, lymphovascular invasion, and perineural invasion (PNI) [25, 29, 31, 32].

In a recent publication, gene expression data of 4151 CRC patients was examined. Five subtypes emerged. The worst subtype was called CSM4 (mesenchymal subtype), where CRC cells partly activate the mesenchymal program at baseline without the need to go into an EMT process. This translated into statistically significant worst overall survival, relapse-free, and survival after relapse compared to all other subtypes. Twenty-three percent of all the CRC specimens were CSM4 and around 24% of CMS4 were located in the rectum [33].

Local recurrence is thought to be due to regrowth of residual microscopic spread after surgical resection. Neoadjuvant treatment helps to sterilize any missed local tumor seeding. R1/R2 resections were a consistent theme among all trials, predicting factors associated with local recurrence. Distal recurrence, on the other hand, is the systematic spread of tumor cells via hematogenous and lymphatic routes. Adjuvant systematic cytotoxic therapy facilitates the elimination of these spreading cancer cells. Over the past few years, multiple bodies of evidence have challenged the dichotomy of EMT hematogenous/lymphatic spread vs. collective local infiltrative migration. An important study by Rahbari et al. [34] investigated the outcomes of metastases at various time intervals after CRC diagnosis. A total of 1027 patients were included, with T4 ($p < 0.0001$) and node-positive tumors ($p < 0.0001$) more frequently in the immediate group to develop metastasis. Lung metastases ($p < 0.0001$) and single-site metastases ($p < 0.0001$) were more prevalent in the late group. The dormancy observed in patients developing late distal metastasis in comparison with patients who develop synchronous distal disease and show a locally advanced primary tumor suggest two distinct biological processes driving the metastatic process.

A third mixed pathway exists where cancer cells spread via collective migration and invasion, but to a much further distance, using pathways of least resistance. An example is PNI, where cancer cells attach to and invade the subspace between the connective tissues surrounding the neurons. In a meta-analysis of 11 studies including 3837 patients with rectal cancer PNI was reported to be present in 25% (range 10–38%) of the patients. PNI was significantly associated with high tumor stage, poor tumor differentiation, incidence of metastasis at time of diagnosis, and lymphatic and venous invasion. PNI was independently associated with poor survival in seven of eleven studies, and three of eleven studies confirmed a positive association on univariate analyses [35].

Similar to PNI, the presence of extranodal tumor deposits (ENTD), as independent entities or part of perivascular, perilymphatic, or perilymphovascular space, were evaluated as part of a meta-analysis involving 19,980 patients [36]. There was a significantly increased odds ratio (OR) of having ENTD if extramural venous invasion was present, with a pooled OR of 2.51 (95% CI 2.27–2.77, $p < 0.001$.) The pooled hazard ratio for adverse overall survival in patients with ENTD was 1.63 (95% CI 1.44–1.61, $p < 0.001$). In a fashion similar to PNI spread, rectal cancer can utilize these available pathways of least resistance to collectively migrate and invade locoregional lymph nodes. A new emerging body of literature is supporting the continuity of the mesentery with its rich lymphatics between the rectum, colon, and small intestine [37]. This concept has the potential to open a new wide highway for rectal cancer to invade in a collective local fashion, but with far outreach to distal lymph nodes. Lymph node metastases can be the result of this inherent tumor phenotype of collective migration as well as EMT.

The autopsies of 1393 patients with metastatic CRC where reviewed for patterns of regional lymph node metastasis. Lymph node-positive and -negative CRC patients were compared. Patients with regional lymph node-positive CRC were more often found to develop peritoneal metastases (28 vs. 21%, $p = 0.003$) and distant lymph node metastases (25 vs. 15%, $p < 0.001$). The incidences of liver and lung metastases were comparable in both groups. Regional lymph node-positive CRC shows a slightly different dissemination pattern, with higher rates of peritoneal and distant lymph node metastases. Comparable incidences of liver and lung metastases support the hypothesis that dissemination to distant organs can occur independently of lymphatic spread [38, 39].

To summarize, LRRC emerges from missed tumor microseeding post-surgical resection. Despite our best efforts, the recurrence rate of rectal cancer, particularly after advancing locally and breaking the TME plane, should motivate the surgical field for better patient stratification to identify patients with a high risk of seeding. Suggested criteria include histopathological markers associated with invasion such as PNI, extramural vascular invasion, tumor budding, and ENTD. In addition, the new molecular subtype with very negative predictor outcome (CSM4) should be further examined. The traditional thinking of the stepwise approach guiding the process of metastasis is over simplistic. Unfortunately, an R0 resection margin does not negate the microseeding of a cancer. The downside of grouping heterogeneous rectal cancer patients, with various biological behavior and varying surgical procedures, in one cohort has the potential to dilute the impact of some of the suggested approaches to reduce the rate of local recurrence.

Oncological Outcomes and Radiation Therapy

Subtotal resection followed by postoperative radiation or chemoradiation was the standard treatment for patients with LARC. The reported failure rates ranged from 40 to 70% and improved with dose escalation [40]. In a Dutch TME trial [41] evaluating short-course radiation therapy, 120 patients in the surgery-alone arm had a positive CRM. The two-year local recurrence rate in positive-margin patients was 17% in those who received postoperative radiation vs. 16% in patients who did not. The local recurrence rate in the preoperative radiation-alone arm among patients with positive resection margin was 9% and not significantly different from the 16% local recurrence rate in the margin positive surgery-alone arm ($p = 0.08$) [41]. In sum, these data suggest that doses in excess of 60 Gy are likely required for control of microscopic disease at least in the postoperative setting. In patients with very locally advanced disease, a number of investigators have evaluated higher doses of radiation in conjunction with fluorouracil (5-FU) as a strategy to improve disease control and survival. Toxicity to the small bowel descending in the pelvis can limit dose escalation for patients with rectal cancer. An alternative strategy is to combine external radiation and chemotherapy preoperatively with an intraoperative radiotherapy (IORT) boost at the time of surgery (Figure 26.3). A number of observational experiences have been published reporting the results of IORT for advanced LARC. Local control rates of 90% or higher are generally

Figure 26.3 IORT to the pelvic sidewall following resection of a locally advanced tumor. *Source:* Awad M. Jarrar and Scott R. Steele.

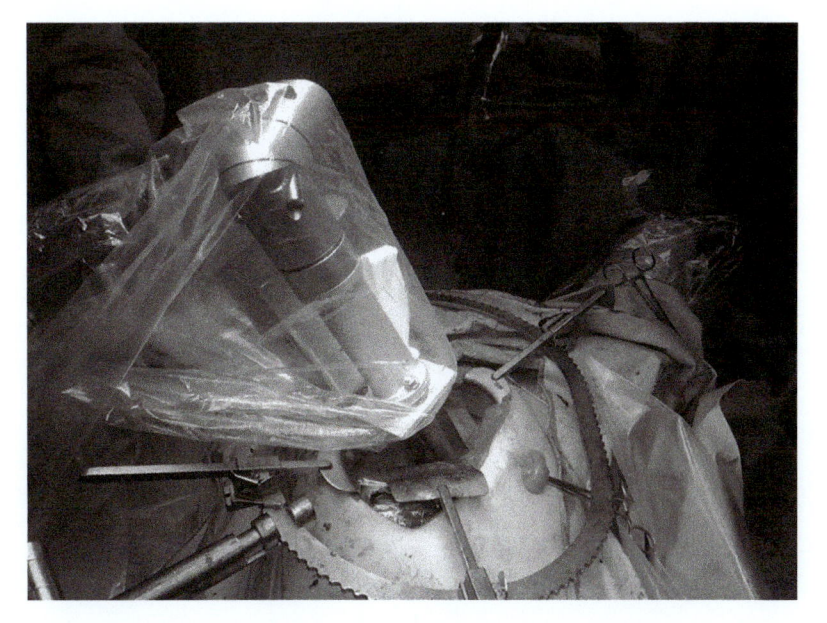

reported with survival at five years in the range of 50–80%. The predominant pattern of relapse is distant disease. The lack of unbiased contemporary controls in most series hampers the ability to draw definitive conclusions regarding the added benefit of IORT despite the excellent results reported. Non-randomized comparisons suggest improvements in local control [42–45]. In a French study [46], there was no difference in local control or survival with the addition of IORT. However, 90% of patients in the study had T3 as opposed to T4 tumors and the local control rate of 93% in the non-IORT arm suggests that most of the patients enrolled did not meet the definition of locally advanced disease.

It has been demonstrated that re-irradiation in the setting of recurrent rectal cancer can be performed with acceptable late toxicities. In a series of 103 patients with recurrent previously irradiated rectal cancer, patients were retreated with 15–49.2 Gy (median 34.8 Gy) with 5-FU followed by surgery in 34 patients [46]. Late complications were observed in 21% of patients, including chronic severe diarrhea (17%), small bowel obstruction (15%), fistula (4%), and skin ulceration (2%). Previous results suggest the utilization of radiation therapy for pelvic field sterilization in patients with rectal cancers and high-risk features.

Outcomes of the Largest Pelvic Exenteration Series in the Literature

Nearly all studies have shown that aggressive resection, including that of extended resections (Figure 26.4), will yield improved long-term survival and disease control in a significant number of patients. The largest two outcome studies of pelvic exenteration for LRRC [18] and LARC [22] are summarized in Table 26.2. The fields marked in blue are significantly different between LARC and LRRC. Interestingly, median overall survival is comparable between node-positive LARC and node-positive LRRC. Patients with node positivity among LARC have a comparable overall survival to node-negative LRRC patients as well. A significant difference in overall survival also exists in node-negative patients with LARC when compared to LRRC. Additionally, the prognostic power of lymph node positivity is lost in LRRC. The deductions we can make

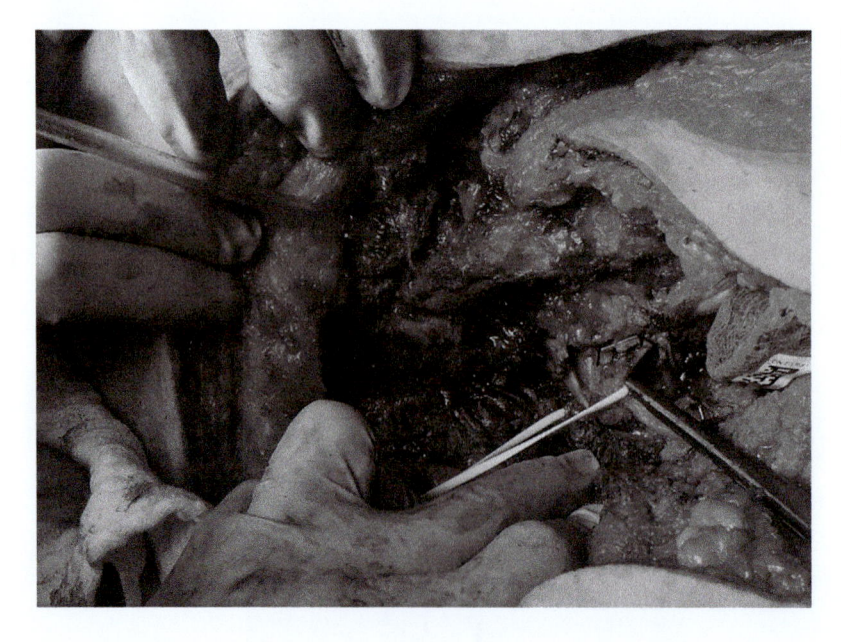

Figure 26.4 En-bloc sacrectomy in the setting of LARC. *Source:* Awad M. Jarrar and Scott R. Steele.

Table 26.2 Outcomes associated with pelvic exenteration for LARC.

	Number of patients	Neoadjuvant therapy	R0 percentage	Mortality rate	Major complications		R0	R1	R2	Bone resection	Node-positive	Node-negative	Factors by multivariante analysis to predict survival
LRRC	1184	51.90%	55.40%	1.80%	32.10%	Median overall survival	36 months	27 months	16 months	36 months vs. 29 months	22 months	29 months	Margin status and bone resection
						Three-year survival	48.10%	33.90%	15%				
LARC	1291	78.10%	79.90%	1.5%	37.80%	Median overall	43 months	21 months	10 months	37 months vs. 29 months	31 months	46 months	Margin and node status
						Three-year survival	56.40%	29.60%	8.10%				

from these significant findings can be summarized as the following take-home points: (i) nodal status in LARC is a segregate for rectal cancers with varying aggressiveness and behavior; (ii) in LRRC, tumor cells have likely already gone through a selection process, and only the strong resistant phenotype survives; and (iii) the biological process leans toward homogeneity and aggressiveness in LRRC.

Mortality and Morbidity

Overall Mortality and Morbidity

The first large cohort of multivisceral resections for locally advanced CRC was published in 1946. The procedure was justified by the fact that 19 of 34 patients who had undergone complete removal of a locally advanced CRC had survived "for considerable periods" [47]. The operation was then described as "the most radical of abdominal operations that have been carried out with some measure of consistency". Similarly, in 1950, Appleby described an operation where he employed "the most radical measures" in order to cure LARC in a smaller series of eight male patients [48]. Historically, the high morbidity and mortality rates associated with pelvic exenteration question the benefit of such radicality [49, 50]. For years it has not been accepted as a standard procedure. Enhanced imaging modalities coupled with the establishment of specialized multidisciplinary teams lead to better selection of surgical candidates. Improvement in surgical techniques and perioperative management translated into improved outcomes. Currently, mortality rates vary between 0 and 5% at one month and 8% at three months [18, 19]. The causes of death are mainly disseminated coagulopathies related to prolonged blood loss, cardiac events, and pulmonary embolism [18, 51, 52]. Morbidity remains significantly high, ranging from 13 to 82% [17, 53–58], and increases with the complexity of resection [3, 59–61].

Intraoperative Complications

Bleeding is the most serious and severe intraoperative complication and occurs in 0.2–9% of cases. It is associated with a high rate of mortality [11–14]. Intraoperative blood loss varies according to the type of exenteration performed, with sacrectomy being the strongest risk factor. Studies report a median of 4200 cc of blood loss for low sacrectomies ($\leq$ S3) and 7500 cc for high ones ($\geq$ S2–S3) [62]. Similar findings have been shown in other series, with sacrectomy procedures (compared with different operations) being associated with a significantly higher mean of blood loss (2854 vs. 1608 cc, $p < 0.001$) [58].

Postoperative Complications

The principal postoperative complications include pelvic abscess and collection (7–50%), sepsis (33%), intestinal obstruction (5–10%), postoperative bleed (8%), enterocutaneous or entero-perineal fistulas (1–3%), perineal wound dehiscence (4–24%), urinary tract infection (14–47%), cardiovascular, renal, and pulmonary complications (1–20%), neuropathic urinary retention (6–33%), postoperative bleeding (8%), and urinary conduit leak (22%) [18–21, 48, 50, 58].

Neoadjuvant Treatment and Postoperative Complications

The effects of neoadjuvant treatment on postoperative complications have been explored in a few large cohorts of pelvic exenterations. The largest contained 1184 patients, of which 614 had neoadjuvant chemoradiotherapy. Patients who received neoadjuvant therapy were 1.5 times more likely to experience a complication within 30 days (OR 1.53, 95% CI 1.19–1.97, $p < 0.001$) and twice more likely to get readmitted within 30 days postoperatively. (OR 2.33, 95% CI 1.18–4.52, $p = 0.013$). Use of neoadjuvant therapy did not affect duration of hospital stay. Patients who had neoadjuvant therapy were no more likely to need surgical reoperation (p = 0.125) but they were more likely to have radiological reintervention (OR 2.12, 95% CI 1.17–3.83, p = 0.012) [18].

Hospital Stay

The median hospital stay after exenteration ranges between 15 and 21 days, with 15% remaining as an inpatient at 30 days postoperatively [14, 18, 58]. The readmission rate ranges between 6 and 10%, with 8–24% of patients requiring surgical or radiological reintervention. In a series of 100 patients undergoing exenterations, sacrectomies (25 vs. 19 days, p = 0.017) and perineal flaps (23 vs. 18 days, p = 0.042) were the only two factors associated with longer hospital course in comparison with patients without. Underlying etiology (LARC and LRRC) did not affect the duration of hospital stay postoperatively [18].

Summary Box

- Despite the morbidity associated with pelvic exenteration, it remains a potential curative surgery for select patients with LARC and LRRC. This is clearly reflected by an improved overall survival following exenteration.
- The complexities in treating LARC and LRRC are due to the heterogeneity in tumor-specific factors dictating the tumor behavior and microseeding behind R0 resection, patient-specific factors, and surgery-specific factors. Failure to appreciate these intricacies will reflect poorly on outcomes.
- R0 resection remains a very important surrogate in predicting oncological outcomes.
- Further biological and histopathological surrogates need to be investigated in order to achieve a better stratification of patients with high risk of recurrence.
- Thorough preoperative evaluation is required to ensure appropriate patient selection, and a multidisciplinary approach is critical to successful outcomes in these patients.

References

1 MacFarlane, J.K., Ryall, R.D.H., and Heald, R.J. (1993). Mesorectal excision for rectal cancer. *Lancet* 341 (8843): 457–460.
Classic paper highlighting the need for initial proper oncological resection to minimize risk of recurrence.

2 Heald, R.J. (1995). Total mesorectal excision is optimal surgery for rectal cancer: a Scandinavian consensus. *Br. J. Surg.* 82 (10): 1297–1299.
Consensus statement on TME as the critical operation for patients with rectal cancer.

3 Heriot, A.G., Byrne, C.M., Lee, P. et al. (2008). Extended radical resection: the choice for locally recurrent rectal cancer. *Dis. Colon Rectum* 51 (3): 284–291.

4 Guillem, J.G., Chessin, D.B., Cohen, A.M. et al. (2005). Long-term oncologic outcome following preoperative combined modality therapy and total mesorectal excision of locally advanced rectal cancer. *Ann. Surg.* 241 (5): 829–838.

5 Weiser, M.R., Landmann, R.G., Wong, W.D. et al. (2005). Surgical salvage of recurrent rectal cancer after transanal excision. *Dis. Colon Rectum* 48 (6): 1169–1175.

6 Birbeck, K.F., Macklin, C.P., Tiffin, N.J. et al. (2002). Rates of circumferential resection margin involvement vary between surgeons and predict outcomes in rectal cancer surgery. *Ann. Surg.* 235 (4): 449–457.

7 Nagtegaal, I.D., CAM, M., Kranenbarg, E.K. et al. (2002). Circumferential margin involvement is still an important predictor of local recurrence in rectal carcinoma. *Am. J. Surg. Pathol.* 26 (3): 350–357.

8 Meyer, J.E., Narang, T., Schnoll-Sussman, F.H. et al. (2010). Increasing incidence of rectal cancer in patients aged younger than 40 years: an analysis of the surveillance, epidemiology, and end results database. *Cancer* 116 (18): 4354–4359.

9 Beyond TME Collabortive (2013). Consensus statement on the multidisciplinary management of patients with recurrent and primary rectal cancer beyond total mesorectal excision planes. *Br. J. Surg.* 100 (8): E1–E33.

10 Sineshaw, H.M., Jemal, A., Thomas, C.R., and Mitin, T. (2016). Changes in treatment patterns for patients with locally advanced rectal cancer in the United States over the past decade: an analysis from the National Cancer Data Base. *Cancer* 122 (13): 1996–2003.

11 Solum, A.M., Riffenburgh, R.H., and Johnstone, P.A.S. (2004). Survival of patients with untreated rectal cancer. *J. Surg. Oncol.* 87 (4): 157–161.

12 Carlsson, U., Lasson, Å., and Ekelund, G. (1987). Recurrence rates after curative surgery for rectal carcinoma, with special reference to their accuracy. *Dis. Colon Rectum* 30 (6): 431–434.

13 Arnott, S.J. (1975). The value of combined 5-fluorouracil and x-ray therapy in the palliation of locally recurrent and inoperable rectal carcinoma. *Clin. Radiol.* 26 (C): 177–182.

14 Radwan, R.W., Jones, H.G., Rawat, N. et al. (2015). Determinants of survival following pelvic exenteration for primary rectal cancer. *Br. J. Surg.* 102 (10): 1278–1284.

15 Milne, T., Solomon, M.J., Lee, P. et al. (2014). Sacral resection with pelvic exenteration for advanced primary and recurrent pelvic cancer: a single-institution experience of 100 sacrectomies. *Dis. Colon Rectum* 57 (10): 1153–1161.

16 Ferenschild, F.T.J., Vermaas, M., and Verhoef, C. (2009). Total pelvic exenteration for primary and recurrent malignancies. *World J. Surg.* 33 (7): 1502–1508.

17 Ishiguro, S., Akasu, T., Fujita, S. et al. (2009). Pelvic exenteration for clinical T4 rectal cancer: oncologic outcome in 93 patients at a single institution over a 30-year period. *Surgery* 145 (2): 189–195.

18 PelvEx Collaborative (2018). Factors affecting outcomes following pelvic exenteration for locally recurrent rectal cancer. *Br. J. Surg* 105 (6): 650–657.

19 Palmer, G., Martling, A., Cedermark, B., and Holm, T. (2006). A population-based study on the management and outcome in patients with locally recurrent rectal cancer. *Ann. Surg. Oncol* 14 (2): 447–454.

20 Habr-Gama, A., Perez, R.O., and Lynn, P. (2011). Current issues on the understanding of locally advanced colorectal cancer. *Arq. Gastroenterol* 48 (4): 223–224.

21 Beyond TME Collaborative (2013). Consensus statement on the multidisciplinary management of patients with recurrent and primary rectal cancer beyond total mesorectal excision planes. *Br. J. Surg* 100 (8): E1–E33.

22 PelvEx Collaborative (2019;269(2): 315–21). Surgical and survival outcomes following pelvic exenteration for locally advanced primary rectal cancer: results from an international collaboration. *Ann. Surg.*

23 Topor, B., Acland, R., Kolodko, V., and Galandiuk, S. (2003). Mesorectal lymph nodes: their location and distribution within the mesorectum. *Dis. Colon Rectum* 46 (6): 779–785.

24 Kalluri, R. and Weinberg, R.A. (2009). The basics of epithelial–mesenchymal transition. *J. Clin. Invest.* 119 (6): 1420–1428.

25 Choi, C.J., Park, K.J., Shin, J.S. et al. (2007). Tumor budding as a prognostic marker in

stage-III rectal carcinoma. *Int. J. Colorectal Dis.* 22 (8): 863–868.

26 Shinto, E., Jass, J.R., Tsuda, H. et al. (2006). Differential prognostic significance of morphologic invasive markers in colorectal cancer: tumor budding and cytoplasmic podia. *Dis. Colon Rectum* 49 (9): 1422–1430.

27 Ohtsuki, K., Koyama, F., Tamura, T. et al. (2008). Prognostic value of immunohistochemical analysis of tumor budding in colorectal carcinoma. *Anticancer Res* 28 (3 B): 1831–1836.

28 Tanaka, M., Hashiguchi, Y., Ueno, H. et al. (2003). Tumor budding at the invasive margin can predict patients at high risk of recurrence after curative surgery for stage II, T3 colon cancer. *Dis. Colon Rectum* 46 (8): 1054–1059.

29 Betge, J., Kornprat, P., Pollheimer, M.J. et al. (2012). Tumor budding is an independent predictor of outcome in AJCC/UICC stage II colorectal cancer. *Ann. Surg. Oncol* 19 (12): 3706–3712.

30 Park, K.J., Choi, J.H., Roh, M.S. et al. (2005). Intensity of tumor budding and its prognostic implications in invasive colon carcinoma. *Dis. Colon Rectum* 48 (8): 1597–1602.

31 Hase, K., Shatney, C., Johnson, D. et al. (1993). Prognostic value of tumor "budding" in patients with colorectal cancer. *Dis. Colon Rectum* 36 (7): 627–635.

32 Wang, L.M., Kevans, D., Mulcahy, H. et al. (2009). Tumor budding is a strong and reproducible prognostic marker in T3N0 colorectal cancer. *Am. J. Surg Pathol* 33 (1): 134–141.

33 Guinney, J., Dienstmann, R., Wang, X. et al. (2015). The consensus molecular subtypes of colorectal cancer. *Nat. Med.* 21 (11): 1350–1356.

34 Rahbari, N.N., Ulrich, A.B., Bruckner, T. et al. (2011). Surgery for locally recurrent rectal cancer in the era of total mesorectal excision. *Ann. Surg.* 253 (3): 522–533.

35 van Wyk, H.C., Park, J., Roxburgh, C. et al. (2015). The role of tumour budding in predicting survival in patients with primary operable colorectal cancer: a systematic review. *Cancer Treat. Rev* 41 (2): 151–159.

36 Lord, A.C., D'Souza, N., Pucher, P.H. et al. (2017). Significance of extranodal tumour deposits in colorectal cancer: a systematic review and meta-analysis. *Eur. J. Cancer* 82: 92–102.

37 Coffey, J.C. and O'Leary, D.P. (2016). The mesentery: structure, function, and role in disease. *Lancet Gastroenterol. Hepatol* 1 (3): 238–247.

38 Knijn, N., van Erning, F.N., Overbeek, L.I.H. et al. (2016). Limited effect of lymph node status on the metastatic pattern in colorectal cancer. *Oncotarget* 7 (22): 31699–31707.

39 Singh, D., Luo, J., Liu, X. et al. (2017). The long-term survival benefits of high and low ligation of inferior mesenteric artery in colorectal cancer surgery: a review and meta-analysis. *Medicine (Baltimore)* 96 (47): e8520.

40 Allee, P.E. et al. (1989). Postoperative radiation therapy for incompletely resected colorectal carcinoma. *Int. J. Radiat. Oncol. Biol. Phys.* 17 (6): 1171–1176.

41 Marijnen, C.A.M., Nagtegaal, I.D., Kapiteijn, E. et al. (2003). Radiotherapy does not compensate for positive resection margins in rectal cancer patients: report of a multicenter randomized trial. *Int. J. Radiat. Oncol. Biol. Phys.* 55 (5): 1311–1320.

42 Willett, C.G., Shellito, P.C., Tepper, J.E. et al. (1991). Intraoperative electron beam radiation therapy for primary locally advanced rectal and rectosigmoid carcinoma. *J. Clin. Oncol* 9 (5): 843–849.

43 Sadahiro, S., Suzuki, T., Ishikawa, K. et al. (2004). Preoperative radio/chemo-radiotherapy in combination with intraoperative radiotherapy for T3-4Nx rectal cancer. *Eur. J. Surg. Oncol.* 30 (7): 750–758.

44 Valentini, V., Coco, C., Rizzo, G. et al. (2009). Outcomes of clinical T4M0 extra-peritoneal rectal cancer treated with preoperative radiochemotherapy and surgery: a prospective evaluation of a single institutional experience. *Surgery* 145 (5): 486–494.

45 Alberda, W.J., Verhoef, C., Nuyttens, J.J. et al. (2014). Intraoperative radiation therapy reduces local recurrence rates in patients with microscopically involved circumferential resection margins after resection of locally advanced rectal cancer. *Int. J. Radiat. Oncol. Biol. Phys.* 88 (5): 1032–1040.

46 Dubois, J.B., Bussieres, E., Richaud, P. et al. (2001). Intra-operative radiotherapy of rectal cancer: results of the French Multi-Institutional Randomized Study. *Radiother. Oncol.* 98 (3): 298–303.

47 Sugarbaker, E.D. (1946). Coincident removal of additional structures in resections for carcinoma of the colon and rectum. *Ann. Surg.* 123: 1036–1046.

48 Appleby, L.H. (1950). Proctocystectomy; the management of colostomy with ureteral transplants. *Am. J. Surg.* 79 (1): 57–60.

49 Dunphy, J.E. (1947). Recurrent cancer of the colon and rectum. *N. Engl. J. Med.* 237 (4): 111–113.

50 Verschueren, R.C.J., Mulder, N.H., Hooykaas, J.A. et al. (1998). Pelvic exenteration for advanced primary rectal cancer in male patients. *Clin. Oncol.* 10 (5): 318–321.

51 Tilney, H.S., Rasheed, S., Northover, J.M., and Tekkis, P. (2009). The influence of circumferential resection margins on long-term outcomes following rectal cancer surgery. *Dis. Colon Rectum* 52 (10): 1723–1729.

52 Khani, M.H. and Smedh, K. (2010). Centralization of rectal cancer surgery improves long-term survival. *Colorectal Dis.* 12 (9): 874–879.

53 Nielsen, M.B., Rasmussen, P.C., Lindegaard, J.C., and Laurberg, S. (2012). A 10-year experience of total pelvic exenteration for primary advanced and locally recurrent rectal cancer based on a prospective database. *Colorectal Dis.* 14 (9): 1076–1083.

54 Gannon, C.J., Zager, J.S., Chang, G.J. et al. (2007). Pelvic exenteration affords safe and durable treatment for locally advanced rectal carcinoma. *Ann. Surg. Oncol.* 14 (6): 1870–1877.

55 Yamada, K., Ishizawa, T., Niwa, K. et al. (2002). Pelvic exenteration and sacral resection for locally advanced primary and recurrent rectal cancer. *Dis. Colon Rectum* 45 (8): 1078–1084.

56 Ike, H., Shimada, H., Yamaguchi, S. et al. (2003). Outcome of total pelvic exenteration for primary rectal cancer. *Dis. Colon Rectum* 46 (4): 474–480.

57 Nishio, M., Sakakura, C., Nagata, T. et al. (2009). Outcomes of total pelvic exenteration for colorectal cancer. *Hepatogastroenterology* 56 (96): 1637–1641.

58 Bhangu, A., Ali, S.M., Brown, G. et al. (2014). Indications and outcome of pelvic exenteration for locally advanced primary and recurrent rectal cancer. *Ann. Surg.* 259 (2): 315–322.

59 Nielsen, M.B., Laurberg, S., and Holm, T. (2009). Current management of locally recurrent rectal cancer. *Colorectal Dis.* 13 (7): 732–742.

60 Harji, D.P., Griffiths, B., DR, M.A., and Sagar, P.M. (2013). Surgery for recurrent rectal cancer: higher and wider? *Colorectal Dis.* 15 (2): 139–145.

61 Wells, B.J., Stotland, P., Ko, M.A. et al. (2006). Results of an aggressive approach to resection of locally recurrent rectal cancer. *Ann. Surg. Oncol.* 14 (2): 390–395.

62 Milne, T., Solomon, M.J., Lee, P. et al. (2013). Assessing the impact of a sacral resection on morbidity and survival after extended radical surgery for locally recurrent rectal cancer. *Ann. Surg.* 258 (6): 1007–1013.

27

Outcomes Following Exenteration for Urological Neoplasms
Frank McDermott, Ian Daniels, Neil Smart, and John McGrath

Exeter Surgical Health Service Research Unit (HeSRU)/University of Exeter Medical School, Exeter, UK

Background

The indications for pelvic exenteration (PE) for urological origin include advanced prostate and invasive bladder cancers. PE can be performed with either curative or palliative intent, but all indications are associated with considerable morbidity and/or mortality [1–4].

The management of urological cancer is complex, with multiple treatment options with varying efficacy. There has been considerable evolution in operative approaches, especially with increased uptake of laparoscopic and robotic techniques to perform extended resection that previously could only be performed with an open approach [6]. In addition, there have been improvements in urological reconstruction and diversion options that have impacted on postoperative quality of life (QoL).

Prostate Cancer

Prostate cancer is common, with 1.4 million cases reported globally in 2016 and 381 000 associated deaths. It ranks as the most common cancer in males and is a leading cause of cancer deaths [7]. Despite earlier diagnosis due to screening programs, patients still present with advanced prostatic disease, and rates of recurrence following radiotherapy are as high as 10% [8].

Locally Advanced Disease

Symptoms from locally advanced disease can be debilitating and include hematuria, obstructive uropathy, severe pelvic pain, and, rarely, bowel obstruction. Management options for locally advanced prostate cancer are dependent on several factors such as the comorbidity of the patient and the adjacent structures that are involved. Many treatment modalities are described and the optimal management is widely debated. In less-fit patients, a conservative (watch and wait) approach may be favored or the use of hormonal therapy. In those fit for radical treatment, neoadjuvant hormones followed by radical radiotherapy is the commonest treatment modality in all age groups. However, there is increasing use of "multimodality" therapy encompassing primary radical prostatectomy followed by adjuvant radiotherapy and/or hormonal therapy, dependent on margins and postoperative prostate-specific antigen (PSA) levels. Wider PE remains an option for the treatment of advanced disease as well as for palliation of severe symptoms that can be experienced by patients.

Surgical Management of Advanced Pelvic Cancer, First Edition.
Edited by Michael E. Kelly and Desmond C. Winter.
© 2022 John Wiley & Sons Ltd. Published 2022 by John Wiley & Sons Ltd.

Advanced Prostate Cancer

In advanced prostate cancer there may be local spread to surrounding structures including seminal vesicles, the bladder, and less commonly the rectum. Multicompartment exenterative surgery is infrequently practised and is reserved for aggressive management of either advanced, symptomatic prostate cancers or, less commonly, synchronous tumors of the rectum and prostate. Essential to improvements in outcomes is patient selection, aided by improvements in cross-sectional imaging, particularly magnetic resonance imaging (MRI) for preoperative planning and prostate-specific membrane antigen–positron emission tomography (PSMA-PET) to exclude distant disease. Exenterative surgery is complex and requires excellent anatomical knowledge outside traditional planes of dissection, the use of multiple techniques, and often the input and collaboration of several consultant-level surgeons. There are limited data on exenterative surgery for prostate specifically, reflecting its infrequent use. One of the largest series details the management of 62 patients who underwent radical prostatectomy [29], anterior exenteration [21], and total exenteration [5]. The median time to progression was 7.5 and 1.3 years for radical prostatectomy and exenterations respectively [9]. The tumors were larger in those patients that required exenterations, but the authors conclude that exenterations are of questionable benefit due to the rapid nature of progression. An unpublished conference presentation details the management of 31 locally advanced castration-resistant prostate cancer patients with median time to death of 2.8 years and time to relapse of 398 days [10]. In addition, 85% of the included patients had severe symptoms attributable to locally advanced disease which were relieved by surgery until time of recurrence [10].

The subgroup of patients being considered for exenterative surgery need to be appropriately consented for the risks and be deemed to be in a cohort that are likely to benefit from aggressive surgical management [11].

Synchronous Prostate and Rectal Cancer

Several different treatment modalities are suggested for the relatively uncommon presentation of synchronous rectal and prostate cancers. It is likely that, with the aging population, these cancers are likely to become more common either synchronously or as metachronous tumors. The treatment options are challenging, on account of not only the normal anatomical constraints of the male pelvis but also the choice of neoadjuvant therapies [12]. Radiotherapy regimens used are often aimed at rectal cancer at doses that are subtherapeutic for the prostate. Prostate-level radiation damages the surgical field even further, destroying natural anatomical planes and worsening the inflammatory reaction.

Due to the high risk of anastomotic leaks in these patients, exenterations offer an alternative solution for R0 resections, albeit with high risks of morbidity. Other options include aggressive chemoradiotherapy regimens, as some patients have complete radiological response and might be suitable for a watch and wait policy, although this is currently subject to multiple studies in rectal cancer only groups.

The studies published for this subgroup have very small numbers and highlight the need for good preoperative staging and collaboration between dedicated advanced disease multidisciplinary team (MDT) meetings or between colorectal and urology MDT [13].

Bladder Cancer

There were 437 000 incident cases of bladder cancer globally in 2016, with 186 000 deaths [7]. Radical cystectomy (RC) is performed for primary tumors of the urinary tract – most commonly for bladder cancer and less frequently for tumors of the prostate, seminal vesicle, or ureters. It can also be a component part of PE for more advanced disease. There are multiple reconstructive options for the urinary tract, with the majority of patients undergoing formation of an ileal conduit (IC) and a lesser proportion being offered orthotopic ileal neobladder reconstruction. A catheterizable pouch (Mitrofanoff) is occasionally performed and there are a small numbers of cases described involving formation of a "wet colostomy" (implanting ureters directly into the large bowel). The complications for patients undergoing more radical surgery are higher [14]. A single high-volume center found that the complications after cystectomy as part of a PE were higher than those for a cystectomy for primary malignancy. In this series of 231 patients (98 cystectomy alone, 133 as part of PE), urological complications were 33% in the cystectomy group compared to 59% in the PE group ($p < 0.001$) [15]. In addition, the complications were higher when the PE was performed for recurrence compared to primary malignancy. Urological leaks occurred in 3%, 6%, and 14% in patients who had cystectomy alone, PE for primary malignancy, and PE for recurrence respectively. Both major blood loss and previous pelvic radiotherapy were independently associated with conduit leak.

Carcinoma of the bladder requires aggressive radical treatment, as the five-year recurrence risk for non-muscle invasive bladder cancer (NMIBC) with poor prognostic factors reaches 45% [16], whilst the five-year survival of patients undergoing RC for potentially curative muscle-invasive bladder cancer remains around 50–60%. Patients with muscle-invasive bladder cancer (MIBC), high-risk NMIBC, or NMIBC refractory to intravesical therapy (mitomycin or BCG) should be considered for radical surgery [17]. Standard radical treatment for localized or locally advanced MIBC is neoadjuvant chemotherapy followed by RC or radical radiotherapy. The decision to offer surgery or radiotherapy is determined by factors such as histological type, comorbidity, patient preference, and concomitant obstruction of the upper urinary tract. Pelvic lymphadenectomy is performed routinely with the addition of total hysterectomy and bilateral salpingo-oopherectomy in females to optimize clearance [18]. In younger female patients, the ovaries may be spared.

A clear distinction must be made between the anterior exenteration that is the standard approach for women with bladder transitional cell carcinoma (TCC) versus a multicompartmental PE. Once a bladder TCC has invaded the colon or rectum it is classified as systemic disease and patients are usually offered palliative chemotherapy rather than aggressive surgical management. However, patients with locally invasive bladder TCC into the prostate, cervix, or vagina are classified as T4 disease but can be offered an RC.

There are now several large series for outcomes of PEs for mixed pelvic disease but less for those of urological origin specifically. One series details the outcomes of 160 female patients who underwent anterior exenteration for urothelial malignancy with a recurrence in 22 patients (13.8%) [19]. Patients who had neoadjuvant chemo- or radiotherapy had higher recurrence rates. They identified trigonal/bladder floor tumors, palpable posterior mass, and clinical lymphadenopathy as associated with pelvic organ involvement.

A series from the National Surgical Quality Program (NSQIP) and Surveillance, Epidemiology, and End Results (SEER) databases [20] provides data on the pre- and intraoperative management of 151 patients who underwent exenteration for bladder cancer (NSQIP) and long-term outcome data on 389 patients (SEER). These data are presented in Table 27.1.

Table 27.1 Outcomes of PE due to bladder cancer.

Variable	Result
Mortality (30 day)	3 (2%)
Overall complication rate	95 (62.9%)
Major complication rate	84 (55.6%)
Early return to theater	11 (7.3%)
Length of stay (days)	9 (7–12)
Operative time (minutes)	366 (262–453.5)

Source: Data from Speicher, P. J., Turley, R. S., Sloane, J. L., Mantyh, C. R., & Migaly, J. (2013). Pelvic Exenteration for the Treatment of Locally Advanced Colorectal and Bladder Malignancies in the Modern Era. Journal of Gastrointestinal Surgery, 18(4), 782–788.
Source: adapted from Speicher et al. [20].

A large series from the British Association of Urological Surgeons details the outcomes of 2537 open radical cystectomies (74% male) [4]. The median operative time was five hours, median 11–20 lymph node harvest, median blood loss of 500–1000 ml, and a transfusion required in 21.8%. The median length of stay was 11 days, with a 30-day mortality rate of 1.58%. The most common indication for RC was MIBC (46%), followed by NMIBC refractory to intravesical therapy (13%) and primary NMIBC (10%). Positive surgical margins were present in 8% of patients, although data were not available on 22%.

Radical cystectomies can be performed robotically with a series detailing the management in 114 consecutive patients. Eighty-two percent were male and an IC was performed in 97 patients and orthoptic bladder in 17 [5]. The procedure was completed robotically in all patients excluding one, with a transfusion rate of 9%, Clavien-Dindo III–IV in 18.4%, and 30-day mortality of 0.9%. Length of stay was 7 days (3–68) compared with 11 days in the open RC study [4].

The preoperative variable identified that predisposed to major postoperative complications was the American Society of Anesthiologists (ASA) classification of >3 (adjusted odds ratio (AOR) 1.66 (1.0–2.76)), and having a normal creatinine preoperatively appeared to be protective (AOR 0.22 (0.04–1.0)). This paper collated data on both rectal and bladder cancer. The overall survival (OS) of rectal cancer patients who had a PE was 48 months (95% CI 38–58) compared with 10 months (95% CI 12–16) in those that declined surgery. The OS of patients with bladder cancer undergoing PE was much worse, with an OS of 14 months (95% CI 12–16) compared with 1.5 months in the non-operative control group (Figure 27.1). This pattern can also be demonstrated on subgroup analysis of the operative or non-operative management of either stage 3 or 4 bladder cancer (Figure 27.2).

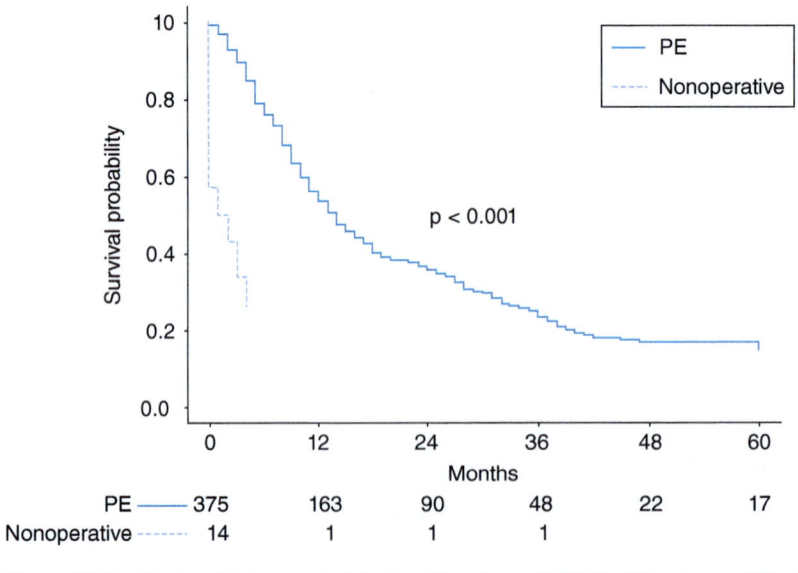

Figure 27.1 Kaplan–Meier survival for locally advanced T4 bladder cancer: PE versus non-operative management. *Source:* adapted from Speicher et al. [20]. *Source:* Speicher, P. J., Turley, R. S., Sloane, J. L., Mantyh, C. R., & Migaly, J. (2013). Pelvic Exenteration for the Treatment of Locally Advanced Colorectal and Bladder Malignancies in the Modern Era. Journal of Gastrointestinal Surgery, 18(4), 782–788.

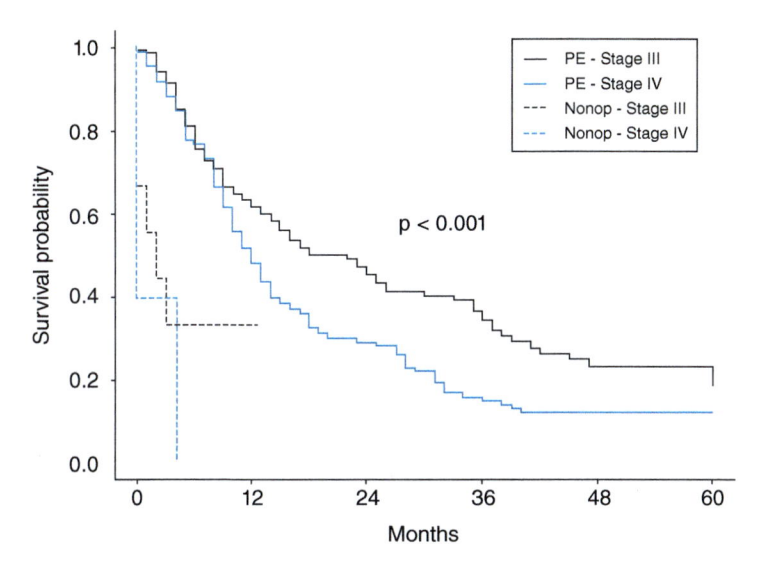

Figure 27.2 Kaplan–Meier survival for locally advanced bladder cancer stratified by disease stage and use of PE. *Source:* adapted from Speicher et al. [20]. *Source:* Speicher, P. J., Turley, R. S., Sloane, J. L., Mantyh, C. R., & Migaly, J. (2013). Pelvic Exenteration for the Treatment of Locally Advanced Colorectal and Bladder Malignancies in the Modern Era. Journal of Gastrointestinal Surgery, 18(4), 782–788.

Complications

Table 27.2 shows general and specific complications of exenterative surgery.

Urological Leaks

Anastomotic leaks are potentially life threatening and highly morbid complications of any intra-abdominal surgery. There are several options for urinary diversion following cystectomy or PE which can be divided into continent – that is, an orthotopic bladder or incontinent, i.e. IC or wet colostomy [21, 22]. For example, an IC necessitates an ileal–ileal anastomosis and anastomosis of both ureters to the conduit. This provides two potential anastomoses that can leak, whereas wet colostomy avoids ileal–ileal anastomosis and only has the two uretero-colic anastomoses [23].

Ileal Conduit

An IC utilizes an approximately 12- to 18-cm portion of ileum as a conduit for the two ureters with a urostomy usually formed in the right iliac fossa. This necessitates a uretero-ileal anastomosis with both ureters stented and an ileal–ileal anastomosis [24]. It remains one

Table 27.2 General and specific complications of exenterative surgery.

General	Specific
Wound infection	*Urological*
Bleeding	Urosepsis
Venous thromboembolism	Urinary conduit leak
	Anastomotic stricture (late)
Seroma	*Gastrointestinal*
Hernias	Bleeding
	Anastomotic leak
	Adhesions/ileus/obstruction
	Stoma complications/parastomal hernia (late)
	Perineal fistula
	Sepsis
	Pelvic abscess
	Reconstruction (depends on type)
	Flap necrosis
	Donor site complications

of the most popular techniques over the last few decades, with low complication rates outside the initial postoperative period when anastomotic leaks may occur.

In a study of 281 patients having different urological diversions, 118 had an IC with a uretero-ileal leakage rate of 0.8% and ileal–ileal leak rate of 0.8% [23]. Overall, early complication rates were high in all urological diversions – 48% for ICs. In addition, there was a high rate of uretero-ileal strictures in 11% of patients, with 17/23 developing irreversible partial loss of renal function. However, other series report higher uretero-ileal leak rates of 7% which they report is more likely due to poor surgical technique, i.e. tension, rotation, or devascularization of the ureters [25]. Conservative management is usually sufficient as the ureters are stented, with management of sepsis, drainage, and adequate nutrition. Occasionally, diversion by nephrostomies is necessary [11]. Most of the published studies comparing the urinary diversion technique are following RC rather than PE. Early and late complications appear to be high in all urinary diversion techniques [26]. A systematic review details the outcome following urinary diversion for bladder cancer [24]. The authors quote early complication rates (< 30 days) with urinary leak 1.8–10%, ureteric obstruction 0–6.3%, and urethral/stomal stricture (2–14.3%). Late complications included ureteral obstruction/stricture 2–30%, renal deterioration 0.4–10.5%, pyelonephritis 3–10%, and bowel obstruction 4–8%.

Orthotopic Bladder

Orthotopic bladder utilizes either a detubularized piece of colon or, more commonly, small bowel to form a neobladder that is anastomosed to the urethra [26]. Other techniques such as the Hautmann bladder utilize 60 cm of terminal ileum in a "W" configuration [27]. These are continent methods and the patient empties the neobladder with a Valsalva maneuver, with the use of intermittent self-catheterization as necessary [28]. Although widely utilized in some centers, the contraindications include tumors that invade the bladder neck/urethra, poor renal function, and inflammatory bowel disease affecting a potential donor site for the reservoir [29]. In addition, like any "pouch" surgery the patient must be appropriately motivated to ensure regular emptying of the reservoir throughout the day and night with or without intermittent self-catheterization.

A large series of orthotopic bladder reconstructions following RC demonstrated complication rates of 58% for 1013 patients [30]. Minor complications occurred in 36% and major in 22%, and complications were infections (24%), genitourinary (17%), gastrointestinal (15%), and wound related (9%). The 90-day mortality rate was 2.3%.

Wet Colostomy

Alexander Brunschwig originally described PE with an end colostomy and bilateral uretero-sigmoidostomy in 1948 [31, 32]. However, this was largely abandoned due to the high complication rates including electrolyte imbalance, ascending urinary infections, and high-volume watery diarrhea. In 1989, double barrel wet colostomy (DBWC) was described which requires only one loop colostomy [33]. This technique uses a double-barreled loop colostomy with both ureters anastomosed to the distal portion of the colon, and therefore urine does not come into direct content with feces. Proponents report lower urinary infection rates and it is a useful technique in patients where the small bowel cannot be used, for example post radiotherapy [34]. Some small retrospective case series comparing DBWC with IC demonstrated either equivalent or improved outcomes with DBWC and the benefit of one stoma [35]. Due to the small numbers and heterogeneity of these studies it is not possible to say that DBWC is superior to other techniques, but it is an option and the preferred technique in some centers [22].

Palliative Exenterations

Both advanced bladder and prostate cancers can cause severe debilitating symptoms including pain, dysuria, hematuria, and outflow obstruction [8]. Chronic outflow obstruction of the bladder or ureters may cause renal failure and necessitate interventions including long-term urethral catheters, stents, or nephrostomies. Locally advanced pelvic malignancies are associated with reduced QoL, and if resectable this can be improved by a PE in addition to long-term survival [36]. However, a PE for palliation is more controversial, with a study of 39 patients who underwent palliative PE demonstrating reduced QoL postoperatively which continued to decline thereafter [37]. Overall median survival was 24 months with a mortality rate of 31% at one year.

There are multiple other treatment options that can be tried to help palliate symptoms in this patient group and this requires a multidisciplinary approach including surgeons, oncologists, and pain specialists. Options include palliative radiotherapy, hormonal treatment, and analgesics. If these options have been tried, then palliative exenterations are an option in a select subgroup who are fit for this extensive surgery with a view to improving QoL [38, 39].

Quality of Life

Traditionally, study outcomes focused solely on clinical outcomes, but there is now a much greater emphasis on patient-reported outcome measures (PROMs). Assessing these factors is challenging for exenterations due to the extensive nature of the surgery and impact on patients across multiple domains including physical, mental, and sexual function. There is a lack of a validated QoL scoring system for exenterations and wide variability in tools reported in studies. Relatively little has been published in terms of PROMs and QoL for urology-specific malignancies. A meta-analysis of 18 non-randomized papers that reported on health-related quality of life (HR-QoL) in patients having urological reconstruction with IC or orthotopic neobladder (ONB) demonstrated higher HR-QoL for ONB over IC [40]. This finding was replicated in a study of patients undergoing urological reconstruction for RC using the European Organization for Research and Treatment of Cancer (EORTC) QoL questionnaire. Patients having ONB had improved physical, social, and global health status [41]. Patients having a PE for any cause of locally advanced pelvic cancer demonstrated improved QoL (Functional Assessment of Cancer Therapy – Colorectal (FACT-C)) compared with those that did not have surgery. Those that underwent PE had reduced QoL at one month postoperatively, which then continually increased and returned to baseline QoL at nine months [42]. Those patients who did not have surgery had reduced QoL at one month, which slowly increased up to six months before declining after nine months. A systematic review of QoL post exenteration for locally and recurrent rectal cancer demonstrated that baseline QoL was the strongest indicator for postoperative QoL [43]. In addition, they identified that female gender, total PE with or without bone resection, and positive surgical margins were associated with a reduced QoL.

A systematic review from 2016 identified 24 studies which included 976 patients having exenterations with data on QoL. However, only six of these studies recorded baseline QoL. They identified nine themes across the literature: body image, social impact, sexual function, treatment expectations, symptoms, communication, psychological impact, relationships, and work and finance [44]. There are collaborative efforts ongoing such as the Association of Coloproctology of Great Britain and Ireland (ACPGBI) "IeMPACT" and PelvEx that plan to validate an exenteration-specific QoL scoring system.

> **Summary Box**
>
> - There has been a significant reduction in morbidity and mortality following PE for urological neoplasms.
> - Multicompartment exenterative surgery is infrequently practised for prostate cancer and is reserved for aggressive management of either advanced, symptomatic prostate cancers or, less commonly, synchronous tumors of the rectum and prostate.
> - Definitions are important, as all females having an RC have an anterior exenteration but this is not the same as a multi-compartment PE.
> - Bladder TCC invading the colon or rectum is classified as systemic disease and treated with palliative chemotherapy. However, patients with locally invasive bladder TCC into the prostate, cervix, or vagina are classified as having T4 disease but can be offered an RC.
> - PE can be used for palliation of symptoms in selective cases of urological neoplasms.

References

1 PelvEx Collaborative (2019). Surgical and survival outcomes following pelvic exenteration for locally advanced primary rectal cancer: results from an international collaboration. *Ann. Surg.* 269 (2): 315–321.
2 PelvEx Collaborative (2018). Factors affecting outcomes following pelvic exenteration for locally recurrent rectal cancer. *Br. J. Surg.* 105 (6): 650–657.
3 Hounsome, L.S., Verne, J., McGrath, J.S., and Gillatt, D.A. (2015). Trends in operative caseload and mortality rates after radical cystectomy for bladder cancer in England for 1998–2010. *Eur. Urol.* 67 (6): 1056–1062.
4 Jefferies, E.R., Cresswell, J., McGrath, J.S. et al. (2018). Open radical cystectomy in England: the current standard of care – an analysis of the British Association of Urological Surgeons (BAUS) cystectomy audit and hospital episodes statistics (HES) data. *BJU Int.* 121 (6): 880–885.
5 Miller, C., Campain, N.J., Dbeis, R. et al. (2017). Introduction of robot-assisted radical cystectomy within an established enhanced recovery programme. *BJU Int.* 120 (2): 265–272.
6 Pomel, C., Rouzier, R., Pocard, M. et al. (2003). Laparoscopic total pelvic exenteration for cervical cancer relapse. *Gynecol. Oncol.* 91 (3): 616–618.
7 Fitzmaurice, C., Akinyemiju, T.F., Al Lami, F.H. et al. (2018;4(11):1553–68). Global, regional, and national cancer incidence, mortality, years of life lost, years lived with disability, and disability-adjusted life-years for 29 cancer groups, 1990 to 2016: a systematic analysis for the global burden of disease study. *JAMA Oncol.*
8 Oefelein, M.G. (2004). Prognostic significance of obstructive uropathy in advanced prostate cancer. *Urology* 63 (6): 1117–1121.
9 Zincke, H. (1992). Radical prostatectomy and exenterative procedures for local failure after radiotherapy with curative intent: comparison of outcomes. *J. Urol.* 147 (3 Pt 2): 894–899.
10 Donahue, T.M.M., Slovin, S., Scher, H. et al. (2015). Pelvic exenteration in patients with non-metastatic, locally advanced castration-resistant prostate cancer. *J. Urol.*: e1038.
11 Pawlik, T.M., Skibber, J.M., and Rodriguez-Bigas, M.A. (2006). Pelvic exenteration for advanced pelvic malignancies. *Ann. Surg. Oncol.* 13 (5): 612–623.
12 Kavanagh, D.O., Quinlan, D.M., Armstrong, J.G. et al. (2012). Management of synchronous rectal and prostate cancer. *Int. J. Color. Dis.* 27 (11): 1501–1508.

13 Seretis, C., Seretis, F., and Liakos, N. (2014). Multidisciplinary approach to synchronous prostate and rectal cancer: current experience and future challenges. *J. Clin. Med. Res.* 6 (3): 157–161.
14 Teixeira, S.C., Ferenschild, F.T., Solomon, M.J. et al. (2012). Urological leaks after pelvic exenterations comparing formation of colonic and ileal conduits. *Eur. J. Surg. Oncol.* 38 (4): 361–366.
15 Brown, K.G., Solomon, M.J., Latif, E.R. et al. (2017). Urological complications after cystectomy as part of pelvic exenteration are higher than that after cystectomy for primary bladder malignancy. *J. Surg. Oncol.* 115 (3): 307–311.
16 Sylvester, R.J., van der Meijden, A.P., Oosterlinck, W. et al. (2006). Predicting recurrence and progression in individual patients with stage Ta T1 bladder cancer using EORTC risk tables: a combined analysis of 2596 patients from seven EORTC trials. *Eur. Urol.* 49 (3): 466–465; discussion 75–7.
17 van den Bosch, S. and Alfred Witjes, J. (2011). Long-term cancer-specific survival in patients with high-risk, non-muscle-invasive bladder cancer and tumour progression: a systematic review. *Eur. Urol.* 60 (3): 493–500.
18 Marshall, F.F. and Treiger, B.F. (1991). Radical cystectomy (anterior exenteration) in the female patient. *Urol. Clin. North Am.* 18 (4): 765–775.
19 Gregg, J.R., Emeruwa, C., Wong, J. et al. (2016). Oncologic outcomes after anterior exenteration for muscle invasive bladder cancer in women. *J. Urol.* 196 (4): 1030–1035.
20 Speicher, P.J., Turley, R.S., Sloane, J.L. et al. (2014). Pelvic exenteration for the treatment of locally advanced colorectal and bladder malignancies in the modern era. *J. Gastrointest. Surg.* 18 (4): 782–788.
21 Hautmann, R.E., de Petriconi, R.C., Pfeiffer, C., and Volkmer, B.G. (2012). Radical cystectomy for urothelial carcinoma of the bladder without neoadjuvant or adjuvant therapy: long-term results in 1100 patients. *Eur. Urol.* 61 (5): 1039–1047.
22 Golda, T., Biondo, S., Kreisler, E. et al. (2010). Follow-up of double-barreled wet colostomy after pelvic exenteration at a single institution. *Dis. Colon Rectum* 53 (5): 822–829.
23 Nieuwenhuijzen, J.A., de Vries, R.R., Bex, A. et al. (2008). Urinary diversions after cystectomy: the association of clinical factors, complications and functional results of four different diversions. *Eur. Urol.* 53 (4): 834–842; discussion 42–4.
24 Lee, R.K., Abol-Enein, H., Artibani, W. et al. (2014). Urinary diversion after radical cystectomy for bladder cancer: options, patient selection, and outcomes. *BJU Int.* 113 (1): 11–23.
25 Colombo, R.N.R. (2010). Ileal conduit as the standard for urinary diversion after radical cystectomy for bladder cancer. *Eur. Assoc. Urol.* 9 (10): 736–744.
26 Studer, U.E. and Turner, W.H. (1995). The ileal orthotopic bladder. *Urology* 45 (2): 185–189.
27 Hautmann, R.E., Egghart, G., Frohneberg, D., and Miller, K. (1987). The ileal neobladder. *Urologe A.* 26 (2): 67–73.
28 Chang, D.T. and Lawrentschuk, N. (2015). Orthotopic neobladder reconstruction. *Urol. Ann.* 7 (1): 1–7.
29 Hautmann, R.E., de Petriconi, R.C., and Volkmer, B.G. (2010). Lessons learned from 1,000 neobladders: the 90-day complication rate. *J. Urol.* 184 (3): 990–994; quiz 1235.
30 Hautmann, R.E., de Petriconi, R.C., and Volkmer, B.G. (2011). 25 years of experience with 1,000 neobladders: long-term complications. *J. Urol.* 185 (6): 2207–2212.
31 Brunschwig, A. (1948). Complete excision of pelvic viscera for advanced carcinoma; a one-stage abdominoperineal operation with end colostomy and bilateral ureteral implantation into the colon above the colostomy. *Cancer* 1 (2): 177–183.
32 Brunschwig, A. and Daniel, W. (1960). Pelvic exenteration operations: with summary of sixty-six cases surviving more than five years. *Ann. Surg.* 151: 571–576.

33 Carter, M.F., Dalton, D.P., and Garnett, J.E. (1989). Simultaneous diversion of the urinary and fecal streams utilizing a single abdominal stoma: the double-barreled wet colostomy. *J. Urol.* 141 (5): 1189–1191.

34 Lopes de Queiroz, F., Barbosa-Silva, T., Pyramo Costa, L.M. et al. (2006). Double-barrelled wet colostomy with simultaneous urinary and faecal diversion: results in 9 patients and review of the literature. *Colorectal Dis.* 8 (4): 353–359.

35 Gan, J. and Hamid, R. (2017). Literature review: double-barrelled wet colostomy (one stoma) versus ileal conduit with colostomy (two stomas). *Urol. Int.* 98 (3): 249–254.

36 Quyn, A.J., Austin, K.K., Young, J.M. et al. (2016). Outcomes of pelvic exenteration for locally advanced primary rectal cancer: overall survival and quality of life. *Eur. J. Surg. Oncol.* 42 (6): 823–828.

37 Quyn, A.J., Solomon, M.J., Lee, P.M. et al. (2016). Palliative pelvic exenteration: clinical outcomes and quality of life. *Dis. Colon Rectum* 59 (11): 1005–1010.

38 Hockel, M. (2003). Laterally extended endopelvic resection. Novel surgical treatment of locally recurrent cervical carcinoma involving the pelvic side wall. *Gynecol. Oncol.* 91 (2): 369–377.

39 Huang, M., Iglesias, D.A., Westin, S.N. et al. (2014). Pelvic exenteration: impact of age on surgical and oncologic outcomes. *Gynecol. Oncol.* 132 (1): 114–118.

40 Cerruto, M.A., D'Elia, C., Siracusano, S. et al. (2016). Systematic review and meta-analysis of non RCTs on health related quality of life after radical cystectomy using validated questionnaires: better results with orthotopic neobladder versus ileal conduit. *Eur. J. Surg. Oncol.* 42 (3): 343–360.

41 Singh, V., Yadav, R., Sinha, R.J., and Gupta, D.K. (2014). Prospective comparison of quality-of-life outcomes between ileal conduit urinary diversion and orthotopic neobladder reconstruction after radical cystectomy: a statistical model. *BJU Int.* 113 (5): 726–732.

42 Young, J.M., Badgery-Parker, T., Masya, L.M. et al. (2014). Quality of life and other patient-reported outcomes following exenteration for pelvic malignancy. *Br. J. Surg.* 101 (3): 277–287.

43 Rausa, E., Kelly, M.E., Bonavina, L. et al. (2017). A systematic review examining quality of life following pelvic exenteration for locally advanced and recurrent rectal cancer. *Colorectal Dis.* 19 (5): 430–436.

44 Harji, D.P., Griffiths, B., Velikova, G. et al. (2016). Systematic review of health-related quality of life in patients undergoing pelvic exenteration. *Eur. J. Surg. Oncol.* 42 (8): 1132–1145.

28

Outcomes Following Exenteration for Gynecological Neoplasms

Päivi Kannisto[1], Fredrik Liedberg[2], and Marie-Louise Lydrup[3]

[1] Department of Obstetrics and Gynecology, Skåne University Hospital, Lund, Sweden
[2] Institution of Translational Medicine, Lund University, Malmö, Sweden; Department of Urology, Skåne University Hospital, Malmö, Sweden
[3] Division of Surgery, Department of Clinical Sciences, Lund University, Skåne University Hospital, Malmö, Sweden

Background

The primary treatment of gynecological malignancies has considerably evolved over the last century, with a move to less aggressive procedures when appropriate [1–3]. However, gynecological malignancies comprise a heterogeneous group, with varying treatment options. In cervical cancer, T1a tumors without risk factors are treated with radical local excision only, whereas T1b1 and T2a1 (≤ 4cm) cervical cancers need a radical hysterectomy and pelvic lymphadenectomy. Chemoradiation is recommended if lymph node involvement is suspected or clear margins around the tumor are threatened [4, 5]. For T2 tumors > 4cm and T3 tumors, treatment with primary chemoradiation is preferable, with improved progression free survival compared to neoadjuvant chemotherapy followed by radical surgery [6].

Small vaginal cancers less than 4cm [7] or early stages of vulva cancer and endometrial cancer are predominantly treated with radical surgery and consolidated with chemoradiation or chemotherapy when indicated. Minor recurrences, like endometrial cancer in the vaginal cuff, are treated with curative chemoradiation [8, 9]. Apart from those situations, pelvic exenteration (PE) is the only procedure to cure women from locally advanced primary or recurrent gynecological cancer. It remains the first-line treatment of advanced vulva cancer with urethral extension (T2–T3 tumor) [10, 11] and advanced endometrial cancer involving the bladder and ureters (T3–T4 tumors) [12, 13]. In addition, resistance to chemoradiation or a relapse after chemoradiation are the most common indications for total exenteration in recurrent cervical cancer [14]. Rarer indications for exenteration include the presence of a frozen pelvis and complications of postradiotherapy (fistulation) [14, 15].

Depending on the localization of the gynecological tumor, anterior, posterior, or total exenteration is performed. Laterally extended endopelvic resection (LEER) and extended pelvic resections (EPR) have been reported in selected cases of advanced gynecological malignancies [16]. The choice of reconstructive method for urinary and fecal diversion is crucial, as most patients have been previously irradiated with high doses or had prior surgery for their primary neoplasm. Table 28.1 lists some absolute [17] and relative [6, 18–21] contraindications.

Surgical Management of Advanced Pelvic Cancer, First Edition.
Edited by Michael E. Kelly and Desmond C. Winter.
© 2022 John Wiley & Sons Ltd. Published 2022 by John Wiley & Sons Ltd.

Table 28.1 Considered contraindications.

Relative contraindication	Absolute contraindication
Involvement of external iliac vessels	Sciatic nerve involvement without prospect of clear margins
Pelvic bone metastasis	Distant metastatic disease or extensive carcinomatosis
Pathological para-aortic lymph nodes	

Further Important Situations

Engagement of Pelvic Sidewalls

Involvement of the external iliac vessels has traditionally been a contraindication for PE, since a radical resection may require grafting. Suspicious pelvic bone metastases should be verified by preoperative magnetic resonance imaging (MRI) or computed tomography–positron emission tomography (CT-PET), or both, if extended en-bloc resection is possible [21]. Höckel et al. (2012) [16] have reported 100% R0 resections using LEER on recurrent cancers of the cervix and vagina with tumors fixed to the lateral pelvic wall. Hydronephrosis is not a contraindication for PE [16, 19, 20].

Para-Aortic Lymph Nodes

It seems evident that the presence of pathological para-aortal lymph nodes significantly worsens survival; nevertheless, most units do not consider para-aortic spread a contraindication for PE in cervical and endometrial cancer [18, 19]. However, finding multiple and bulky nodes above the origin of the inferior mesenteric artery probably indicates a non-curable situation where surgery is questionable [17, 20].

Age and Comorbidity

Due to the long duration, the complexity of the surgical procedure, and the risk of substantial blood loss, the patient's comorbidity must be thoroughly evaluated. If performance status is evaluated according to Eastern Cooperative Oncology Group (ECOG) the score should be between 0 and 2 when considering PE [22]; thus ECOG = 3 and above should be considered as a relative contraindication. Conflicting results concerning the influence of age on postoperative mortality have been reported. Baiocchi et al. [23] reported a postoperative mortality of 42% in patients aged > 70 compared to 5% in younger patients. In patients > 70 years of age with comorbidities corresponding to American Society of Anesthesiologists (ASA) class III, the risk of postoperative death was reported as high as 64%. On the contrary, Huang et al. [24] did not observe any major difference in complications or survival when comparing younger and elderly patient cohorts; however, these survival differences are probably mainly related to selection bias between the series.

The impact of body mass index (BMI) on overall complication rates and survival has been reported by Huang et al. [24] and by Iglesias et al. [25] without any association between BMI and complication rates or worse survival outcomes. Whereas advanced age or high BMI should not be interpreted as contraindications for PE, special attention should be paid to the patient's nutritional status and kidney function. Low albumin levels are associated with impaired outcome [26]. The patient's quality of life (QoL) preoperatively must also be considered [27]. Postoperative QoL after PE due to recurrent colorectal malignancy can be predicted from baseline QoL before surgery [28].

Preoperative Workup Specific to Gynecological Neoplasms

The most important issue for successful surgery and survival is a complete resection [15, 29]. CT-PET and MRI are both suitable methods for imaging primary, persistent, and recurrent pelvic disease but also to differentiate between active disease and post-radiation artifacts. This is crucial for evaluation if PE is manageable and if pelvic sidewalls are involved. Moreover, it is of great importance to predict the extent of the surgery and the possibility to obtain clear margins [21]. Further, quantitative metrics of fludeoxyglucose (FDG) uptake metabolic tumor volume have been shown to predict progression-free and overall survival [30]. However, Meads et al. [31] showed no evidence supporting a superior diagnostic accuracy of CT-PET in recurrent or persisting cervical cancer compared to MRI and CT. Neither could Sardain et al. [32] find a preoperative procedure that could confirm free margins at the end of the operation.

Cystoscopy, colonoscopy, and gynecological examination under anesthesia should be performed to tailor treatments. Diagnostic laparoscopy is only indicated in cases with suspected peritoneal carcinomatosis on preoperative imaging.

Preoperative Planning and Counseling

Urinary Diversion

The type of urinary diversion should be discussed with the patient preoperatively, preferably based on information on long-term functional outcomes and complications [33–35]. Patient characteristics, such as age and comorbidity, also affect the choice of urinary diversion, especially when opting for a continent reconstruction in the setting of an anterior exenteration for a gynecological cancer. Continence after orthotopic neobladder surgery is worse in females compared to in males [36, 37]. As preservation of the uterus and performing nerve-sparing surgery is not feasible with PE, the functional outcome is further reduced [38]. The need for simultaneous posterior exenteration affects whether a continent reconstruction is a suitable option.

Previous pelvic radiation increases the risk of short-term complications after urinary diversion [39], and probably puts the patient at an increased risk of late diversion-related complications such as ureteroenteric strictures [40]. Consequently, a selected bowel segment outside the irradiated field is recommended [41]. Ileal conduit is the most common form of urinary diversion in conjunction with anterior exenteration for gynecological cancers. An increased use of ileal conduit in recent years is a consequence of performing surgery in elderly and comorbid patients more frequently and accumulating evidence of decreased need of reoperations from a population-based survey [35], but also decreased in-hospital complications at long-term follow-up [42], compared to a continent reconstruction. The indications for a continent reconstruction are related to patient preferences, but require intact mental status, manual dexterity, and glomerular filtration rate (GFR) > 40 ml/min/1.73 m^2 and the willingness to accept an increased risk of complications and reoperations compared to conduit diversion.

For patients with advanced gynecological tumors requiring both urinary and fecal diversion, i.e. two stomas, a double-barreled colostomy has been popularized [43]. The rationale for this type of diversion is to offer the patient one instead of two stomas. So far, the experience of the method is limited and the stoma appliances is a challenge, and until now appliances for terminal ileostomies have been used. The optimal localization of the urinary stoma is an integral part of the preoperative preparation and of critical importance to avoid postoperative difficulties with stoma accessories or emptying a continent cutaneous diversion. Thus, marking the site of the stoma should be done in close cooperation with the stoma-therapists.

Bowel Continuity

In the case of supralevator PE, bowel continuity could be restored with low colorectal or coloanal anastomosis. Successful restoration of bowel continuity was reported by Schmidt et al. [19] in 97% of patients having PE for cervical cancer and in 75% of patients with advanced or recurrent endometrial cancer [13] However, anastomotic complications, especially leakages, have been reported to occur in up to 54% of such patients [19, 20, 44, 45].

Decision regarding low anterior resection syndrome (LARS) and tailoring of the bowel reconstruction should be based on a thorough patient discussion.

Neovagina

After vaginectomy, a neovagina can be constructed using either myocutanous grafts or interposed bowel. Berek et al. [46] reported construction of neovagina in 54/75 patients (72%) after PE and in 45/54 using gracilis myocutaneous pedicle grafts, rectus abdominis pedicle flaps, or split or full-thickness skin graft. Also, transverse and vertical rectus abdominis myocutaneous (TRAM and VRAM) flaps have been shown to be reliable alternatives for neovaginal reconstructions, with a similar distribution of flap-specific complications [47]. The deep inferior epigastric perforator (DIEP) flap has been shown to give promising results compared to TRAM [48]. Generally, problems such as chronic stenosis, lack of lubrication, intravaginal hair growth, and inadequate length are described when using myocutaneous grafts. To overcome these shortcomings, enterocolpoplasties using the right or descending colon have been reported by Ferrari et al. [49] and Bridoux et al. [50]. Construction of a neovagina from a colonic segment after PE due to cervical cancer recurrence was also successfully performed in 249/282 patients by Schmidt et al. [19].

Pelvic Floor Reconstruction

In order to fill the empty pelvis and prevent small intestinal descent, herniation, or obstruction, the rectus abdominis muscle, gluteus maximus, and/or gracilis flaps may be used as space fillers (with/without omentum) [51–53] (see Chapter 17).

Complications

Most published work on postoperative complications are based on single-center retrospective cohort studies. Due to the absence of uniform definitions of complications and early vs. late diagnosis of complications, comparison between studies is difficult. The reported complication rates reviewed in Table 28.2 should thus be regarded as examples of the complication panorama. Early postoperative mortality has decreased from 23% [1] in historical series to 0% in some recent studies [2, 3]. According to our review in Table 28.2, early complications are reported in 30–78% of patients and late complications in 41–49%. The high complication rate can be explained by the high percentage of patients having a recurrent or radioresistant cervical cancer. Infections, urinary complications, intestinal complications (fistulas, ileus, anastomotic leak), and wound complications are the commonest complications.

Severe late complications after PE are related to the urinary diversion. Indeed, the incidence of complications correlates with the length of follow-up [62]. Long-term follow-up reports diversion-related complications including metabolic dysfunction, infections, and urolithiasis, as well as conduit and bowel/stoma complications, and renal dysfunction. Vitamin B12 deficiency relating to decreased intestinal uptake from the ileum may arise in a minority of patients.

Table 28.2 Complications after PE for gynecological malignancies.

Authors, year	n	Surgical details					Complications				
		Type of PE: percentage colorectal anastomosis	Urinary diversion	Vaginal reconstruction	Perineal reconstruction	Early complications	Type of complication	Late complications	Type of complication	Early reoperations	Late reoperations	Mortality, 30 days
Fleisch et al. 2007 [54]	203	TPE: 67/203 = 33% APE: 91/203 = 45% PPE: 45/203 = 22% Colorectal anastomosis: 59/112 = 53%, colostomy: 53/112 = 47%	77% 49% conduit 28% pouch 8% neobladder 11% ureterocutaneostomy 14% bladder augment	X	X	< POD 180	Urinary 61/156 = 39% Intestinal 28/112 = 25%		X		35/203 = 16% < POD 180	1%
Maggioni et al. 2009 [55]	106	TPE: 48/106 = 45% APE: 53/106 = 50% PPE: 6/106 = 5.7% Colorectal anastomosis: 17/54 = 32%	95% 48% non-continent ileoconduit 52% continent ileoconduit	18%	23%	45% < POD 30	Intestinal 12/106 = 11% Urinary 9/101 = 9% Other 33/106 = 30% AL 3/17 = 18% Rectoneovaginal fistula 2 cases	49% ≥ POD 30	Intestinal 8/106 = 7% Urinary 42/101 = 41% Other 13/106 = 12% Rectoneovaginal fistula 2 cases Ureterocolic stricture 1 case	14/106 = 13%	11/106 = 10%	0%

(*Continued*)

Table 28.2 (Continued)

Authors, year	n	Type of PE: percentage colorectal anastomosis	Urinary diversion	Vaginal reconstruction	Perineal reconstruction	Early complications	Type of complication	Late complications	Type of complication	Early reoperations	Late reoperations	Mortality, 30 days
		Surgical details				**Complications**						
Fotopoulou et al. 2010 [56]	47	TPE: 32/47 = 68% APE: 12/47 = 26% PPE: 3/47 = 6.4% No information concerning colorectal anastomosis	64% 23% ureterocutaneostomy 62% incontinent ileoconduit 4% continent ileoconduit	4%	X	No definition of early and late	Wound 6% Urinary leak 6% AL 30% Ileus 8% Cardiovascular and thromboembolic events 7% Other 6%		X	14/47 = 30%	X	8.5%
Baiocchi et al. 2012 [23]	107	TPE: 56/107 = 52% APE: 31/107 = 29% PPE: 10/107 = 9.3% Lateral extended resection: 10/107 = 9.3% Colorectal anastomosis: 12/56 = 21% (of TPE)	91% 45% DBWC Orthotopic bladder: 1 patient	X	X	53%	Wound infection 26% Intestinal fistula 14% Urinary fistula 9% Pelvic floor infection 30% Bleeding 5% DVT 5%	45%	Urinary obstruction 33% Urinary fistula 10% Intestinal fistula 6% Ileus 19% Pelvic floor infection 17% DVT 6%	33%	29%	8.4%

Study	N	Procedure	R0	Morbidity	Major complications		Minor complications		Mortality
Kaur et al. 2012 [2]	36	TPE: 28/36 = 78%	92%	X	78%	Wound 9/36 = 25%		Wound 7/36 = 19%	14/36 = 38%	0%
		APE: 5/36 = 14%	52% incontinent conduit		< POD 30	Urinary 9/36 = 25%		Urinary 13/36 = 36%	No information on early or late	
		PPE: 3/36 = 8.3%	48% continent conduit			Intestinal 1/36 = 2.8		Intestinal 4/36 = 3%		
		Colorectal anastomosis: 18/31 = 58%				Rectovaginal fistula 1/36 = 3%		Rectovaginal fistula 4/36 = 11%		
								Vesicovaginal fistula 1/36 = 3%		
						Other 8/36 = 22%		Other 5/36 = 14%		
Khoury-Collado et al. 2012 [57]	21	No information concerning colorectal anastomosis	95%	29%	< POD 30	Infection 13/21 = 62%	POD 31–90	Infection 6/21 = 29%	1/21 = 5%	0%
						Thromboembolism 1/21 = 5%		Thromboembolism 3/21 = 14%	< POD 30	
						Enterocutaneous fistula 1/21 = 5%		Enterocutaneous fistula 3/21 = 14%	POD 31–90	
						Urinary leak 1/21 = 5%		AL 1/21 = 5%		
								Vesicovaginal fistula 1/21 = 5%		
								Ureteroenteral stricture 1/21 = 5%		
								Urostomy retraction 1/21 = 5%		
						Psychiatric 4/21 = 19%		Psychiatric 1/21 = 5%		
Yoo et al. 2012 [58]	61	TPE: 42/61 = 69%	97%	7%	18%	Wound infection 4/61 = 7%	25/61 = 41%	Wound infection 1/61 = 1.6%	X	X
		APE: 17/61 = 11%			30%	Wound dehiscence 3/61 = 5%	≥ POD 30			
		PPE: 2/61 = 3.3%			< POD 30	Ileus 1/61 = 2%		Ileus 10/61 = 16%		

(*Continued*)

Table 28.2 (Continued)

Authors, year	n	Surgical details				Complications				Early reoperations	Late reoperations	Mortality, 30 days
		Type of PE: percentage colorectal anastomosis	Urinary diversion	Vaginal reconstruction	Perineal reconstruction	Early complications	Type of complication	Late complications	Type of complication			
		Colorectal anastomosis: 6/45 = 13%					Enterocutaneous fistula 1/61 = 1.6%		Enterocutaneous fistula 1/61 = 1.6%			
							Ureteroenteral fistula 1/61 = 1.6%		Ureteroenteral fistula 7/61 = 11%			
							Rectovaginal fistula 2/61% = 3.3%		Rectovaginal fistula 2/61 = 3.3%			
									Pelvic abscess 1/61 = 1.6%			
									Incisional hernia 1/61 = 1.6%			
									DVT 1/61 = 1.6%			
									Urostomy obstruction 1/61 = 1.6%			
Jäger et al. 2013 [3]	28	TPE: 11/28 = 39%	46%	14%	21%	< POD 30	CDIIIa and above 8/28 = 29%	≥ POD 30	CDIIIb and above 10/28 = 36%	3/28 = 11% < POD 30	10/28 = 36% ≥ POD 30	0%
		APE: 2/28 = 7%					Pelvic abscess 3/28 = 11%		Ileus 4/28==14%			
		PPE: 15/28 = 54%					Urinary leak 1/28 = 4%		Fistula 2/28 = 7%			
		Colorectal anastomosis: 20/26 = 38%					Vaginal stricture 1/28 = 4%		Urostomy necrosis 1/28 = 3.6%			
							Pleural effusion 1/28=4%					
							AL 1/28 = 4%		Wound infection 1/28 = 3.6%			

Study	N	Procedure			Complications	
Chiantera et al. 2014 [59]	230	TPE: 131/230 = 57%	86%	10%	Massive bleeding 1/28 = 4%	5%
		APE: 68/230 = 30%	24% continent conduit		Stoma prolapse 1/28 = 3.6%	
		PPE: 31/230 = 13%	4% neobladder		Anastomotic stricture 1/28 = 3.6%	3%
		Colorectal anastomosis: 93/162 = 57%	72% non-continent conduit		Early and late complications not seperated	X
			ureterocutaneo stomy: 4 patients		Infection 66/230 = 29%	X
					Other 15/230 = 6.5%	
					Wound dehiscence 39/230 = 17%	
					Vaginal stump dehiscence 11/239 = 4.8%	
					AL 19/93 = 20%	
					Small intestinal perforation 8/230 = 3.5%	
					Neovaginal complication 5/24 = 21%	
Chiantera et al. 2014 [60]	21	TPE: 10 = 48%	76%	0%	AL 3/8 = 38%	0%
		APE: 6/21 = 29%	Incontinent conduit: 15 patients			4.8%
		PPE: 5/21 = 24%	Continent conduit: 1 patient			
		Colorectal anastomosis: 8/15 = 53%				

(*Continued*)

Table 28.2 (Continued)

Authors, year	n	Surgical details				Complications					
		Type of PE: percentage colorectal anastomosis	Urinary diversion	Vaginal reconstruction	Perineal reconstruction	Early complications	Type of complication	Late complications	Type of complication	Early reoperations	Late reoperations	Mortality, 30 days
Huang et al. 2014 [24]	161	TPE: 103 (64%) APE: 35 (22%) PPE: 23 (14%) No information concerning colorectal anastomosis	89% 29% continent conduit 71% incontinent conduit	0%	67%	< POD 60	Wound 47/161 = 29% Intestinal 27/161 = 17% Urinary stricture 5/161 = 3% Ureteric lesion 9/161 = 5.6% Renal insufficiency 6/161 = 3.7% Urostomy complication 42/161 = 26% Infection 64/161 = 40% Cardiology 4/161 = 2.5%	≥ POD 60	Wound 3/161 = 2% Intestinal 17/161 = 11% Urinary stricture 11/161 = 7% Ureteric lesion 15/161 = 9% Renal insufficiency 8/161 = 5% Urostomy complication 21/161 = 13% Kidney stones 15/161 = 9.3% Infection 12/161 = 8% Cardiology 9/161 = 6%	15/161 = 9%	3/161 = 2%	X
Westin et al. 2014 [61]	160	TPE: 110/160 = 69% APE: 34/160 = 21% PPE: 16/160 = 10%	89% 68% incontinent conduit	68%	X	< POD 60	Wound 47/160 = 29% Infection 55/160 = 34% Urinary 76/160 = 47%	≥ POD 60	Wound 3/160 = 1.9% Infection 12/160 = 8% Urinary 55/160 = 34%	< POD 60 15/160 = 9%	≥ POD 60 3/160 = 1.9%	1.3%

Study	N							Complications		
		No information concerning colorectal anastomosis						Fistula 14/160 = 9% Ileus 16/160 = 10% Colostomy complication 11/106 = 7% Flap 25/160 = 16% Other 4/160 = 2.5%	X	Fistula 14/160 = 9% Ileus 14/160 = 9% Colostomy complication 3/160 = 1.9% Flap 9/160 = 6% Other 9/106 = 6%	X	7%
Schmidt et al. 2016 [13]	40	TPE: 34/40 = 85% APE: 2/40 = 5% PPE: 4/40 = 10% Colorectal anastomosis: 37/38 = 97%	90%	83% continent conduit	75%	X	X			

X Information not given; TPE, total pelvic exenteration; APE, anterior pelvic exenteration; PPE, posterior pelvic exenteration; DBWC, double-barrelled wet colostomy; AL, anastomotic leakage; POD, postoperative day; DVT, deep vein thrombosis; CD, Clavien-Dindo.

Number of patients with restored bowel continuity is indicated as a percentage of total number of patients operated on with TPE or PPE. Concerning complications and reoperations, varying specifications of early and late in the different studies are indicated in the table.

In the Cochrane Database of Systematic Reviews on exenterative surgery for recurrent gynecological malignancies, Ang et al. [63] states there is no evidence currently available from which to determine whether exenterative surgery is better than, equivalent to, or worse than non-surgical treatment in terms of prolonged survival, treatment-related complications, and impact on QoL.

Survival and Quality of Life

The reported five-year survival rate in patients with mixed diagnosis varies between 21 and 70% (Table 28.3). In addition, Graves et al. [65] reported an overall survival of 73 months after PE in women with node-negative cervical cancer. The PelvEx Collaborative [66] further reported three-year survival rates of 44, 48, and 49% in women with vaginal, endometrial, and cervical cancer respectively. Patients with endometrial cancer seem to have a better survival after PE compared to those with cervical cancer.

Negative resection margins are uniformly reported in more than 70% of patients. Complex complications have been associated with shorter survival [67].

Information on QoL after PE for gynecological malignancies is scarce. However, a recent study on prospective assessment of patient-reported outcomes showed a persistent low body image, decrease in physical functions, and declining sexual pleasure/function during 12 months after PE [68]. Body image worsened over time whereas sexual discomfort was unchanged during follow-up. Mental functioning remained stable and there were no significant changes in stoma-related QoL. Still, 79% of the women stated after one year that they would undergo PE again. On the other hand, the QLQ C30 gradually decreased, compared to baseline, from one month postoperatively and did not reach the baseline level until one year postoperatively. Elderly patients never regained their social and physical activities after PE [26].

Table 28.3 Survival after PE for gynecological malignancies.

Author, year Type of cancer	Number of patients	R0 (%)	Five-year survival (%)
Fleisch et al. 2007 [54]	203		
Cervical	133		
Endometrial	26		
Vaginal/vulval	33		
Other	11		
All types	203	X	21
Maggioni et al. 2009 [55]			
Cervical	62		52
Endometrial	10		35
Vulval	9		X
Vaginal	21		19
Other	4		X
All types	106	93	X
Forner and Lampe 2011 [18]			
Cervical	35	86	43

Table 28.3 (Continued)

Author, year Type of cancer	Number of patients	R0 (%)	Five-year survival (%)
Baiocchi et al. 2012 [23]			
Cervical	73		23
Endometrial	14		64
Vaginal/vulval	17		X
Other	3		X
All types	107	92	27
Kaur et al. 2012 [2]			
Cervical	18		44
Endometrial	9		80
Vaginal/vulval	8		57
Other	1		X
All types	36	83	
Khoury-Collado et al. 2012 [57]			
Endometrial	17		
Other	4		
All types	21	90	40
Schmidt et al. 2012 [19]			
Cervical	282	65	41
Yoo et al. 2012 [58]			
Cervical	61	85	56
Jäger et al. 2013 [3]	28	82	70
Cervical	10		
Endometrial	4		
Vaginal/vulval	7		
Other	9		
All types	28	82	70
Chiantera et al. 2014 [20]			
Cervical	167	72	38
Chiantera et al. 2014 [59]			
Cervical	177	72	38
Endometrial	28	86	40
Vaginal/vulval	25	X	X
All types	230		

(Continued)

Table 28.3 (Continued)

Author, year Type of cancer	Number of patients	R0 (%)	Five-year survival (%)
Chiantera et al. 2014 [60]			
Endometrial	21	86	40
Huang et al. 2014 [24]			
Cervical	86		
Endometrial	15		
Vaginal/vulval	59		
Other	1		
All types	161	84	X
Westin et al. 2014 [61]			
Cervical	86		
Endometrial	15		
Vaginal/vulval	58		
Other	1		
All types	160	X	40
Arians et al. 2016 [64]			
Cervical	18		6
Endometrial	12		50
Vulval	6		17
All types	36	42	22
Schmidt et al. 2016 [13]			
Endometrial	40	92	61

The contribution of different gynecological malignancies in each study is presented. In most of the studies, survival for the whole group is presented, while in a few, survival for each of the different diagnoses is presented.
X, Information not given.

Summary Box

- PE is the only procedure to cure selected patients from locally advanced primary or recurrent gynecological cancer.
- The complications due to PE are frequent, especially in women previously treated with primary radiotherapy.
- The most important issue for successful surgery is a complete resection.
- The type of urinary diversion should be discussed with the patient before surgery.
- When complete PE is planned, an ileal conduit instead of continent reconstruction might be an advantage, with less short- and long-term complications.
- Information on QoL after PE in patients with gynecological malignancies is scarce and indicates persistent low body image and sexual discomfort. More studies should concentrate on measuring QoL in this group of patients.

References

1 Brunschwig, A. (1948). The surgical treatment of cancer of the cervix uteri; a radical operation for cancer of the cervix. *Bull. N. Y. Acad. Med.* 24: 672–683.

2 Kaur, M., Joniau, S., D'Hoore, A. et al. (2012). Pelvic exenterations for gynecological malignancies. A study of 36 cases. *Int. J. Gynecol. Cancer* 22: 889–896.

3 Jäger, L., Nilsson, P., and Flöter Rådestad, A. (2013). Pelvic exenteration for recurrent gynecologic malignancy. A study of 28 consecutive patients at a single institution. *Int. J. Gynecol. Cancer* 23: 755–762.

4 Kinney, W., Alvarez, R., Reid, G. et al. (1989). Value of adjuvant whole-pelvis irradiation after Wertheim hysterectomy for early-stage squamous carcinoma of the cervix with pelvic nodal metastasis: a matched-control study. *Gynecol. Oncol.* 34: 258–262.

5 Rotman, M., Sedlis, A., Piedmonte, M. et al. (2006). A phase III randomized trial of postoperative pelvic irradiation in stage IB cervical carcinoma with poor prognostic features: follow-up of a gynecologic oncology group study. *Int. J. Radiat. Oncol. Biol. Phys.* 65 (1): 169–176.

6 Gupta, S., Maheshwari, A., Parab, P. et al. (2018). Neoadjuvant chemotherapy followed by radical surgery versus concomitant chemotherapy and radiotherapy in patients with stage IB2, IIA, or IIB squamous cervical cancer: a randomized controlled trial. *J. Clin. Oncol.* 12: JCO2017759985.

7 Shah, C., Goff, B., Lowe, K. et al. (2009). Factors affecting risk of mortality in women with vaginal cancer. *Obstet. Gynecol.* 113: 1038–1045.

8 Nout, R., Smit, V., Putter, H. et al. (2010). Vaginal brachytherapy versus pelvic external beam radiotherapy for patients with endometrial cancer of high-intermediate risk (PORTEC-2): an open-label, non-inferiority, randomised trial. *Lancet* 375: 816–823.

9 Creutzberg, C., Nout, R., Lybeert, M. et al. (2011). Fifteen-year radiotherapy outcomes of the randomized PORTEC-1 trial for endometrial cancer. *Int. J. Radiat. Oncol. Biol. Phys.* 81: e631–e638.

10 Forner, M. and Lampe, B. (2012). Exenteration in the treatment of stage III/IV vulvar cancer. *Gynecol. Oncol.* 124: 87–91.

11 Di Donato, V., Bracchi, C., Cigna, E. et al. (2017). Vulvo-vaginal reconstruction after radical excision for treatment of vulvar cancer: evaluation of feasibility and morbidity of different surgical techniques. *Surg. Oncol.* 26: 511–521.

12 Andikyan, V., Khoury-Collado, F., Sonoda, Y. et al. (2012). Extended pelvic resections for recurrent or persistent uterine and cervical malignancies: an update on out of the box surgery. *Gynecol. Oncol.* 125: 404–408.

13 Schmidt, A., Imesch, P., Fink, D., and Egger, H. (2016). Pelvic exenterations for advanced and recurrent endometrial cancer: clinical outcomes of 40 patients. *Int. J. Gynecol. Cancer* 26: 716–721.

14 Höckel, M. and Dornhöfer, N. (2006). Pelvic exenteration for gynaecological tumours: achievements and unanswered questions. *Lancet Oncol.* 7: 837–847.

15 Hope, J. and Pothuri, B. (2013). The role of palliative surgery in gynecologic cancer cases. *Oncologist* 18: 73–79.

16 Höckel, M., Horn, L., and Einenkel, J. (2012). (Laterally) extended endopelvic resection: surgical treatment of locally advanced and recurrent cancer of the uterine cervix and vagina based on ontogenetic anatomy. *Gynecol. Oncol.* 127: 297–302.

17 Kaur, M., Joniau, S., D'Hoore, A., and Vergote, I. (2014). Indications, techniques and outcomes for pelvic exenteration in gynecological malignancy. *Curr. Opin. Oncol.* 26: 514–520.

18 Forner, M. and Lampe, B. (2011). Exenteration as a primary treatment for locally advanced cervical cancer: longterm results and prognostic factors. *Am. J. Obstet. Gynecol.* 205 (148): e1–e6.

19 Schmidt, A.M., Imesch, P., Fink, D., and Egger, H. (2012). Indications and long-term clinical outcomes in 282 patients with pelvic exenteration for advanced or recurrent cervical cancer. *Gynecol. Oncol.* 125: 604–609.

20 Chiantera, V., Rossi, M., De Iaco, P. et al. (2014). Survival after curative pelvic exenteration for primary or recurrent cervical cancer a retrospective multicentric study of 167 patients. *Int. J. Gynecol. Cancer* 24: 916–922.

21 Lakhman, Y., Nougaret, S., Miccò, M. et al. (2015). Role of MR imaging and FDG PET/CT in selection and follow-up of patients treated with pelvic exenteration for gynecologic malignancies. *Radiographics* 35: 1295–1313.

22 Chew, M., Yeh, Y., Toh, E. et al. (2017). Critical evaluation of contemporary management in a new pelvic exenteration unit: the first 25 consecutive cases. *World J. Gastrointest. Oncol.* 15: 218–227.

23 Baiocchi, G., Guimaraes, G., Oliveira, R. et al. (2012). Prognostic factors in pelvic exenteration for gynecological malignancies. *Eur. J. Surg. Oncol.* 38: 948–954.

24 Huang, M., Iglesias, D., Westin, S. et al. (2014). Pelvic exenteration: impact of age on surgical and oncologic outcomes. *Gynecol. Oncol.* 132: 114–118.

25 Iglesias, D., Westin, S., Rallapalli, V. et al. (2012). The effect of body mass index on surgical outcomes and survival following pelvic exenteration. *Gynecol. Oncol.* 125: 336–342.

26 Tobert, C., Hamilton-Reeves, J., Norian, L. et al. (2017). Emerging impact of malnutrition on surgical patients: literature review and potential implications for cystectomy in bladder cancer. *J. Urol.* 198: 511–519.

27 Martinez, A., Filleron, T., Rouanet, P. et al. (2018). Prospective assessment of first-year quality of life after pelvic exenteration for gynecologic malignancy: a French multicentric study. *Ann. Surg. Oncol.* 25: 535–541.

28 Choy, I., Badgery-Parker, T., Masya, L. et al. (2017). Baseline quality of life predicts pelvic exenteration outcome. *ANZ J. Surg.* 87: 935–939.

29 Marnitz, S., Köhler, C., Müller, M. et al. (2006). Indications for primary and secondary exenterations in patients with cervical cancer. *Gynecol. Oncol.* 103: 1023–1030.

30 Burger, I., Vargas, H., Donati, O. et al. (2013). The value of 18F-FDG PET/CT in recurrent gynecologic malignancies prior to pelvic exenteration. *Gynecol. Oncol.* 129: 586–592.

31 Meads, C., Davenport, C., Małysiak, S. et al. (2014). Evaluating PET-CT in the detection and management of recurrent cervical cancer: systematic reviews of diagnostic accuracy and subjective elicitation. *Br. J. Obstet. Gynecol.* 121: 389–407.

32 Sardain, H., Lavoue, V., Redpath, M. et al. (2015). Curative pelvic exenteration for recurrent cervicalcarcinoma in the era of concurrent chemotherapy and radiation therapy. *Eur. J. Surg. Oncol.* 41: 975–985.

33 Liedberg, F., Gudjonsson, S., Xu, A. et al. (2017a). Long-term third-party assessment of results after continent cutaneous diversion with Lundiana pouch. *BJU Int.* 120: 530–536.

34 Liedberg, F., Ahlgren, G., Baseckas, G. et al. (2017b). Long-term functional outcomes after radical cystectomy with ileal bladder substitute: does the definition of continence matter? *Scand. J. Urol.* 51: 44–49.

35 Liedberg, F., Holmberg, E., Holmäng, S. et al. (2012). Long-term follow-up after radical cystectomy with emphasis on complications and reoperations: a Swedish population-based survey. *Scand. J. Urol. Nephrol.* 46: 14–18.

36 Anderson, C., Cookson, M., Chang, S. et al. (2012). Voiding function in women with orthotopic neobladder urinary diversion. *J. Urol.* 88: 200–204.

37 Bartsch, G., Daneshmand, S., Skinner, E.C. et al. (2014). Urinary functional outcomes in female neobladder patients. *World J. Urol.* 32: 221–228.

38 Gross, T., Meierhans Ruf, S., Meissner, C. et al. (2015). Orthotopic ileal bladder substitution in women: factors influencing urinary incontinence and hypercontinence. *Eur. Urol.* 68: 664–671.

39 Eisenberg, M., Dorin, R., Bartsch, G. et al. (2010). Early complications of cystectomy after high dose pelvic radiation. *J. Urol.* 184: 2264–2269.

40 Meijer, R., Mertens, L., Meinhardt, W. et al. (2015). The colon shuffle: a modified urinary diversion. *Eur. J. Surg. Oncol.* 41: 1264–1268.

41 Stolzenburg, J., Schwalenberg, T., Liatsikos, E. et al. (2007). Colon pouch (Mainz III) for continent urinary diversion. *BJU Int.* 99: 1473–1477.

42 Van, Hemelrijck, M., Thorstenson, A., Smith, P. et al. (2013). Risk of in-hospital complications after radical cystectomy for urinary bladder carcinoma: population-based follow-up study of 7608 patients. *BJU Int.* 112: 1113–1120.

43 Gan, J. and Hamid, R. (2017). Literature review: double-barrelled wet colostomy (one stoma) versus Ileal conduit with colostomy (two stomas). *Urol. Int.* 98: 249–254.

44 Angioli, R., Benedetti Panici, P., Mirhashemi, R. et al. (2003). Continent urinary diversion and low colorectal anastomosis after pelvic exenteration. Quality of life and complication risk. *Crit. Rev. Oncol. Hematol.* 48: 281–285.

45 Husain, A., Akhurst, T., Larson, S. et al. (2007). A prospective study of the accuracy of 18Fluorodeoxyglucose positron emission tomography (18FDG PET) in identifying sites of metastasis prior to pelvic exenteration. *Gynecol. Oncol.* 106: 177–180.

46 Berek, J., Howe, C., Lagasse, L., and Hacker, N. (2005). Pelvic exenteration for recurrent gynecologic malignancy: survival and morbidity analysis of the 45-year experience at UCLA. *Gynecol. Oncol.* 99: 153–159.

47 Soper, J., Havrilesky, L., Secord, A. et al. (2005). Rectus abdominis myocutaneous flaps for neovaginal reconstruction after radical pelvic surgery. *Int. J. Gynecol. Cancer* 15: 542–548.

48 Qiu, S., Jurado, M., and Hontanilla, B. (2013). Comparison of TRAM versus DIEP flap in total vaginal reconstruction after pelvic exenteration. *Plast. Reconstr. Surg.* 132: 1020–1026.

49 Ferrari, J., Hemphill, A., and de Jesus, R. (2013). Modified rotational bowel vaginoplasty after total pelvic exenteration. *Ann. Plast. Surg.* 70: 335–336.

50 Bridoux, V., Kianifard, B., Michot, F. et al. (2010). Transposed right colon segment for vaginal reconstruction after pelvic exenteration. *Eur. J. Surg. Oncol.* 36: 1080–1084.

51 Sinna, R., Alharbi, M., Assaf, N. et al. (2013). Management of the perineal wound after abdominoperineal resection. *J. Visc. Surg.* 150: 9–18.

52 Campbell, C. and Butler, C. (2011). Use of adjuvant techniques improves surgical outcomes of complex vertical rectus abdominis myocutaneous flap reconstructions of pelvic cancer defects. *Plast. Reconstr. Surg.* 128: 447–458.

53 Creagh, T., Dixon, L., and Frizelle, F. (2012). Reconstruction with vertical rectus abdominus myocutaneous flap in advanced pelvic malignancy. *J. Plast. Reconstr. Aesthet. Surg.* 65: 791–797.

54 Fleisch, M., Pantke, P., Beckmann, M. et al. (2007). Predictors for long-term survival after interdisciplinary salvage surgery for advanced or recurrent gynecologic cancers. *J. Surg. Oncol.* 95: 476–484.

55 Maggioni, A., Roviglioni, G., Landoni, F. et al. (2009). Pelvic exenteration: ten-year experience at the European Institute of Oncology in Milan. *Gynecol. Oncol.* 114: 64–68.

56 Fotopoulou, C., Neumann, U., Kraetschell, R. et al. (2010). Long-term clinical outcome of pelvic exenteration in patients with advanced gynecological malignancies. *J. Surg. Oncol.* 101: 507–512.

57 Khoury-Collado, F., Einstein, M., Bochner, B. et al. (2012). Pelvic exenteration with curative intent for recurrent uterine malignancies. *Gynecol. Oncol.* 124: 42–47.

58 Yoo, H., Lim, M., Seo, S. et al. (2012). Pelvic exenteration for recurrent cervical cancer: ten year experience at National Cancer Center in Korea. *J. Gynecol. Oncol.* 23: 242–250.

59 Chiantera, V., Rossi, M., De, Iaco, P. et al. (2014). Morbidity after pelvic exenteration for gynecological malignancies a retrospective multicentric study of 230 patients. *Int. J. Gynecol. Cancer* 24: 156–164.

60 Chiantera, V., Rossi, M., De, Iaco, P. et al. (2014). Pelvic exenteration for recurrent endometrial adenocarcinoma: a retrospective multi-institutional study about 21 patients. *Int. J. Gynecol. Cancer* 24: 880–884.

61 Westin, S., Rallapalli, V., Fellman, B. et al. (2014;134). Overall survival after pelvic exenteration for gynecologic malignancy. *Gynecol. Oncol.*: 546–551.

62 Shimko, M., Tollefson, M., Umbreit, E. et al. (2011). Long-term complications of conduit urinary diversion. *J. Urol.* 185: 562–567.

63 Ang, C., Bryant, A., Barton, D.P.J. et al. (2014). Exenterative surgery for recurrent gynaecological malignancies. *Cochrane Database Syst. Rev.* ((2): CD010449.

64 Arians, N., Foerster, R., Rom, J. et al. (2016). Outcome of patients with local recurrent gynecologic malignancies after resection combined with intraoperative electron radiation therapy (IOERT). *Radiat. Oncol.* 11: 44.

65 Graves, S., Seagle, B., Strohl, A. et al. (2017). Survival after pelvic exenteration for cervical cancer: a National Cancer Database study. *Int. J. Gynecol. Cancer* 27: 390–395.

66 PelvExCollaborative (2019). Pelvic exenteration for advanced nonrectal pelvic malignancy. *Ann. Surg.* 270: 899–905.

67 Benn, T., Brooks, R., Zhang, Q. et al. (2011). Pelvic exenteration in gynecologic oncology: a single institution study over 20 years. *Gynecol. Oncol.* 122: 14–18.

68 Armbruster, S., Sun, C., Westin, S. et al. (2018). Prospective assessment of patient-reported outcomes in gynecologic cancer patients before and after pelvic exenteration. *Gynecol. Oncol.* 149: 484–490.

29

Mesenchymal and Non-Epithelial Tumors of the Pelvis

Eugenia Schwarzkopf and Patrick Boland

Orthopaedic Service, Department of Surgery at Memorial Sloan Kettering Cancer Center, New York; City, USA

Background

Tumors arising from tissue of the primitive mesenchymal mesenchyme comprise a heterogeneous group of benign and malignant neoplasms [1]. They involve muscles, tendons, adipose tissues, lymphatics, blood vessels, synovium, and bone. Supporting soft tissues of the visceral organs of the abdomen and pelvis may also be involved. Peripheral neurogenic tumors which are of ectodermal origin are also included since their behavior is similar, they are treated like soft tissue tumors.

The pathologic classification is largely based on recognition of the tissues origin, such as chondrosarcoma neoplasms arising from cartilage, or merely descriptive, e.g. spindle cell tumors or small round cell tumors when the origin is not clear. Traditionally, these tumors are divided into soft tissue and bone tumors, or benign versus malignant.

Incidence

The true incidence of benign lesions is unknown since the majority are asymptomatic. It is estimated that sarcomas account for 1% of all invasive neoplasms excluding skin cancers [2]. The relative incidence of sarcomas in children and young adults is higher than in older patients [3].

Soft tissue sarcomas are more common than primary malignant bone tumors. The majority of sarcomas occur in the limbs, but soft tissue sarcomas are not uncommon in the pelvis [4]. Chondrosarcoma and Ewing's sarcoma frequently involve the bony pelvis. The low incidence of sarcomas should not diminish their importance, their early detection, and their treatment to improve survival and limb salvage rates.

Etiology

The cause of most benign and malignant mesenchymal tumors is unknown. Cancers are caused by mutations and alterations in genes. These alterations in DNA result from inherited predispositions to such mutations or exposure to carcinogens, or can result from sporadic DNA replication [5]. Examples of tumors associated with genetic susceptibility include neurofibromatosis type 1 (NF1), familial adenomatous popyposis (FAP), and Li-Fraumeni syndrome (germline mutation in TP 53) [6, 7]. Autosomal dominant

---

Surgical Management of Advanced Pelvic Cancer, First Edition.
Edited by Michael E. Kelly and Desmond C. Winter.
© 2022 John Wiley & Sons Ltd. Published 2022 by John Wiley & Sons Ltd.

retinoblastoma is associated with osteosarcoma. In addition, prior radiation therapy is associated with development of bone and soft tissue sarcomas, and some chronic inflammatory states such as Paget's disease and chronic osteomyelitis can result in the development of bone sarcomas.

Specific Diagnostics

The diagnostic process begins with a complete history and physical examination. Deep pelvic pain, an antalgic gait, or sciatica can be the presenting features of pelvic tumors. Deep pelvic tumors are rarely palpable; however, the presence of lower limb swelling can occasionally occur in pelvic sarcomas due to direct invasion or extrinsic pressure on deep pelvic vasculature.

Imaging

Plain film X-ray is the initial first step in imaging. A soft tissue shadow or bone erosion may be noted in soft tissue tumors. X-rays may be very informative in primary bone neoplasms, but cross-sectional imaging is often required. Computed tomography (CT) scans are particularly useful in detecting cortical bone damage, and useful in outlining soft tissue anatomy. Magnetic resonance imaging (MRI) is undoubtedly the most useful imaging modality when imaging bone and soft tissue tumors. In some cases, MRI may be diagnostic, especially in low-grade fatty tumors and chondrosarcomas. It is useful for outlining the pelvic anatomy and relationship of tumor to the normal structures, for operative planning. Bone scans (with methylene diphosphonate (MDP Tc)) and positron-emission tomography (PET) scans are also useful in characterizing the primary tumor, with the added benefit of assessing the presence of metastatic disease. In addition, they are often used post neoadjuvant therapy to assess response to treatment.

Biopsy

In order to make a definitive diagnosis, microscopic examination of a tumor specimen obtained by biopsy is necessary. In the pelvis we favor a core or Tru-cut biopsy carried out using image-guidance (CT, MRI, or ultrasound). This avoids damaging vital structures and reduces the risk of contamination. Fine needle biopsies are usually inadequate. If image-guided biopsy proves inconclusive a careful open biopsy should be done. At the time of definitive surgery, biopsy tracts should be excised en bloc with the tumor. In addition to routine histologic examination, immunohistochemical staining and molecular studies are often carried out in order to confirm a diagnosis and provide information for targeted systemic therapy. Based on the histology, tumors are graded as benign or malignant, low-grade (G1) or high-grade (G2 + 3). Based on this and the clinical staging, a prognostic assessment can be made.

There are tumors that are both a mix of soft tissue and bony, that are not by definition malignant, and that are locally aggressive but do not metastasize. Examples include desmoid tumors of soft tissue and giant cell tumors of bone.

Staging Systems

Two main staging systems are used for sarcomas. One is described by Enneking et al. and adapted by the Musculoskeletal Tumor Society (MSTS); it is most commonly used for staging bone sarcomas (Table 29.1) [8]. The second is proposed by the American Joint Committee on Cancer (AJCC) (Table 29.2) [9]. Soft tissue sarcomas are staged using the AJCC system (Table 29.3) [9].

Distant metastases of bone and soft tissue sarcomas usually occur in the lungs, but can also spread to the bone (spine) and soft tissues (like in myxoid liposarcomas). Sarcomas with epitheliod features often involve regional lymph nodes.

Table 29.1 Musculoskeletal Tumor Society (MSTS) [8] staging system for bone sarcomas.

Stage	Grade	Local extent of disease
IA	Low	Intracompartmental
IB	Low	Extracompartmental
IIA	High	Intracompartmental
IIB	High	Extracompartmental
III	Any	Any

Source: Enneking, W. F., Spanier, S. S., & Goodman, M. A. The Classic: A System for the Surgical Staging of Musculoskeletal Sarcoma. Clinical Orthopaedics and Related Research, 415, 4–18. © 2003 Wolters Kluwer.

Treatment

Treatment methods used in the management of musculoskeletal tumors of the pelvis include observation, surgery, radiation, and systemic therapy. Occasionally, minimally invasive cryotherapy or radiofrequency ablation is done. However, surgery is the most common active treatment modality used. Surgical procedures are classified as followed: (i) intralesional, (ii) marginal, (iii) wide, or (iv) radical resections. Intralesional resection is indicated for benign tumors. Marginal resection describes a shelling-out procedure where the margin is the tumor

Table 29.2 American Joint Committee on Cancer (AJCC 8th Edition) [9] staging system for bone sarcomas.

Stage	Primary tumor (T)	Regional lymph node (N)	Distant metastasis (M)	Histologic grade (G)
IA	≤ 8 cm	No	No	G1 or Gx
IB	> 8 cm or discontinuous tumors in primary bone site	No	No	G1 or Gx
IIA	≤ 8 cm	No	No	G2 or G3
IIIB	≤ 8 cm	No	No	G2 or G3
III	Discontinuous tumors in primary bone site	No	No	G2 or G3
IVA	Any T	Yes	Yes (lung)	Any G
IVB	Any T	Any N	Yes (extrapulmonary)	Any G

Source: Tanaka, K., & Ozaki, T. New TNM classification (AJCC eighth edition) of bone and soft tissue sarcomas: JCOG Bone and Soft Tissue Tumor Study Group. Japanese Journal of Clinical Oncology. © 2018 Oxford University Press

Table 29.3 American Joint Committee on Cancer (AJCC 8th Edition) [9] staging system for soft tissue sarcomas.

Stage	Primary tumor (T)	Regional lymph node (N)	Distant metastasis	Histologic grade (G)
IA	≤ 5 cm	No	No	G1 or Gx
IB	> 5 cm and ≤ 10 cm	No	No	G1 or Gx
II	≤ 5 cm	No	No	G2 or G3
IIIA	> 10 cm and ≤ 15 cm	No	No	G2 or G3
IIIB	> 15 cm	No	No	G2 or G3
IV	Any T	Yes	No	Any G
	Any T	Any N	Yes	Any G

Source: Based on Tanaka, K., & Ozaki, T. (2018). New TNM classification (AJCC eighth edition) of bone and soft tissue sarcomas: JCOG Bone and Soft Tissue Tumor Study Group. Japanese Journal of Clinical Oncology.

capsule. It is indicated for removal of benign non-invasive tumors of soft tissue and bone. Intralesional or marginal excisions are not appropriate for oncological resections. Wide resections are the most common procedure used in the management of soft tissue and bone sarcomas and are indicated for some benign aggressive tumors. Surgeons attempt to achieve a clear margin of at least 2 cm. Radical resection involves removal of an entire anatomic compartment and is indicated in high-grade tumors.

Radiation therapy may be used in both a neoadjuvant and adjuvant setting. The former is often used as an attempt to shrink the tumor preoperatively in order to improve the chances of achieving a negative margin and to treat local microscopic metastases. Postoperative or adjuvant radiation is often used following resection of large tumors (> 5 cm) especially when the resection margins are close. Radiation therapy can be administered as a photon beam or as particle therapy (carbon ion therapy).

Neoadjuvant and adjuvant chemotherapy is routinely used in chemotherapy-sensitive tumors like osteosarcoma, Ewing's sarcoma, and embryonal rhabdomyosarcomas [10]. While chemotherapy is also used in other sarcomas, its efficacy is debated. Chemotherapy is occasionally used for palliation when tumors are unresectable or as definitive treatment in certain large tumors. Tyrosine kinase inhibitors including imatinib have proven to be effective in advanced gastrointestinal stromal tumors (GIST) of the colon and rectum [11].

Cryotherapy administered under image guidance can be effective in eliminating small recurrent sarcoma nodules. Radiofrequency ablation is very effective in the management of osteoid osteoma.

Benign Soft Tissue Tumors of the Pelvis

Lipoma/Pelvic Lipomatosis

Lipoma is the most common mesenchymal tumor in adults [12]. These tumors are usually asymptomatic and have a homogeneous well-marginated appearance on MRI scan. They may be observed or marginally excised.

Pelvis lipomatosis is a diffuse overgrowth of mature adipose tissue which in the pelvis can surround the bladder and rectum [13]. It is most common in black males. Rarely, these patients develop hydronephrosis or bowel obstruction, requiring debulking of the fatty mass. Recurrence occurs frequently.

Schwannoma

Pelvic schwannomas (Figure 29.1) usually occur in the presacral area arising from presacral nerve roots commonly at the S2 foramen. They may cause presacral pressure erosion of bone. MRI scan shows enlargement of the involved foramen and may show a characteristic target sign [14]. The diagnosis can be confirmed with core biopsy. If asymptomatic, schwannomas can be safely observed. Symptomatic lesions can be successfully excised by enucleation of the tumor, retaining the peripheral nerve fibers. In neurofibromas, separation of the tumor from the nerve fibers can be extremely difficult and in symptomatic cases resection of the nerve root may be necessary. Removal of a solitary lower sacral nerve root rarely results in significant disability. Malignant change of these tumors

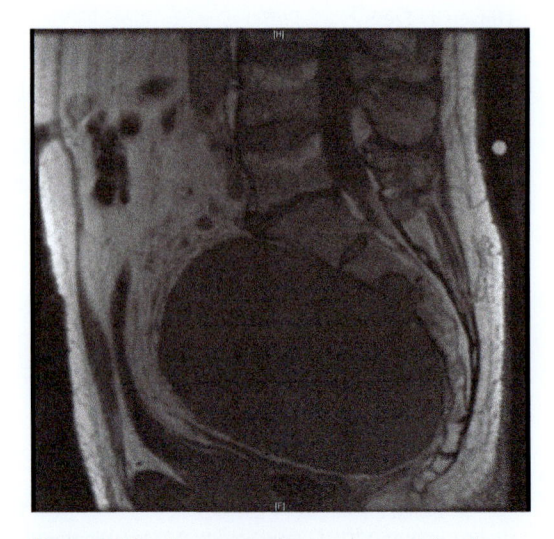

Figure 29.1 Presacral schwannoma arising from the S2 root. *Source:* Eugenia Schwarzkopf and Patrick Boland.

is extremely rare except in the setting of multiple NF1 [15].

Desmoid-Type Fibromatosis

Desmoid-type fibromatoses are benign but locally aggressive fibroblastic tumors. Based on the anatomic location, three types are described: abdominal wall, extra-abdominal, and intra-abdominal tumors. Intra-abdominal desmoids frequently occur in the sidewall of the pelvis or in the mesentery. They are common in women of childbearing age and may be misdiagnosed as malignant ovarian tumors [16]. They are usually slow-growing. Mesenteric desmoids account for up to 15% of all desmoid tumors and may be associated with Gardner's syndrome [17].

It should be noted when planning treatment that desmoid tumors never metastasize, but they can be locally aggressive. Many desmoid tumors remain indolent and may regress with time. Traditionally, the standard treatment was surgery, attempting to achieve a negative margin without causing morbidity. It should be noted that while resection with negative margins has the lowest incidence of recurrence, a significant proportion of these tumors are resected with positive margins. Following surgery, recurrence rates are higher in large tumors, young patients, and extremity locations. Based on the experience of the Memorial Sloan Kettering Cancer Centre, we recommend the following algorithm:

- Primary disease: (i) observation; (ii) consider resection if procedure is not morbid; (iii) systemic therapy for locally advanced disease.
- Recurrent disease: (i) observation; (ii) systemic therapy including anti-estrogens, pegylated liposomal doxorubicin, or doxorubicin/dacarbazine.

Soft Tissue Sarcomas of the Pelvis

It is estimated that 18% of abdomino-pelvic sarcomas arise in the pelvis, with many more extending from the retroperitoneum into the pelvis [18]. Extension through the sciatic notch and obturator foramen is not uncommon. Invasion of the bony pelvis in primary sarcomas is extremely rare. Tumors not directly involving pelvic viscera, nerves, or blood vessels can usually be resected without sacrificing these structures. Wide surgical resection achieving negative margins must be attempted in all cases in order to reduce the incidence of local recurrence. If it is necessary, due to direct tumor invasion, resection of all or part of the pelvic viscera (pelvic exenteration), nerves, or vessels should be done. Tumors surrounding or infiltrating major arteries including the common iliac or external iliac artery require vascular grafting following resection, while no such reconstruction is necessary following major vein resection. These patients are managed with postoperative elevation and use of compression stockings.

Sacrifice of the obturator nerve causes little dysfunction, unlike resection of the femoral or sciatic nerves. However, following resection of the femoral or sciatic nerves, patients can function satisfactorily with rehabilitation. Involvement of both femoral and sciatic nerves is probably an indication for amputation (hemipelvectomy). Partial resection of the bladder or ureter can usually be repaired, requiring specialist input of urology. Sarcomas such as rhabdomyosarcoma or epithelioid sarcomas may arise in the prostate, seminal vesicles, or paratesticular areas, requiring resection of those organs.

Surgery can usually be done through a midline transperitoneal approach with or without inguinal or perineal extension, or through an ilioinguinal or retroperitoneal method. In rare instances, pelvic bone resection with or without skeletal reconstruction will be necessary. Tumors that extend through the sciatic notch into the buttock may require both an anterior and posterior approach. The posterior incision is best done in a longitudinal fashion in the midline over the lower sacrum and posterior iliac crest, elevating the gluteus maximus muscle and reflecting it anteriorly, exposing the sciatic notch, nerve, and gluteal vessels.

Liposarcoma

Liposarcoma is one of the most common pelvic sarcomas. There are three biologic subtypes:

i) well-differentiated liposarcoma and its high-grade variant, dedifferentiated liposarcoma;
ii) myxoid (low grade) and round cell (high grade) liposarcoma; and (iii) pleomorphic liposarcoma (the most malignant subtype but rarely occurring in the pelvis) [19].

Well-differentiated liposarcoma is a non-metastasizing tumor that is not uncommon in the retroperitoneum and pelvis but can transform into a undifferentiated tumor. Dedifferentiated liposarcoma often occurs following resected pelvic or retroperitoneal well-differentiated liposarcoma, but can develop de novo. These two subtypes have different appearances on MRI scan. Myxoid liposarcoma and high-grade round cell type are often very large at the time of diagnosis. These occur more frequently in the proximal thigh but may extend into the pelvis. This subtype has a predilection to metastasize to unusual sites such as the retroperitoneum or bones, especially the spine. Staging studies should be carried out with this in mind.

As with all sarcomas, complete gross resection is the aim. Myxoid liposarcoma is sensitive to radiation therapy and chemotherapy, which may be used as neoadjuvant or adjuvant therapy.

Leiomyosarcoma

Leiomyosarcoma usually occurs in the retroperitoneum and pelvis. Within the pelvis it commonly arises from the uterus, but also it can be derived from around the ureter, prostate, or pelvic sidewall structures [20–23]. Early wide resection is the treatment of choice. Uterine leiomyosarcoma is treated with hysterectomy. In young women, when tumors are confined to the uterus alone, the ovaries can be spared.

Rhabdomyosarcoma

Rhabdomyosarcoma is a malignant tumor featuring skeletal muscle cells. Several histological variants exist:

- Embryonal rhabdomyosarcoma: this is the most common type and occurs in patients from infancy to 15 years of age. Common locations include the retroperitoneum and pelvis [23]. Patients aged one to nine years have better outcomes than adolescents or infants [24].
- Spindle cell rhabdomyosarcoma: this is a rare subtype of rhabdomyosarcomas. It affects children and adults, with a male predominance [25]. Anatomical locations include the paratesticular region and retroperitoneum [26–28].
- Alveolar rhabdomyosarcoma: this is a high-grade malignant tumor, composed of undifferentiated, small, round-oval cells. It is prevalent in adolescents and young adults.
- Pleomorphic rhabdomyosarcoma: these high-grade, aggressive sarcomas are most common in the sixth to seventh decade of life.

Malignant Peripheral Nerve Sheath Tumors

Malignant peripheral nerve sheath tumors (MPNSTs) arise from the cellular components of nerves, the Schwann and perineural cells. These are highly aggressive tumors, with a high tendency to metastasize, and have poor prognosis [29]. MPNSTs occur in three settings: (i) sporadic, (ii) post radiation exposure, and (iii) associated with NF1. While MPNSTs are more common in the extremities, they can also occur in the pelvis. Fifty percent of patients with MPNST have NF1 [25]. These tumors normally involve large nerves in the sciatic and lumbosacral plexus, causing significant symptoms. Treatment is primarily surgical, requiring wide resection. Since the lumbosacral plexus is a common place for involvement of these tumors in the pelvis, a significant neurologic deficit can result from radical surgery. However, this should not deter the surgeon from doing a wide resection. Patients can be rehabilitated following resection of major pelvic nerves. Radiation therapy in addition to surgery is used for tumors > 5 cm, especially if the resection margin is close.

Solitary Fibrous Tumor

Solitary fibrous tumor is defined as a ubiquitous mesenchymal tumor arising from fibroblasts and containing a hemangiopericytoma-like branching vascular pattern. Large tumors are associated with hypoglycemia because of secretion of an insulin-like growth factor (Doege–Potter syndrome) [30]. Eighty-five percent of these tumors are benign, but the remaining 15% are malignant and can metastasize to the lung, liver, or bone. Marginal resection is adequate for benign solitary fibrous tumors, whereas the malignant variant requires wide resection with or without radiation therapy.

Epithelioid Sarcoma

Epithelioid sarcomas are a rare malignant mesenchymal neoplasm where the cell of origin is unknown. There are two subtypes: the conventional type which arises in acral sites, and the proximal type which occurs in perineal and groin areas. This latter type is characterized by pleomorphic epithelioid carcinoma-like cells. They can grow to large sizes and tend to be infiltrative [31]. In addition to metastasizing to the lung, they frequently metastasize to the lymph nodes. Treatment consists of wide resection and sentinel node mapping, with lymphadenectomy if indicated. Chemotherapy is rarely effective.

Undifferentiated Pleomorphic Sarcomas

Formally known as malignant fibrous histiocytomas, undifferentiated pleomorphic sarcomas consist of tumor cells with diffuse pleomorphism and no identifiable line of differentiation. They represent 20% of all soft tissue sarcomas, occur in older adults, and can be found in any location, including the pelvis [32]. While the etiology is unknown, there is evidence that at least 25% of them are radiation-associated tumors. Wide resection is the recommended treatment and adjuvant radiation therapy is effective in 50% of cases [32].

Benign Bone Tumors Involving the Pelvis

The pelvis skeleton is composed of two innominate bones and the sacrum connected by bilateral sacroiliac joints and the symphysis pubis. It is estimated that benign tumors outnumber malignant ones by a factor of 100. Most benign tumors are asymptomatic, discovered incidentally, and require no intervention.

Enneking et al. proposed a system for staging benign bone tumors using Arabic numbers 1, 2, and 3 (latent, active, and aggressive) [8]. Observation or intralesional intervention with or without the use of physical adjuvant therapies are usually the management modalities of choice depending on symptoms or radiographic appearances. Marginal or wide resection may be indicated for aggressive benign bone tumors, especially as they are located in expandable portions of the pelvis.

Osteochondroma

The most common benign pelvic tumor is an osteochondroma, usually in the iliac bone. Excision is indicated if they are symptomatic or increasing in size in an adult. Multiple hereditary osteochondromatosis is an autosomal dominant condition characterized by development of multiple osteochondromas with mutations in EXT1 and/or EXT2 genes [33]. Malignant degeneration occurs in 5% of cases [34]. Malignant change occurs more often in pelvic lesions and is suspected with onset of pain and growth of the cartilage over 1.5 cm.

Ganglion Cyst

Supra-acetabular bone cysts are associated with degenerative hip disease. Treatment is directed at the underlying arthritis if symptomatic.

Aneurysmal Bone Cyst

Aneurysmal bone cyst (ABC) can be active or aggressive. Symptoms may include local pain, antalgic gait, and rarely radiculopathy depending on the tumor location. Imaging usually shows an expansible lesion. MRI scan classically reveals fluid–fluid levels (Figure 29.2). These tumors usually occur in iliac bone or the posterior elements of the sacrum. Histology shows a benign histiocytic stroma with blood-filled spaces and giant cells. ABC may be secondary to other benign tumors. ABC is a true tumor resulting from translocation of ubiquitin-specific-peptidase 6 (USP6) [35]. Treatment includes arterial embolism, open intralesional curettage, cryosurgery, and bone grafting. Recurrence occurs in up to 25% of cases. ABC of the sacrum can often be managed with marginal resection.

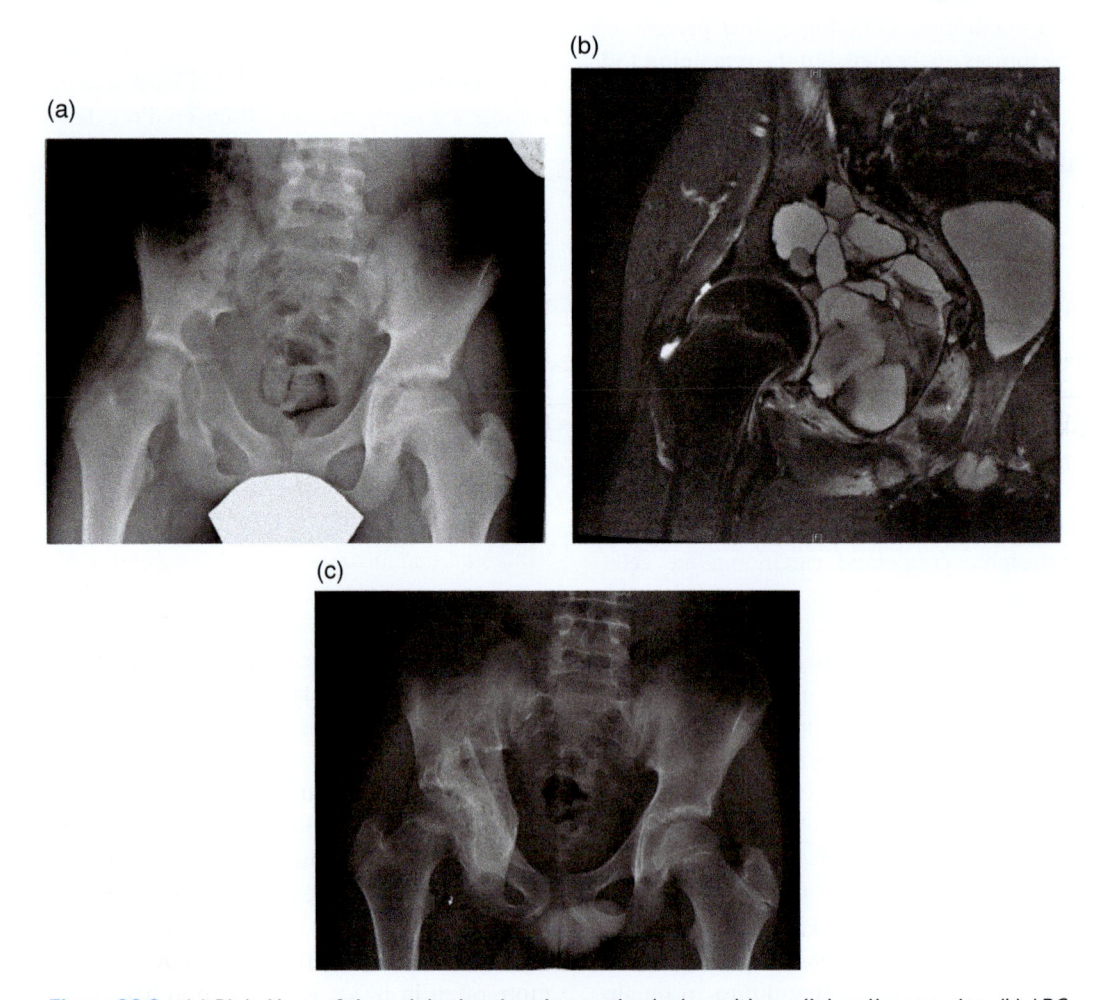

Figure 29.2 (a) Plain X-ray of the pelvis showing destructive lesion with medial wall expansion. (b) ABC arising from the inner wall of the pelvis with fluid–fluid levels in the cystic lesion. (c) Healed ABC one year postoperatively. *Source:* Eugenia Schwarzkopf and Patrick Boland.

Giant Cell Tumor

Giant cell tumor (GCT) is an example of an aggressive benign tumor. While it most commonly occurs in the epiphysis of long bones, it can occur in the pelvis or sacrum. In the sacrum, it frequently involves the body of the second sacral segment, making treatment complicated.

GCT may be associated with aneurysmal bone cysts resulting in a higher incidence of local recurrence following treatment. It is more common in females, with a peak incidence in the third and fourth decades [36]. The cell of origin is unknown, but histologically GCT consists of multinucleated giant cells and benign spindle cells, the latter being the true tumor cells.

For pelvic GCT, recommended treatment includes intralesional curettage and adjuvant cryosurgery. The defect maybe filled with methyl methacrylate which is also an adjuvant therapy. In the sacrum, tumors occurring below the third sacral roots should be excised. Tumors that extend higher have been successfully treated with low sacrectomy preserving the S3 roots and radiation to the higher sacral levels, followed by intralesional curettage. The sacral nerve roots should be preserved [37]. Denosumab reduces the size of the tumor. It eliminates the giant cells but has no effect on the true tumor component, i.e. spindle cells, so aggressive recurrence is almost inevitable. The use of denosumab in the management of GCT has not been determined [38].

Osteoid Osteoma

Osteoid osteoma is usually a very painful benign bone lesion characterized by the radiographic presence of a small central lucent area (< 1.5 cm) representing fibro-osseous tissue surrounded by reactive bone. It occurs in childhood and adolescence [39]. The pain is usually relieved by non-steroidal anti-inflammatory drugs. In the pelvis it often occurs in the acetabulum, causing hip pain. In the sacrum it occurs in the posterior bony elements.

While excision of the nidus was the traditional treatment, most are now successfully treated with percutaneous radiofrequency ablation of the central nidus.

Osteoblastoma

Osteoblastoma is a rare fibro-osseous tumor of bone with similar histologic features as osteoid osteoma, but it is larger and more aggressively destructive, and the pain is not usually relieved by non-steroidal anti-inflammatory drugs. Radiographically, it is larger than osteoid osteoma (2–10 cm) [40]. While rare, the sacrum is a favored anatomic location. Osteoblastoma classically involves the sacral lamina. On MRI, the tumor is frequently surrounded by an area of high signal change representing reactive changes, making this tumor appear larger. Treatment requires complete excision.

Malignant Bone Tumors of the Pelvis

While metastatic malignancy is the most common malignant tumor in the pelvis, four malignant neoplasms account for the vast majority of primary tumors of the pelvis and are briefly described. They include osteosarcoma, Ewing's sarcoma, chondrosarcoma, and sacral chordoma.

Osteosarcoma and Ewing's sarcoma occur most commonly in children and adolescents, while chondrosarcoma and chordoma are diseases of the older age group. Osteosarcoma and Ewing's sarcoma are managed with multimodality treatment including chemotherapy and surgery, and in the case of Ewing's sarcoma radiation may be employed. Chondrosarcoma is resistant to radiation and chemotherapy, while the primary treatment for chordoma is wide surgical resection, and modern forms of radiation therapy are being used as adjuvants. Wide resection with negative margins is essential for all these pelvic and sacral malignancies.

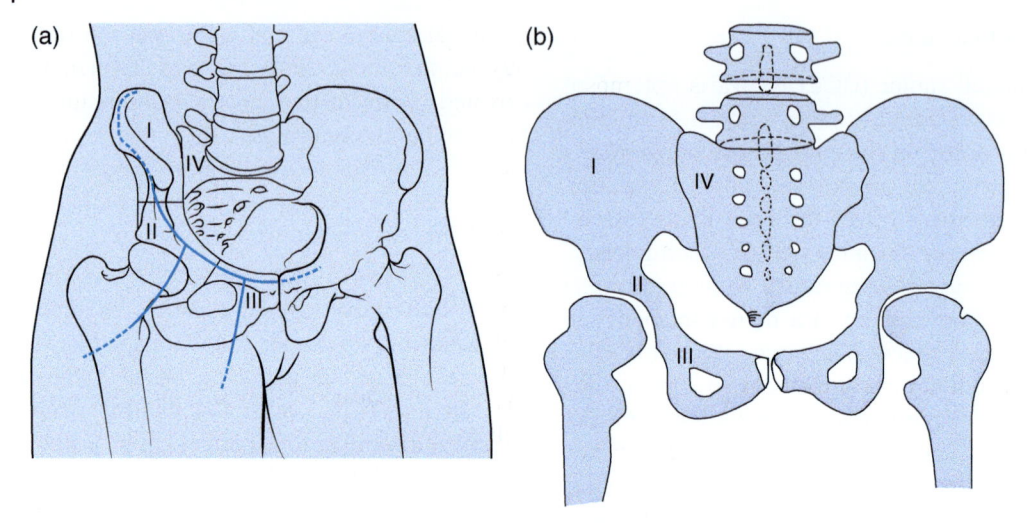

Figure 29.3 Incisions for internal hemipelvectomy.

Wide resection of pelvic tumors is challenging but usually possible. Hemipelvectomy was the traditional surgical treatment; however, studies have shown that local control and survival are equivalent in the management of soft tissue and bone sarcomas, assuming wide margins are achieved. Involvement of the common iliac or external iliac artery can be dealt with by arterial resection and reconstruction. Major vein vessels do not require reconstruction. In cases where it is necessary to resect both the sciatic and femoral nerve, an external hemipelvectomy is probably indicated.

The incision for internal hemipelvectomy used by the authors was described by Enneking et al. and is shown in Figure 29.3a. Any part or all of these incisions are used depending on the extent of the resection. Four types of resections are described and shown in Figure 29.3b.

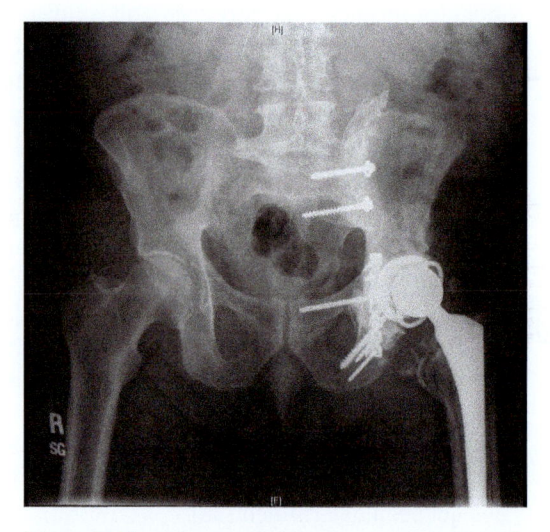

Figure 29.4 Reconstruction using a pelvic allograft and hip prosthesis following type 1/2 and partial type 3 resection. *Source:* Eugenia Schwarzkopf and Patrick Boland.

Types of Resections

Reconstruction is recommended when resection includes type II (acetabular and hip) excisions. Type III when done alone does not require stabilization. Type I resection is usually reconstructed, but function can be satisfactory without repair. Resection of the total innominate bone can be reconstructed using a custom prosthesis (Figure 29.4) or occasionally the leg can be left flail. Since there is a very high postoperative complication rate with allograft or prostheses, some surgeons often omit reconstruction.

Radiation therapy may be given in an adjuvant setting preceding or following surgical resection. It is occasionally used instead of surgery in pelvic Ewing's sarcoma. Occasionally it is given as definitive treatment for non-operable tumors or for palliation.

Osteosarcoma

High-grade classic osteosarcoma is the most common primary bone tumor and affects adolescents most commonly. A second peak in incidences occurs in older people and these are frequently secondary to radiation therapy, Paget's disease, fibrous dysplasia, or osteomyelitis [41]. Osteosarcoma usually arises in the appendicular skeleton but does occur in the pelvis and sacrum. The prognosis for pelvic and sacral osteosarcoma is poor.

Treatment consists of neoadjuvant chemotherapy, followed by surgery, followed by six months of postoperative systemic treatment. Wide surgical resection is essential. Reconstruction is usually carried out as indicated.

Ewing's Sarcoma

Ewing's sarcoma is a high-grade malignant round cell tumor and is the second most common bone malignancy in young people. In the trunk, the most common location is the pelvis, followed by the sacrum [42].

Imaging reveals a lytic lesion usually associated with a large soft tissue mass. Clinically it presents with pain or sciatica in pelvic sacral lesions. It is often accompanied by fever. As in the case of osteosarcoma, treatment consists of neoadjuvant chemotherapy, surgery, and/or radiation therapy followed by adjuvant chemotherapy. Radiation should be reserved for inoperable tumors or as an adjuvant when resection resulted in positive margins. The use of radiation therapy in Ewing's sarcoma is associated with a low but significant incidence of radiation-associated tumors.

Chondrosarcoma

The pelvis is the most common location of occurrence for conventional chondrosarcoma [43]. It is composed of malignant chondrocytes which may be low, intermediate, or high-grade. The higher the grade, the worse the prognosis. Chondrosarcomas of the pelvis are usually more aggressive than their histology would indicate, so a diagnosis of a benign cartilage tumor of the pelvis should be interpreted with caution. Due to the anatomy, pelvic chondrosarcomas are often very large when diagnosed. Pain deep in the pelvis or radicular is the most common presenting feature.

Undifferentiated chondrosarcoma is a subtype common in the pelvis. It arises in a low-grade tumor and is characterized by sudden onset of pain or a rapid growth of a pre-existing mass. Secondary chondrosarcomas of the pelvis or sacrum arise in pre-existing benign tumors, including enchondroma and Ollier's disease (multiple enchondromatosis), and in osteochondromas usually in the setting of pelvic multiple hereditary osteochondromas.

Chondrosarcoma is radioresistant and there is no proven effective systemic treatment. Wide surgical resection of these tumors is the treatment of choice.

The recent discovery of mutation in isocitrate dehydrogenase 1 (IDH1) is important in diagnosis [44]. Monoclonal antibodies developed against these mutations may lead to effective targeted therapy.

Chordoma

Chordoma is a slow-growing locally destructive malignant tumor thought to arise from vestigial notochordal tissue. It accounts for 20% of all primary malignant bone tumors, making it the fourth most common bone neoplasm. It occurs almost exclusively in the spine; 50% of the tumors arise in the sacrum [45].

Patients typically present with a long-standing history of low back pain or sciatica. In advanced cases, patients present with loss of bowel, bladder, and sexual function due to destruction of the higher sacral nerves, S3 and above.

Although the tumor is lytic, the area of destruction may be subtle on plain X-ray and bone scan is frequently normal. MRI is the imaging modality of choice and shows a tumor arising from the center of the vertebral

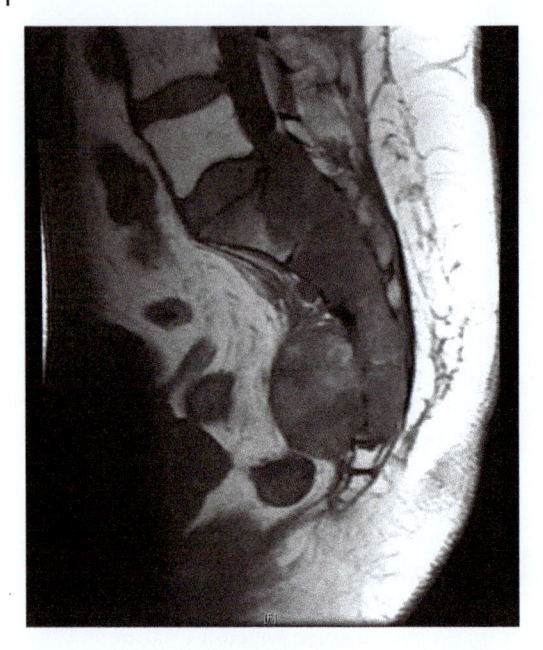

Figure 29.5 Sacral chordoma extending proximally to the L5–S1 level. *Source:* Eugenia Schwarzkopf and Patrick Boland.

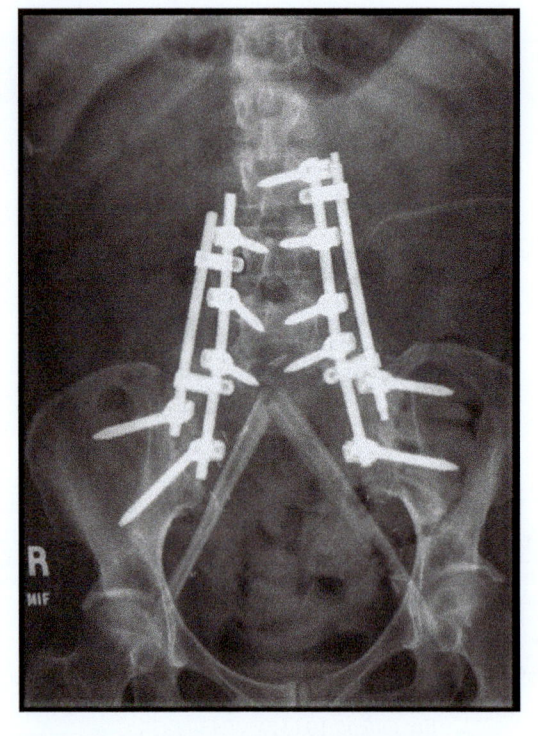

Figure 29.6 Typical reconstruction following sacrectomy; fibular strut graft was used anteriorly, and posterior spinal-pelvic stabilization was achieved with screws and rods. *Source:* Eugenia Schwarzkopf and Patrick Boland.

body, with a soft tissue mass extending anteriorly and posteriorly (Figure 29.5). Microscopic examination reveals large vacuolated cells with vacuolated cytoplasm (physaliferous cells). Immunohistochemistry staining for S100, epithelial markers, and Brachyury transcription factors expressed by notochordal cells is positive [46].

Wide resection with negative margins is the treatment of choice. Resection of both S3 roots usually results in loss of bowel, bladder, and sexual function. Sacropelvic stabilization is recommended when the resection is carried out at or above the level of the first sacral foramen (Figure 29.6). When large tumors have been removed, a vertical rectus abdominis musculocutaneous (VRAM) flap is strongly recommended.

Summary Box

- Tumours arising from tissue of the primitive mesenchymal mesenchyme comprise a heterogeneous group of benign and malignant neoplasms. The pathologic classification is largely based on recognition of the tissues of origin.
- Treatment methods used in the management of musculoskeletal tumours of the pelvis include observation, surgery, radiation, and systemic therapy.
- Neoadjuvant and adjuvant chemotherapy is routinely used in chemotherapy-sensitive tumors like osteosarcoma, Ewing's sarcoma, and embryonal rhabdomyosarcomas.
- Surgical options can require extensive reconstruction to restore function in most instances. Clear preoperative counseling is vital to manage patient expectations.

References

1. Yang, J., Ren, Z., Du, X. et al. (2014). The role of mesenchymal stem/progenitor cells in sarcoma: update and dispute. *Stem Cell Invest.* 1: 18.
2. Herzog, C.E. (2005). Overview of sarcomas in the adolescent and young adult population. *J. Pediatr. Hematol. Oncol.* 27 (4): 215–218.
3. Ferrari, A., Sultan, I., Huang, T.T. et al. (2011). Soft tissue sarcoma across the age spectrum: a population-based study from the surveillance epidemiology and end results database. *Pediatr. Blood Cancer* 57 (6): 943–949.
4. Morrison, B.A. (2003). Soft tissue sarcomas of the extremities. *Proc. (Bayl. Univ. Med. Cent.)* 16 (3): 285–290.
5. Fletcher, C.D., Gustafson, P., Rydholm, A. et al. (2001). Clinicopathologic re-evaluation of 100 malignant fibrous histiocytomas: prognostic relevance of subclassification. *J. Clin. Oncol.* 19 (12): 3045–3050.
6. Widemann, B.C. (2009). Current status of sporadic and neurofibromatosis type 1-associated malignant peripheral nerve sheath tumors. *Curr. Oncol. Rep.* 11 (4): 322–328.
7. Hisada, M., Garber, J.E., Fung, C.Y. et al. (1998). Multiple primary cancers in families with Li-Fraumeni syndrome. *J. Natl Cancer Inst.* 90 (8): 606–611.
8. Enneking, W.F., Spanier, S.S., and Goodman, M.A. (1980). A system for the surgical staging of musculoskeletal sarcoma. *Clin. Orthop. Relat. Res.* 153: 106–120.
9. Tanaka, K. and Ozaki, T. (2019). New TNM classification (AJCC eighth edition) of bone and soft tissue sarcomas: JCOG bone and soft tissue tumor study group. *Jap. J. Clin. Oncol.* 49 (2): 103–107.
10. Gurria, J.P. and Dasgupta, R. (2018). Rhabdomyosarcoma and extraosseous Ewing sarcoma. *Children (Basel)* 5 (12): 165.
11. Zhu, R., Liu, F., Grisotti, G. et al. (2018). Distinctive features of gastrointestinal stromal tumors arising from the colon and rectum. *J. Gastroint. Oncol.* 9 (2): 231–240.
12. Weiss, S.W. (1996). Lipomatous tumors. *Monogr. Pathol.* 38: 207–239.
13. McKusick, V.A. (2007). Mendelian inheritance in man and its online version, OMIM. *Am. J. Human Genet.* 80 (4): 588–604.
14. Koga, H., Matsumoto, S., Manabe, J. et al. (2007). Definition of the target sign and its use for the diagnosis of schwannomas. *Clin. Orthop. Relat. Res.* 464: 224–229.
15. Walker, L., Thompson, D., Easton, D. et al. (2006). A prospective study of neurofibromatosis type 1 cancer incidence in the UK. *Br. J. Cancer* 95 (2): 233–238.
16. Merchant, N.B., Lewis, J.J., Woodruff, J.M. et al. (1999). Extremity and trunk desmoid tumors. *Cancer* 86 (10): 2045–2052.
17. Mishra, D.P. and Rout, S.S. (2016). Desmoid tumors: a clear perspective or a persisting enigma? A case report and review of literature. *World J. Oncol.* 7 (1): 21–27.
18. Gronchi, A., Lo Vullo, S., Fiore, M. et al. (2009). Aggressive surgical policies in a retrospectively reviewed single-institution case series of retroperitoneal soft tissue sarcoma patients. *J. Clin. Oncol.* 27 (1): 24–30.
19. Peterson, J.J., Kransdorf, M.J., Bancroft, L.W., and O'Connor, M.I. (2003). Malignant fatty tumors: classification, clinical course, imaging appearance and treatment. *Skelet. Radiol.* 32 (9): 493–503.
20. Ricci, S., Stone, R.L., and Fader, A.N. (2017). Uterine leiomyosarcoma: epidemiology, contemporary treatment strategies and the impact of uterine morcellation. *Gynecol. Oncol.* 145 (1): 208–216.
21. Fung, T.M.K., Wong, W.-s., Lam, Y.-h., and Lau, J.Y.W. (2005). Resection of leiomyosarcoma arising from the iliac vein. *J. Am. Coll. Surg.* 200 (1): 136–137.
22. Griffin, J.H. and Waters, W.B. (1996). Primary leiomyosarcoma of the ureter. *J. Surg. Oncol.* 62 (2): 148–152.

23 Raney, R.B., Walterhouse, D.O., Meza, J.L. et al. (2011). Results of the Intergroup Rhabdomyosarcoma Study Group D9602 protocol, using vincristine and dactinomycin with or without cyclophosphamide and radiation therapy, for newly diagnosed patients with low-risk embryonal rhabdomyosarcoma: a report from the Soft Tissue Sarcoma Committee of the Children's Oncology Group. *J. Clin. Oncol.* 29 (10): 1312–1318.

24 Joshi, D., Anderson, J.R., Paidas, C. et al. (2004). Age is an independent prognostic factor in rhabdomyosarcoma: a report from the Soft Tissue Sarcoma Committee of the Children's Oncology Group. *Pediatr. Blood Cancer* 42 (1): 64–73.

25 Kamil M Amer, Jennifer E Thomson, Dominick Congiusta, Andrew Dobitsch, Ahmed Chaudhry, Matthew Li, Aisha Chaudhry, Anthony Bozzo, Brianna Siracuse, Mahmut Nedim Aytekin, Michelle Ghert, Kathleen S Beebe et al. (2019). Epidemiology, Incidence, and Survival of Rhabdomyosarcoma Subtypes: SEER and ICES Database Analysis. *J Orthop Res.* Oct;37(10):2226-2230. doi: 10.1002/jor.24387.

26 Leuschner, I., Newton, W.A., Schmidt, D. et al. (1993). Spindle cell variants of embryonal rhabdomyosarcoma in the paratesticular region. A report of the Intergroup Rhabdomyosarcoma Study. *Am. J. Surg. Pathol.* 17 (3): 221–230.

27 Cavazzana, A.O., Schmidt, D., Ninfo, V. et al. (1992). Spindle cell rhabdomyosarcoma. A prognostically favorable variant of rhabdomyosarcoma. *Am. J. Surg. Pathol.* 16 (3): 229–235.

28 Nascimento, A.F. and Fletcher, C.D.M. (2005). Spindle cell rhabdomyosarcoma in adults. *Am. J. Surg. Pathol.* 29 (8): 1106–1113.

29 Yuan, Z., Xu, L., Zhao, Z. et al. (2017). Clinicopathological features and prognosis of malignant peripheral nerve sheath tumor: a retrospective study of 159 cases from 1999 to 2016. *Oncotarget* 8 (62): 104785–104795.

30 Doege, K.W. (1930). Fibro-sarcoma of the mediastinum. *Ann. Surg.* 92 (5): 955–960.

31 Hasegawa, T., Matsuno, Y., Shimoda, T. et al. (2001). Proximal-type epithelioid sarcoma: a clinicopathologic study of 20 cases. *Mod. Pathol.* 14 (7): 655–663.

32 Picci, P., Manfrini, M., Fabbri, N. et al. (eds.) (2014). Atlas of Musculoskeletal Tumors and Tumorlike Lesions: The Rizzoli Case Archive. Cham: Springer International Publishing.

33 Ishimaru, D., Gotoh, M., Takayama, S. et al. (2016). Large-scale mutational analysis in the EXT1 and EXT2 genes for Japanese patients with multiple osteochondromas. *BMC Genet.* 17: 52.

34 Murphey, M.D., Choi, J.J., Kransdorf, M.J. et al. (2000). Imaging of osteochondroma: variants and complications with radiologic-pathologic correlation. *Radiographics* 20 (5): 1407–1434.

35 Oliveira, A.M., Hsi, B.-L., Weremowicz, S. et al. (2004). USP6 (Tre2) fusion oncogenes in aneurysmal bone cyst. *Cancer Res.* 64 (6): 1920–1923.

36 Verschoor, A.J., Bovée, J.V.M.G., Mastboom, M.J.L. et al. (2018). Incidence and demographics of giant cell tumor of bone in the Netherlands: first nationwide pathology registry study. *Acta Orthop.* 89 (5): 570–574.

37 Domovitov, S.V., Chandhanayingyong, C., Boland, P.J. et al. (2016). Conservative surgery in the treatment of giant cell tumor of the sacrum: 35 years' experience. *J. Neurosurg. Spine* 24 (2): 228–240.

38 Agarwal, M.G., Gundavda, M.K., Gupta, R., and Reddy, R. (2018). Does denosumab change the giant cell tumor treatment strategy? Lessons learned from early experience. *Clin. Orthop. Relat. Res.* 476 (9): 1773–1782.

39 Hakim, D.N., Pelly, T., Kulendran, M., and Caris, J.A. (2015). Benign tumours of the bone: a review. *J. Bone Oncol.* 4 (2): 37–41.

40 de Souza Dias, L. and Frost, H.M. (1974). Osteoid osteoma—osteoblastoma. *Cancer* 33 (4): 1075–1081.

41 Ottaviani, G. and Jaffe, N. (2009). The etiology of osteosarcoma. *Cancer Treatm. Res.* 152: 15–32.

42 Sucato, D.J., Rougraff, B., McGrath, B.E. et al. (2000). Ewing's sarcoma of the pelvis: long-term survival and functional outcome. *Clin. Orthop.Relat. Res.* 373: 193–201.

43 Deloin, X., Dumaine, V., Biau, D. et al. (2009). Pelvic chondrosarcomas: surgical treatment options. *Orthop. Traumatol. Surg. Res.* 95 (6): 393–401.

44 Amary, M.F., Bacsi, K., Maggiani, F. et al. (2011). IDH1 and IDH2 mutations are frequent events in central chondrosarcoma and central and periosteal chondromas but not in other mesenchymal tumours. *J. Pathol.* 224 (3): 334–343.

45 Radaelli, S., Stacchiotti, S., Ruggieri, P. et al. (2016). Sacral chordoma: long-term outcome of a large series of patients surgically treated at two reference centers. *Spine* 41 (12): 1049–1057.

46 Meis, J.M. and Giraldo, A.A. (1988). Chordoma. An immunohistochemical study of 20 cases. *Arch. Pathol. Lab. Med.* 112 (5): 553–556.

Index

a

ABC. *see* aneurysmal bone cyst (ABC)
abdominal compartment 178
abiraterone acetate 219–220
adjuvant radiation therapy (ART) 218
adjuvant therapy 198–201
ADT. *see* androgen deprivation therapy (ADT)
advanced pelvic malignancies 68
Alexis™ wound retractor 60
anastomosis 154
androgen deprivation therapy (ADT) 219
anemia management 50–51
anesthesia 78, 96–97
aneurysmal bone cyst (ABC) 294
anterior pelvic exenteration
   background 77
   complications 82–83
   diagnostics 77
   morbidity 82
   mortality 82
   quality of life 83
   surgical procedure 77–82
   survival 83
anterior pubic resection 103
ART. *see* adjuvant radiation therapy (ART)

b

benign bone tumors
   ABC 294
   ganglion cyst 294
   GCT 295
   osteoblastoma 295
   osteochondroma 293
   osteoid osteoma 295
bipolar devices 61
bladder cancer 260–263
   chemotherapy 221
   immunotherapy 221
   radiotherapy 221–222
bony exenteration
   anatomical considerations 102–103
   background 101–102
   indications and contraindications 102
   MDM 106
   neoadjuvant treatment 106–107
   operative technique 107–109
   outcomes 110–111
   patient workup
      anesthetic assessment 105–106
      history and examination 103–104
      radiology 104–105
bowel continuity 272
bowel reconstruction
   anastomosis 154
   colonic pouch 154
   double-staple anastomosis 153–154
   endoanal coloanal anastomosis 154
   hand-sutured anastomosis 153
   single-staple anastomosis 153
brachytherapy 219
Brunschwig's operation 2

c

cabazitaxel 220
cancer anatomy
   case study 25–30
   MRI 23–30
   and resectability 22
   roadmap approach 26–27
   tumor categorization 23–24
cardiopulmonary exercise testing (CPET) 50
castration-resistant prostate cancer (CRPC) 219
cervical cancer 210–211
chemoradiation 9
chemoradiotherapy techniques
   regimen 9
   re-irradiation 9–10
chemotherapy 40, 220, 221
chondrosarcoma 297
chordoma 297–298
circumferential resection margin (CRM) 22
colon conduit. *see* urinary diversion
colonic pouch 154
colonoscopy 96–97
colorectal peritoneal metastases 132
compartment syndrome 60
complex pelvic cancer 16–17
composite bone resection 5–8
computed tomography (CT) 22
continent urinary diversions
   vs. incontinent urinary diversions 146–147
   Indiana pouch 145
   Miami pouch 145
   orthotopic neobladder 146
   uretero-ileocecal appendicostomy 145–146
core operating teams 67–68

CPET. *see* cardiopulmonary exercise testing (CPET)
crisis management
　background　174
　intraoperative management　175–177
　postoperative management　178
　surgery　174–175
CRM. *see* circumferential resection margin (CRM)
CRPC. *see* castration-resistant prostate cancer (CRPC)
CT. *see* computed tomography (CT)
cytoreductive surgery　132–133
cytoreductive surgery and hyperthermic intraperitoneal chemotherapy (CRS-HIPEC)　131

d

DBWC. *see* double barrel wet colostomy (DBWC)
desmoid-type fibromatosis　291
direct cutaneous ureterostomy　144
distal colon urinary diversion　143–144
docetaxel　220
double barrel wet colostomy (DBWC)　148, 264
double-staple anastomosis　153–154

e

early salvage radiation therapy (esRT)　219
ELAPE. *see* extra-levator abdomino-perineal resection (ELAPE)
electrothermal bipolar vessel sealing (EBVS)　175
en-bloc cystectomy　5
endoanal coloanal anastomosis　154
endometrial cancer　212–213
endorectal ultrasound (ERUS)　22
enoxaparin and cancer (ENOXACAN)　53
enzalutamide　220
epithelioid sarcoma　293
ERUS. *see* endorectal ultrasound (ERUS)
esRT. *see* early salvage radiation therapy (esRT)
European Society of Parenteral and Enteral Nutrition (ESPEN)　51
Ewing's sarcoma　297
exenterative resections
　anatomy
　　gynecologic structure　116–117
　　muscular　117
　　neurologic　116
　　urologic structure　116–117
　　vascular　116
　background　114–115
　intraoperative management
　　equipment　119
　　operative approach　119–121
　　preparation and positioning　119
　postoperative management　121–122
　preoperative evaluation
　　functional status　118
　　imaging　117–118
　　informed consent　118–119
extended bony resections　98
extended exenterative resection　124
extra-levator abdomino-perineal resection (ELAPE)　137

f

FACT-C. *see* Functional Assessment of Cancer Therapy (FACT-C)
fasciocutaneous flaps　158–160
FDG. *see* fluorodeoxyglucose (FDG)
fecal diversion　147
femoral nerve　177
5-fluorouracil (5-FU)　36
flexible sigmoidoscopy　96–97
fluorodeoxyglucose (FDG)　30
free flaps　160
Functional Assessment of Cancer Therapy (FACT-C)　50

g

ganglion cyst　294
GCT. *see* giant cell tumor (GCT)
general health　84
general room setup　57
giant cell tumor (GCT)　295
gonadotropin-releasing hormone (GnRH)　219
gynecological approach　79
gynecological neoplasms
　age and comorbidity　270
　background　269
　complications　272, 280
　para-aortic lymph nodes　270
　pelvic sidewalls　270
　preoperative planning
　　bowel continuity　272
　　neovagina　272
　　pelvic floor reconstruction　272
　　urinary diversion　271–272
　preoperative workup　271
　quality of life　280–282
　survival　280–282

h

hand-sutured anastomosis　153
hemipelvectomy　103
hemorrhage　166
　control　175–176
high sacrectomy *vs.* low sacrectomy　102–103
hyperthermic intraperitoneal chemotherapy (HIPEC)　132–133

i

ileal conduit, 142–143, 263–264. *see also* urinary diversion
immunotherapy　41–42, 221
incontinent urinary diversions *vs.* continent urinary diversions　144
　direct cutaneous ureterostomy　144
　distal colon urinary diversion　143–144
　ileal conduit　142–143
　transverse colon urinary diversion　143
Indiana pouch　145
intraoperative management
　crisis management
　　femoral nerve　177
　　hemorrhage control　175–176
　　nerve damage　176–177
　　obturator nerve　177
　　postoperative hemorrhage　176
　　sacralplexus　177
　　urinary tract　177
　pelvic exenteration
　　general considerations　163–165
　　intraoperative considerations　166–169
　　preoperative considerations　166
　　surgical considerations　166

intraoperative radiotherapy (IORT) 99, 109, 210
intraoperative stage
  checklist 69
    external examination 70
    general laparotomy 70–73

j
jackknife prone position 60

k
Koenig–Rutzen bag 4–5

l
laboratory tests 49
lateral compartment 79–80
laterally extended endopelvic resection (LEER) 21
lateral pelvic recurrences 98–99
lateral pelvic resection 103
lateral pelvic sidewall resection 8
LEER. *see* laterally extended endopelvic resection (LEER)
leiomyosarcoma 292
lipoma/pelvic lipomatosis 290
liposarcoma 292
locally advanced rectal cancer (LARC)
  background 247–248
  morbidity 254–255
  mortality 254–255
  pelvic exenteration 252–254
  radiation therapy 251–252
  tumor biology 248–251
local recurrent rectal cancer (LRRC) 42
  background 227, 247–248
  morbidity 254–255
  mortality 254–255
  pelvic exenteration 252–254
  radiation/radiotherapy 251–252
    characteristics 228
  re-irradiation
    morbidity 228–229
    primary outcome 229–230
  treatment 227–228
  tumor biology 248–251
Lone Star™ retractor 61

m
magnetic resonance imaging (MRI)
  cancer anatomy 23–30
malignant bone tumors
  chordoma 297-298
  Ewing's sarcoma 297
  osteosarcoma 297
  resections 296
malignant peripheral nerve sheath tumors (MPNSTs) 292–293
massive transfusion 178
MBP. *see* mechanical bowel preparation (MBP)
mCRPC. *see* metastatic castration-resistant prostate cancer (mCRPC)
MDT. *see* multidisciplinary team (MDT)
MDTMs. *see* multidisciplinary team meetings (MDTMs)
mechanical bowel preparation (MBP) 52–53
mental health 84
mesenchymal tumors
  background 287
  diagnostics
    biopsy 288
    imaging 288
    staging systems 288–289
  etiology 287–288
  incidence 287
  treatment 289–290
mesh 156
metastatic castration-resistant prostate cancer (mCRPC) 219
metastatic disease 30–31
Miami pouch 145
MIBC. *see* muscle invasive bladder cancer (MIBC)
minimally invasive pelvic exenteration
  background 136
  history 136–137
  outcomes 139
  reconstruction 138
  robotic approach 137–139
  surgical planning 138
mobilization
  left colon and upper rectum 90
  uterus including adnexa 90–91
modified Lloyd-Davies approach 59
monopolar devices 61
morbidity 49–50
  re-irradiation 228–229
MPNSTs. *see* malignant peripheral nerve sheath tumors (MPNSTs)
MRI. *see* magnetic resonance imaging (MRI)
multidisciplinary meeting (MDM)
  bony exenteration 106
multidisciplinary team (MDT) 66
multidisciplinary team meetings (MDTMs)
  complex pelvic cancer 16–17
  pathological assessment 18
  restaging 18
  staging 17–18
muscle invasive bladder cancer (MIBC) 220
myocutaneous flaps 160

n
neoadjuvant chemotherapy (NAC) 220
neoadjuvant therapy 97
  anatomical considerations 102–103
neovagina 272
nerve
  damage 176–177
  injuries 60–61
nonvitamin K oral anticoagulants (NOACs) 175
novel chemotherapeutic agents 40–41
Nutritional Risk Screening 2002 (NRS-2002) 52
nutritional status 51–52

o
obturator nerve 177
omentum 156
operating room setup
  adjuncts 57–58
  general room setup 57
  robotic room setup 58–59
oral antibiotic prophylaxis 52–53
organ preservation 39–40
orthotopic bladder 264
orthotopic neobladder 146
osteoblastoma 295
osteochondroma 293
osteoid osteoma 295
osteosarcoma 297
ostomy placement 99
ovarian cancer 213–214

p
palliative pelvic exenterative surgery (PPES)
  background 234
  definition 235–236
  history 234–235

indications   236–237
morbidity   237
mortality   237
quality of life   242
survival   242
symptom relief   237–242
parastomal hernia   148–149
partial cystectomy   80
partial exenteration   5
partial prostatectomy   80–81
pathological assessment   18
patient positioning
  complications   60–61
  jackknife prone   60
  modified Lloyd-Davies   59
patient-reported outcome measures (PROMs)   265
PCI. see Peritoneal Cancer Index (PCI)
pedicle flaps   156–158
pelvic exenteration   132–133
  morbidity
    background   162
    intraoperative management   163–169
    postoperative complications   169–171
    postoperative management   169
    risks   162–163
  QOL
    gynecological malignancies   184–190
    mixed malignancies   192
    palliative exenteration   192
    patient-reported outcome   193–194
    rectal malignancy   190–192
  reconstructive techniques
    background   153
    bowel reconstruction   153–154
    perineum   155–160
    urinary tract reconstruction   154–155
pelvic exenterative surgery
  composite bone resection   5–8
  evolution   6
  Koenig–Rutzen bag   4–5
  lateral pelvic sidewall resection   8
  partial exenteration   5
  perineal reconstruction   8–9
  subspecialization   5
  uretero-ileal conduit   5
  urinary reconstruction   2–4

pelvic floor reconstruction   272
pelvis
  benign bone tumors   293–295
  malignant bone tumors   295–298
  soft tissue sarcomas   291–293
  soft tissue tumors   290–291
perineal reconstruction   8–9
perineum
  fasciocutaneous flaps   158–160
  free flaps   160
  mesh   156
  myocutaneous flaps   160
  omentum   156
  pedicle flaps   156–158
Peritoneal Cancer Index (PCI)   31
peritoneal metastases
  background   131–132
  colorectal cancer   132
PET. see positron-emission tomography (PET)
plastic-reconstructive techniques   68
positron-emission tomography (PET)   22
posterior compartment   98
posterior pelvic exenteration
  background   89
  intraoperative decision-making   89–91
  postoperative outcome   91–92
  preoperative assessment   89
  prognosis   91–92
  surgical technique   90–91
postoperative complications, pelvic exenteration
  early complications   169–170
  long-term complications   170–171
postoperative hemorrhage   176
postoperative management
  crisis management
    abdominal compartment   178
    massive transfusion   178
    urinary tract injury   178
  pelvic exenteration
    critical care   169
    enhanced recovery after surgery   169
    VTE   169
PPES. see palliative pelvic exenterative surgery (PPES)
preoperative optimization
  anemia management   50–51
  background   49

clinical examination   49
laboratory tests   49
nutritional status   51–52
preoperative phase
  core teams   67–68
  multidisciplinary team   66
  occasional contributors   69
  operating environment   67
  personnel   67
  regular participants   69
PROMs. see patient-reported outcome measures (PROMs)
prostate cancer
  abiraterone acetate   219–220
  advanced   260
  brachytherapy   219
  chemotherapy   220
  enzalutamide   220
  GnRH   219
  locally advanced disease   259
  radiation therapy   218–219
  rectal cancer   260
  second-line treatment   220
  synchronous   260

q

quality of life (QOL)   83
  background   181
  gynecological neoplasms   280–282
  palliative pelvic exenterative surgery (PPES)   242
  patient-reported outcomes instruments   181–184
  pelvic exenteration
    gynecological malignancies   184–190
    mixed malignancies   192
    palliative exenteration   192
    patient-reported outcome   193–194
    rectal malignancy   190–192
  postoperative   193
  urological neoplasms   265

r

radiation/radiotherapy therapy   202–205, 218–219, 221–222
radiological assessment
  cancer anatomy   23–25
  metastatic disease   30–31
radium-223   220
rectal cancer   79, 137
re-irradiation   9–10, 228–229
rhabdomyosarcoma   292

robotic approach
   minimally invasive pelvic exenteration 137–139
   room setup 58–59

s

sacralplexus 177
sacral resection 102
sacrectomy
   laparoscopic sacrectomy 110
   partial anterior sacrectomy 109–110
sacrum
   tackling recurrent tumors
      high sacrectomy 125–127
      low sacrectomy 124–125
      perineal closure 127
schwannoma 290
sexual dysfunction 83–84
sexual function 99
short-term outcomes 38–39
single-staple anastomosis 153
soft tissue tumors
   desmoid-type fibromatosis 291
   lipoma/pelvic lipomatosis 290
   schwannoma 290
solitary fibrous tumor 293
staging systems 17–18, 288–289
stoma
   background 142
   developments 149
   education 53
   urinary diversion 142
surgical subspecialization 5

t

tackling involvement of recurrent tumors
   anterior compartment 129
   background 124
   pelvic sidewall 127–129
   posterior compartment
      high sacrectomy 125–127
      low sacrectomy 124–125
      perineal closure 127
thromboprophylaxis 53
total mesorectal excision (TME) 137
total neoadjuvant therapy (TNT)
   advantages 37
   background 36–37
   developments 42–43
   disadvantages 37
   long-term oncological outcomes 39
total pelvic exenteration (TPE)
   anesthesia 96–97
   background 94
   colonoscopy 96–97
   fitness for surgery 96
   flexible sigmoidoscopy 96–97
   indications 94–95
   preoperative planning 96
   specialist centers 95–96
   surgical technique 97–99
transverse colon urinary diversion 143

u

ultrasonic energy devices 62
undifferentiated pleomorphic sarcomas 293
ureter dissection 79
uretero-ileal conduit 5
uretero-ileocecal appendicostomy 145–146
urinary catheters 165

urinary diversion 81–82, 142, 271–272
urinary dysfunction 84
urinary function 99
urinary tract 177
   injury 178
   reconstruction 2–4
      diversion, conduit and uretostomy 155
      ureteric reimplantation 154
urological approach 78–79
urological leaks 147, 263
urological neoplasms
   background 259
   bladder cancer 260–263
   complications 263–264
   palliative exenterations 265
   prostate cancer 259–260
   quality of life 265
uterus 81
   involvement 98

v

vagina
   involvement 98
   wall 81
vascular endothelial growth factor (VEGF) 40
venous thromboembolism (VTE) 53, 61, 163, 169
vertical rectus abdominis myocutaneous (VRAM) 107
visualization 61
VTE. see venous thromboembolism (VTE)
vulval cancer 211–212

w

wet colostomy 3, 147–148, 264